THE

CITIZEN-PATIENT

in Revolutionary and Imperial Paris

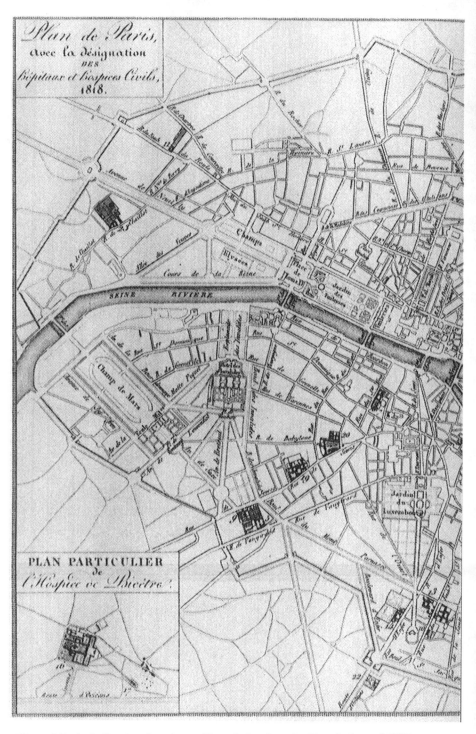

Plan of Paris indicating location of hospitals after the Revolution of 1789, adapted from "Plan de Paris avec la désignation d'hôpitaux et hospices civils"

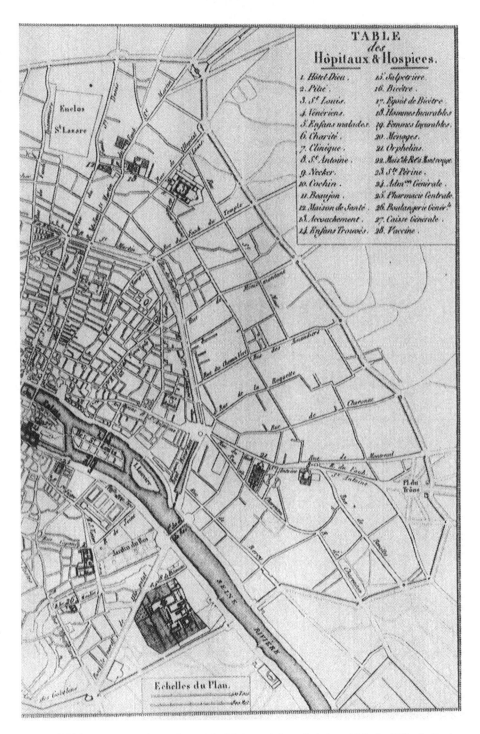

TABLE
des
Hôpitaux & Hospices.

1. Hôtel-Dieu.	15. Salpêtrière.
2. Pitié.	16. Bicêtre.
3. St Louis.	17. Egout de Bicêtre.
4. Vénériens.	18. Hommes Incurables.
5. Enfans malades.	19. Femmes Incurables.
6. Charité.	20. Ménages.
7. Clinique.	21. Orphelins.
8. St Antoine.	22. Mais de Rét St Antoine.
9. Necker.	23. St Périne.
10. Cochin.	24. Admn Générale.
11. Beaujon.	25. Pharmacie Centrale.
12. Maison de Santé.	26. Boulangerie Généralt.
13. Accouchement.	27. Caisse Générale.
14. Enfans Trouvés.	28. Vaccine.

Echelles du Plan.

(1818), in A. Malo and N. M. Maine, *Atlas administratif de la Ville de Paris*
(Paris: Lottin de St. Germain, 1821).

THE HENRY E. SIGERIST SERIES
IN THE HISTORY OF MEDICINE
Sponsored by The American Association
for the History of Medicine and The
Johns Hopkins University Press

*The Development of American Physiology:
Scientific Medicine in the Nineteenth
Century*
by W. Bruce Fye

*Save the Babies: American Public Health
Reform and the Prevention of Infant
Mortality, 1850–1929*
by Richard A. Meckel

*Politics and Public Health in Revolutionary
Russia, 1800–1918*
by John F. Hutchinson

*Rocky Mountain Spotted Fever: History of a
Twentieth-Century Disease*
by Victoria A. Harden

*Quinine's Predecessor: Francesco Torti and
the Early History of Cinchona*
by Saul Jarcho

*The Citizen-Patient in Revolutionary and
Imperial Paris*
by Dora B. Weiner

THE
CITIZEN-PATIENT

in Revolutionary and Imperial Paris

Dora B. Weiner

The Johns Hopkins University Press   *Baltimore and London*

This book has been brought to publication with the generous
assistance of the American Association for the History of Medicine.

The Johns Hopkins University Press
2715 North Charles Street
Baltimore, Maryland 21218-4319
The Johns Hopkins Press Ltd., London

Library of Congress Cataloging-in-Publication Data

Weiner, Dora B.
    The citizen-patient in revolutionary and imperial Paris / Dora B.
Weiner.
        p.   cm. — (The Henry E. Sigerist series in the history of
medicine)
    Includes bibliographical references and index.
    ISBN 0-8018-4483-5 (hc : alk. paper)
    1. Medicine—France—Paris—History—18th century.
2. Medicine—France—Paris—History—19th century.
I. Title. II. Series.
    [DNLM: 1. Delivery of Health Care—history—Paris.
2. Health Policy—history—Paris.   3. Public Health—history—
Paris.   WA 11 GF7 W4c]
R506.P3W45   1993
362.1'0944'3609033—dc20
DNLM/DLC
for Library of Congress   92-49007

A catalog record for this book is available from the British Library.

To the Memory of
Emma, 1889–1990

Contents

Illustrations

Tables

xiii

Preface and Acknowledgments

During the long gestation of this book, my thoughts about illness and health, and about the historic evolution of the relationships among patients, doctors, society, and the government, have gradually matured. I have come to view the French experience during the great Revolution and in the Napoleonic era as the first modern attempt to grapple with the daunting problem of providing health care for an entire needy population.

The list of books and scholars that have challenged, criticized, enriched, or clarified my thoughts stretches back many years to Richard H. Shryock, a friend of France and a reassuring figure to those of us then interested in the social history of medicine but lacking the M.D. degree. The trail toward my theme was blazed by Erwin H. Ackerknecht, Pierre Huard, and George Rosen, three experts generous with their time, helpful support, and critical input. Sadly, I add the name of our colleague William Coleman to the list of departed scholars who believed that the history of medicine in eighteenth- and nineteenth-century France holds special interest and special lessons for the contemporary world.

Among my own and the younger generation and my students, I have incurred debts of a special nature, too numerous to recount in detail. For comments, criticism, information, and help I thank Evelyn Ackerman, Nancy Frieden, Nina Gelbart, Thierry Gineste, Marie-José Imbault-Huart, George Rousseau, Charles E. Rosenberg, and Rob Valkenier.

Three scholars who read the manuscript had a special hand in refining my image of the "citizen-patient": Isser Woloch, who suggested that the Revolutionary decade implied forward movement toward a more perfect "man"; Ann LaBerge, who emphasized that half of those indigent and sick "men" were women; and Herbert Weiner, who is committed to the belief that a good doctor achieves results by working

xv

with patients, rather than by doing things *to* them. Their judicious comments have become part of my thinking.

But study, advice, critique, and consultation here at home could not have come to life in a book had I not been able to spend much time in Paris. For the means to do so, I am beholden to the National Library of Medicine, U.S. Public Health Service, for support as a "Distinguished Scholar" in 1972–1975 and for a research grant in 1989–1992; to the National Endowment for the Humanities for support as a "Senior Humanist Fellow" in 1972; to the American Philosophical Society for a stipend in 1977; and to the University of California Senate for travel grants in 1988 and 1990. At the moment I am honored to hold a Charles E. Culpeper Scholarship in the Medical Humanities. I herewith acknowledge this support with sincere thanks.

The treasures of the archives and libraries in the United States and abroad used for this book are analyzed in the Bibliographic Essay. I should like to record my special thanks to the staff of the Louise M. Darling Biomedical Library at UCLA, Katharine Donahue, Victoria Steele, Tia Choo, and Cynthia Becht. The expertise of the reference staff and the rare books in the History and Special Collections Division make this one of the outstanding libraries in our field.

In appearance and style, this book has benefited from the guidance of my editors, Barbara B. Lamb, Jacqueline Wehmueller, and Lee C. Sioles, and the text owes improved clarity and consistency to the persistence and good taste of the copy editor, Peter Dreyer. I gratefully acknowledge their help and that of my indexer, Alexa Selph.

The hospitality extended over the years by my friends made long stays in Paris affordable. I wish to thank Eva and Pierre Aschheim; Dominique and Pierre Marçais; Elisabeth, Delphine, and the late Philippe Hervé; Marie-José and Roger Imbault-Huart; and Pascaline, Thierry, and Victoire Gineste. They gave me leisure to turn into a Parisian in tune with the French past. As such, I studied and photographed the buildings and gardens of the St. Louis and Laënnec Hospitals, explored the grounds of the Salpêtrière and Bicêtre Hospices, persisted until I gained access to the cellars and manuscripts of the National Institution for the Young Deaf and of the Quinze-Vingts Hospice, and spent hours exploring the surroundings of the old Hôtel-Dieu, the area of the rue de la Bûcherie and St. Julien-le-Pauvre. Only there can one glimpse a towering spire of Notre-Dame cathedral as a poor patient might have done two hundred years ago and feel the grandeur of the Catholic religion, overpowering, real, and nearby. Those feelings were a force in health care for the poor in Paris, which was challenged by the French Revolution. That challenge is the topic of this book.

THE

CITIZEN-PATIENT

in Revolutionary and Imperial Paris

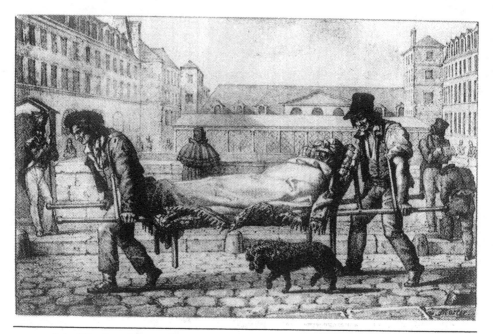

FIGURE I.1. *The Poor Patient Carried to the Hospital.* Lithograph by Jean Henri Marlet, *Tableaux de Paris* (1821). Bibliothèque historique de la Ville de Paris.

The Patient as Citizen and Paris as Model

Public welfare owes the ailing poor assistance that is prompt, free, assured, and complete.

> François Alexandre Frédéric, duc de la
> Rochefoucauld-Liancourt, 1790

The enjoyment of the highest attainable standard of health is one of the fundamental rights of every human being without distinction of race, religion, political belief, economic or social condition.

> Preamble to the Constitution of the
> World Health Organization, 1945

When the French Revolutionaries proclaimed equality as an inalienable right of man in August 1789, they gave no thought to health. Yet within six months of that declaration, thousands of unemployed poor, many of them sick, beleaguered the National Assembly clamoring for aid. The assembly's Poverty Committee (Comité pour l'extinction du paupérisme) soon targeted illness as one major cause of poverty and its chairman, the duc de la Rochefoucauld-Liancourt, proclaimed that society owes the ailing poor assistance that is "prompt, free, assured, and complete."[1] This scion of the old aristocracy and champion of liberal causes spoke with the voice of the Enlightenment. He defined a social obligation that stems from the ancient moral principle that man is his brother's keeper and from the philosophic doctrine of the natural rights of man. This obligation led logically to political concern with the citizens' health. Indeed, sick persons are neither "free" nor equal to healthy persons if they are unable to earn a living. And if nature makes "sad mistakes" at birth, as Pierre Louis Prieur de la Marne argued in the National Assembly, then a responsible society must compensate for these imperfections.[2] Thus a nation for the first time collectively confronted this obligation; her elected national rep-

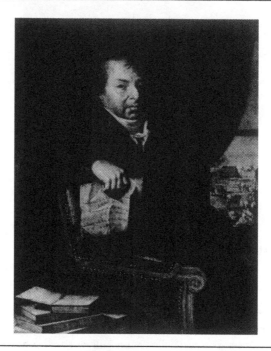

FIGURE I.2. François Alexandre Frédéric, duc de La Rochefoucauld-Liancourt (1747–1827) Engraving by Monsaldi. Bibliothèque nationale, Paris, Cabinet des estampes.

resentatives debated the task; then they attempted to shoulder the burden. This book is an analysis of their enterprise. It surveys the politics of health in France during the Revolution and under Napoleon from the perspective of that compelling obligation.[3]

When the Poverty Committee explored the citizens' claim to health care in 1790 and 1791, it defined health as the ability to work and poverty as income below a fixed sum. The committee's conception of ill health even encompassed the deaf, the blind, and the mentally ill, further extending the nation's responsibilities. In thus delimiting a comprehensive program of aid, the Revolutionaries sought to save their neediest ailing compatriots from acute deprivation. They even felt that the government must compensate handicapped citizens for inequalities caused by nature. We should note that these eighteenth-century leaders here conceived of nature as imperfect—capricious, if not malevolent—a point of view that contrasts with the Enlightenment's usual reverence.

The commissioners soon realized that the rights of "man" they sought to implement applied to an equal number of sick women, and also to babies and children who required custody as well as medical therapy. These were patients to whom doctors had hitherto paid little heed. But, owing to the growing importance of bedside observation in the hospital, the doctor now saw hundreds of patients whose health needs stemmed from age, genetic defects, or gender. Thus grew the doctor's perception that he must serve diverse categories of patients with special needs. The illnesses and problems of women patients attracted a great deal of medical attention—perhaps the only true equality that women attained during that era. This study will also explore the role of women as health care providers and administrators as a contribution to a more balanced view of French Revolutionary history than has hitherto prevailed, especially in the history of medicine.

Medical concerns received national attention soon after the initial political crises of the Revolution subsided. By the time the National Assembly disbanded in September 1791, it had mapped two programs for health care. One was essentially the work of the Poverty Committee's chairman, assisted by his right-hand man, the physician Michel Augustin Thouret. This program encompassed medical therapy, health maintenance, and disease prevention. It targeted the acutely sick worker without neglecting either the chronically disabled poor or those dependent on aid because of their age. The committee projected a national network of doctors, pharmacists, midwives, and nurses and a pyramidal organization rising from provincial general hospitals to specialized research institutions in the nation's capital.[4]

Revolutionary reformers and contemporary physicians believed that the recipients of public medical benefits had not only rights but also duties, in and out of the hospital or hospice. The patients' obligations began with their participation in extensive and repeated admitting interviews. These became routine with the establishment of a central system of triage aimed at the selection of patients for specialized hospitals. When bedside teaching evolved into a crucial part of medical education, the patients' duties broadened to helping elaborate their own case histories and tolerating repeated physical examinations, not only by physicians and surgeons, but by pharmacists, midwives, and students as well. Furthermore, patients were expected punctually to fulfill doctors' orders and to practice thoughtful behavior toward other patients and frugal use of public resources. The Poverty Committee did not discuss the growing expectation among clinical investigators that hospitalized patients serve research and even experiment, and that, as we shall see later, these patients could expect their cadavers to undergo autopsy. The consensus among doctors was that this participation was the citizen's duty in exchange for free and excellent care. The doctors frequently crossed swords with administrators who defended past hospital routine as well as the patients' peace and privacy—a tug-of-war that continues to our own day. As for the patients' feelings, they must be left to the historian's conjecture.

If patients recovered, still other obligations awaited them in the home, especially the practice of hygiene in their personal habits and living quarters. In the public sphere, and particularly after the government instituted a public health program under the Consulate, the reformers expected these citizens to help preserve and protect common resources such as water, undergo preventive measures such as vaccination, show vigilance regarding health hazards in the environment, and report infractions to the police. The Poverty Committee thus looked upon indigent patients as citizens in the full meaning of the term: responsible participants in caring for their own and the public health, reasonable, dedicated, and knowledgeable. The reformers in fact pinned their hopes for success on these model patients of the new era—on the women and men whom this book calls "citizen-patients."

In rivalry with the Poverty Committee's grand design, the National Assembly's Health Committee (Comité de salubrité), chaired by Dr. Joseph Ignace Guillotin, focused narrowly on medical training. The Health Committee's debates had a direct bearing on the curriculum for the new Health Schools of Paris, Montpellier, and Strasbourg, created by the Law of 4 December 1794 (14 Frimaire, Year III).[5] The Health Committee also influenced the creation of a two-tiered system of medical practitioners: physicians for the well-to-do and less-qualified health officers for the poor. That system was established in 1803 but abolished in 1892. It represented an unsatisfactory answer to the perennial problem of training competent personnel who would willingly practice medicine for the poor both in the inner city and in the countryside. The system eventually failed because the health officers received little official acknowledgment of their services and insufficient remuneration. The Revolutionary reformers learned that equal health care for all cannot be established in a market ecomony. Equal access for the poor to therapy, health maintenance, and protection against disease demands control of the public purse and may require the government's authority to impose equality.[6]

The extension of equal rights was an essential goal of the Revolution in matters of health care. In contrast, under the old regime, it was the Christian concept of charity that had inspired the Catholic Church and the monarchy to care for the poor. Traditionally, charity meant giving alms in the form of money and food. Charity for the sick might include medications as well as shelter and nursing care. In fact, the nursing sisters remained a comforting presence throughout our era,

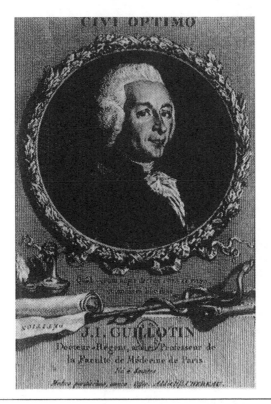

FIGURE I.3. Joseph Ignace Guillotin (1738–1814), chairman of the Health Committee of the National Assembly. Bibliothèque nationale, Paris, Cabinet des estampes.

for they stayed at the patients' bedside even at the price of donning civilian dress during the height of anticlerical hostility. Many returned to the hospital in the guise of domestics so as to fulfill their professional commitment to their patients. While the reformers acknowledged the sisters' dedication, they criticized the women for clinging to Catholic ritual and tradition. Had the Revolutionaries been more aware of these women's valuable contributions, they might have proceeded with greater circumspection and less haste in dissolving the nursing orders.

The monarchy had long shared the religious approach to medical charity by giving alms, but in the eighteenth century, the king also listened to medical advisers. With royal help, the medical care of soldiers set high standards, and disabled veterans lived in the palatial Hôtel des Invalides. Louis XVI bought up unused religious structures

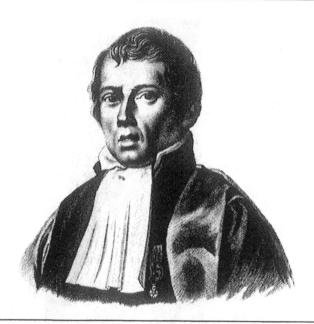

FIGURE I.4. Michel Augustin Thouret (1748–1810), leading physician member of the Poverty Committee of the National Assembly. Académie nationale de médecine, Paris.

and donated them for transformation into hospitals. The king also kept endowing single hospital beds, still a luxury for the poor.

The patients experienced the reformers' attempts to wean them from reliance on charity—to transform them from Christians who meekly accepted pain and suffering into citizens aware of rights and duties when they were sick. Against the old religious ideals of Faith, Hope, and Charity, the philosophes and reformers pitted the Platonic virtue of Justice and the Revolutionary goal of Equality. They argued that charity should make way for "welfare" (*bienfaisance*), a lay concept based on the poor man's entitlement to aid, on a realistic assessment of need and on encouragement to the poor to help themselves. They denounced the preference granted to "respectable paupers" (*pauvres honteux*), tradesmen and artisans who had fallen on hard times but were ashamed to accept charity. They frowned on special favors bestowed on the "deserving poor" (*bons pauvres*), indigents of the parish known to the priest or to the prosperous burghers as law-abiding churchgoing folk. The Revolution abolished these invidious distinctions.

But in attacking Catholic charity, which they considered demeaning, the reformers undermined the motivation of the well-to-do for charitable giving and choked off the main source of alms, endowments, and volunteer work. Having confiscated and nationalized the wealth of the Church, which was derived from bequests, donations, and alms, the reformers planned to dispense these funds for the benefit of the poor, as the Church had not. They considered the providing of health care an optimal use for these riches. They soon discovered how limited the funds would be, and that health care for all the needy entailed enormous financial burdens. Faced with seemingly insuperable problems of staffing and funding, the reformers soon realized that the ultimate solution to the people's claim to health care could only be attained through the active participation of the citizen-patients themselves in health maintenance, disease prevention, and public health.

In the complex activities that constitute the delivery of health care, the hospital plays a central role. Under the old regime, the hospital had functioned as much more than just a building where inpatients received a physician's care and the nurse's and pharmacist's attention. Rather, the hospital had also served as the font of free advice and a place of shelter and ultimate refuge in times of distress. In popular parlance, "going to the hospital" meant giving up and preparing to die. Contemporaries often used *hospital* to connote either an institution designed for the treatment of acute illness or a place of lifelong charitable custody for the ailing poor, more properly called a *hospice*. Compounding the confusion, Louis XIV created the "General Hospital" (*Hôpital général*), an umbrella organization that grouped the hospices of Bicêtre for men and Salpêtrière for women as well as the institutions belonging to the "Great Poorhouse" (*Grand bureau des pauvres*). Beginning in the 1650s, the government herded vagrants and deviants, many of them sick, into these hospices, in what has been called the Great Confinement (*grand renfermement*). While it is not possible to discriminate exactly between the two terms in every instance—for example, when a hospice included a hospital unit—this book distinguishes as clearly as possible between the two institutions, because they served different purposes, one, therapeutic, the other, custodial.

While hospitals and hospices gradually adapted to new purposes, problems of staffing and funding plagued them all. Before long, the deep disruptions of social strife, the drain of war on the economy, and the staunch opposition of the king and the pope to the Revolution grew into daunting obstacles to reform. Heightening these hurdles, the medical profession evidenced unexpected reluctance to serve nationalized medicine: the doctors did not wish to be turned into civil employees. Thus manpower, money, and religion proved to be major national problems on the path to health care reform. There was, moreover, no consensus regarding the pursuit of three contradictory goals: therapeutic medicine, preventive medicine, and education of the citizenry in the practice of health maintenance. This book studies the arguments, achievements, and shortcomings in these three fields.

◆◆◆

The rapid course of Revolutionary events soon overwhelmed the Poverty Committee's humane projects. This has led historians such as Jacques Léonard to argue that these were but "noble utopias . . . the grandiose plans of powdered and sincere reformers."[7] Such a judgment wrongly confines these developments to the early 1790s; it ignores their democratic message and their long-range influence. True, the dramatic political upheavals of 1792–1795 foiled an orderly and quick implementation of these projects. But the definitions, guidelines, and draft legislation elaborated by the Poverty and Health Committees remained standards and reference points for the emergence of the citizen-patient. Just as the Declaration of the Rights of Man and the Citizen could not immediately create citizens who were free and equal but served rather to set that goal for future governments, so the declaration of the citizen's right to health care set a target toward which our societies have striven since the French Revolution. Thus the Poverty Committee's program "failed," but only in the sense that the American Bill of Rights failed, in the short run. When American and French Revolutionaries formulated their belief in man's rights, they implied faraway goals for women and men that democratic societies since the late eighteenth century have felt compelled to pursue.

Léonard's argument also ignores the Revolutionaries' considerable achievements, which consisted, first, in investigating and documenting the hospitalized patients' condition and culling medical problems from general want. This allowed qualified professionals to treat medical patients, replacing the charitable volunteers who had indiscriminately lavished assistance on paupers in need. Second, the Revolutionaries reorganized, modernized, multiplied, and varied the institutions where the citizen found health care; and, third, they collaborated with the professionals trained to dispense medical aid to create orderly and solvent networks. These developments paralleled the evolution of contemporary legal, religious, educational, social, and political change. Just as the Civil Code, the Concordat, or the metric system meant a break with the old regime while incorporating past values and achievements and setting the stage for the future, so the Hospital and Health Councils of the Seine promoted the citizen-patients' emergence. The crucial problem was to educate the patient to behave like a citizen. Henry Sigerist asserted over fifty years ago that "the people's health . . . is the concern of the people themselves. They must want health."[8] To instill that motivation meant to create citizen-patients.

Citizens became active participants in such increasingly important health issues as hygiene, nutrition, and the protection of the environment. These issues had preoccupied the reformers of the 1770s and 1780s, some of whom became the leaders of the 1790s and beyond. Prominent among them ranked Thouret, who was a member of the Royal Society of Medicine (*Société royale de médecine*) and dean of the Paris Health School from 1794 to 1810; the pharmacist Antoine Augustin Parmentier, who devoted a lifetime to the improvement of nutrition; and Jean Noël Hallé, a pioneer in the new field of hygiene. Many such men kept out of sight during the violent phase of the Revolution but resumed leadership under the Consulate. Thus they crossed a symbolic bridge, bringing the outlook and talents of the Enlightenment to the nineteenth century. True, some outstanding scientists, thinkers, and reformers lost their lives or their spirit during the Revolution: the chemist Antoine Laurent Lavoisier perished under the guillotine; the anatomist Félix Vicq d'Azyr died "of a broken heart"; the philosopher J. M. A. de Caritat, marquis de Condorcet, committed suicide; the health inspector Jean Colombier died of "overwork." But others, foremost the physician-chemist François Fourcroy, delved into Revolutionary politics, and the Revolution opened careers for new men whose talents the restrictive laws of the old regime had held at bay. The physician and industrial chemist Jean Antoine Chaptal served as minister of internal affairs during the Consulate; the prominent Ideologue physician Georges Cabanis entered politics; Philippe Pinel, professor of internal medicine at the Paris Health School, presided over Salpêtrière Hospice as physician-in-chief for thirty years. The new leadership stood for secular efficiency and for the use of medical science in the service of the patient.

A centralized administrative health care network evolved in Paris and served as a model for other towns. It focused on ways to promote the citizen-patients' partnership in the improvement of their health. The Hospital Council of the Seine Department, established in 1801, amalgamated traditional paternalism with encouragement of self-help. A central admitting office practiced a stern medical triage: malingerers (*faux malades*) now found themselves blacklisted; applicants judged admissible were referred to hospitals and hospices, or—and this is noteworthy—to an array of new alternative facilities such as outpatient clinics, infirmaries, dispensaries, and nursing homes, whose success depended on the citizen-patients' collaboration, as did that of the national Vaccination Institute. These initiatives succeeded when they targeted specific medical complaints or health hazards. They were designed to alleviate illness as a cause of poverty, as La Rochefoucauld-Liancourt had proposed. They thus helped a little to reduce the general misery of the poor.

Health care thus became more efficient, discriminating, diversified, and appropriate. Patients now found a number of hospitals equipped to cope with their diseases to the best of contemporary knowledge, while the attending physicians evolved into specialists. We can watch dermatology, psychiatry, geriatrics, pediatrics, and even neonatology begin to take shape (for the sake of convenience, we shall commit the anachronism of calling these specialties by their present-day names.) In related developments, hospitals like those for venereal diseases or mental illness spun off small establishments for private care at modest fees. Meantime the National Assembly created public establishments for deaf and blind children and attempted to cull young citizen-patients from among them. The Directory moved the lying-in service and the Foundlings' Hospice from the overcrowded Hôtel-Dieu and its vicinity to the salubrious outskirts of town in the hope of salvaging more babies, and the Consulate opened the world's first children's hospital in 1802. Wherever appropriate, provision was made to render the children literate and to teach them a trade. The Hospital Council of the Seine Department orchestrated these efforts. Half a century later, on 10 January 1849, Louis Napoleon Bonaparte, president of the Second French Republic, transformed the Hospital Council, a pilot organization, into the Public Assistance of Paris (*Assistance publique à Paris*), a permanent part of the municipal government.[9]

◆◆◆

This book analyzes the interplay of adherence and resistance to health care reforms and their impact on the population during the Republic and Empire. It is meant to complement the pioneering work by Erwin H. Ackerknecht, Pierre Huard, and George Rosen and to explore the topic further, together with likeminded colleagues such as Matthew Ramsey and Ann LaBerge. This book remains focused on illness as a cause of destitution, on the experience of citizen-patients, and on their changing relationships to the health professions and the administrative powers, in the light of evolving cultural, economic, and social conditions and of the contemporary revolution in medicine.

It is particularly informative to study the politics of health in Paris, because here powerful forces of the medical Enlightenment had since midcentury been transforming the professions, hospitals, and education. Toby Gelfand, Marie-José Imbault-Huart, and Jean Pierre Goubert have studied important aspects of this theme; a recent book by

Jean Imbert and associates, *La protection sociale sous la révolution française* (Social Protection under the French Revolution), discusses the context in which health care for the needy evolved.[10] Whenever the Revolutionary legislators faced a lack of national facts and figures on health matters, they scrutinized Parisian institutions and then projected national needs on the basis of Parisian (and some foreign) data. Thus, owing to a lack of national information, Paris set the tone and the targets for national medical policy, education, research, and publication. The major schools, laboratories, academies, journals, and publishers were all located in Paris. For a Frenchman success could only be attained in the capital.[11]

When this book follows the Revolutionary reformers on their site visits to Paris hospitals and shares their insistence on single beds, cleanliness, order, and appropriate medical and nursing care, it does more than pursue relevant detail. Rather, we investigate exactly how the reformers attempted to uncover the intimate personal, material, demeaning aspects of charitable care that poor persons had to endure in the past. We observe the reformers' insistence on the creation of a dignified environment for patient care: walls were to be repainted, debris removed, foul odors curbed, sheets properly dried, promenoirs built, and occupational therapy such as needlework or gardening provided for. A stint as patients in the renovated hospital would, the reformers believed, motivate paupers to become citizen-patients.

Paris not only was a magnet but put her imprint on the whole country. Parisian reformers assumed that provincials would follow their lead. And when France conquered a considerable part of Europe and overthrew the old regime in foreign lands, her soldiers and diplomats replaced antiquated structures and methods with French exports ranging from the metric system and the Civil Code to new curricula for medical education and a modernized pharmacopoeia. Paris set the pattern for the continent until the rise of laboratory medicine at midcentury.[12]

♦♦♦
The time frame 1789–1815 has been adhered to in this book because profound and lasting changes occurred in French health care at the turn of the nineteenth century. The year 1789 matters in French politics of health because the national legislature then declared its responsibility for the needy citizens' physical well-being. But in the history of medical ideas, it is not 1789 that stands out but the last third of the eighteenth century. Nor did Bonaparte's coup d'état of November 1799 interrupt the evolution of health care and medical education in France, or change the circumstances of the sick and the handi-

capped, although the restoration of law and order naturally affected everyone. Similarly, the date 1815 is of scant significance in the history of medicine beyond marking the end of a quarter century of war. It meant little, for example, to Catholic professional nurses, who regained their corporate identity in 1808, or to the orphans and foundlings of France, whose fate was sealed by the law of 1811.

Within the era under study, Revolutionary and Napoleonic developments are so intimately connected that they should be seen as phases of one single story. To argue with Colin Jones that hospital policy made a U-turn is to stop short at the time of the Directory.[13] David Vess adopted the same truncated perspective.[14] On the other hand, to extend one's study to 1848, as does Ackerknecht, sacrifices the focus on dramatic Revolutionary change. By limiting the canvas to 1789–1815, the historian can watch Enlightenment thought mature in the early nineteenth century. This framework has been used by Pierre Huard and Jean Imbert in their studies of medical science and hospital law.

After exploring "Enlightened Innovation" under the old regime and following the reformers on their site visits to the "Grim Reality" of the Paris hospitals in Part 1 of the book, we study the subsequent "Reform and Resistance" in Part 2. The argument then focuses on "The Citizen-Patient and the Hospital"—namely the experience of outpatients and inpatients and the impact of specialization; this section encompasses the aged, new mothers, infants, and young children, as well as the multi-pronged efforts to encourage and nurture the ailing or ill among the disadvantaged. In Part 4, entitled "Outreach: The Impaired Citizen-Patient," we follow the Revolutionary reformers' lead and explore their achievements on behalf of the handicapped and the mentally ill. In Part 5, "Prospects," we return to the theme of the citizen-patient's duties, particularly as regards the environment and disease prevention. The Revolutionary and Napoleonic military campaigns had provided veterans with experience in hygiene, and the health officer returning home to civilian practice in Paris found an active public Health Council there and a chair in hygiene at the medical school, where the subject had been taught since 1795. After 1815, France became the leading European nation in public health.[15]

◆◆◆

Not all historians see the physicians of the Revolution as well-intentioned purveyors of health care. For the past quarter of a century, distrust of doctors has pervaded the historical discourse on this topic. Critics such as Robert Castel, Michel Foucault, R. D. Laing, Thomas Szasz, and Andrew Scull have made it fashionable to charge that physicians misused the power they derived from knowledge of their patients' illnesses, particularly in the case of hospitalized poor patients, whom physicians are said to have used indiscriminately for the advancement of their science. According to this argument, doctors turned the hospitals into "curing machines"; a depersonalization of the patient set in, the profession becoming increasingly absorbed with diseases, while "the sick-man gradually disappeared from the doctor's consciousness."[16] Foucault's brilliant concept of the medical *"gaze,"* with its implications of surveillance, investigation of "archeologic" depths of behavior, and contempt for and manipulation of individual human beings, led him to equate the physician with the military commander, the prison warden, and the factory owner. Having endowed the doctor with the class interests of the exploiters, Foucault sees him as a bourgeois dedicated to the production of knowledge, or, in the case of the asylum, as the "medical personage" who sits in perpetual judgment over the inmates.[17] Foucault's world has room neither for patient-oriented treatment of the physically and mentally ill nor for any recognition that patients do need guidance and doctors have expertise that enables them to diagnose an illness correctly and propose an appropriate therapeutic regimen.

While acknowledging the stimulating impact of this critique, this book frequently shows the doctor in roles not envisaged by Foucault: as a humane clinician, a therapist striving to reeducate a handicapped child, an administrator trying to spread vaccination or to salvage part of the annual crop of four to five thousand abandoned babies. Gathering knowledge is not necessarily achieved at the expense of the patient. And while there is no gainsaying that medicine has become more and more physicalist and technologic since the time of the French Revolution, and that some physicians fit Foucault's analysis, many others do not. Foucault's views, when checked against archival sources and printed evidence, prove partial in both senses of the term—they are incomplete and they are biased.

◆◆◆
Fundamental problems explored in this book were illuminated long ago by Alexis de Tocqueville when he argued in *The Old Regime and the French Revolution* (1856) that the institutions of the old regime were already changing in the eighteenth century, so that violent revolution merely cleared away barriers, making social evolution possible. We shall see that the plans and achievements of the Revolution and Napoleonic era in health care did indeed grow out of the Enlightenment, and that the Revolution leveled the field by removing antiquated structures and producing some new leaders. New relations

among patients, doctors, society, and the government resulted from the more orderly administration and management introduced by the Consulate, from the effects of de-Christianization and the subsequent Concordat on patient care, from the impact of the new medical education on doctors and patients, and from the transformation of the lessons in hygiene and prevention garnered on military campaigns into the citizen-patients' ability to maintain their own health.

Various governing bodies held differing views about the citizen-patient's role in health care. Where the Poverty Committee envisioned impoverished patients gladly collaborating in pursuit of the general health, neither the Jacobins nor Napoleon (nor the Utopian Socialists of the nineteenth century) hesitated to impose compliance with rules and obligations. As Jean Jacques Rousseau put it, they "forced the people to be free." This book will remain alert to the nuances of citizen-patients' collaboration in efforts to improve their own and the general health. Their political right to health care would only be won at the ballot box in a democratic future.

When François Furet argues that "the French Revolution is over,"[18] he means that the period of seeing the French upheaval as a rehearsal of the Russian Revolution of 1917 is now past. But that does not mean that in our study of that momentous French event we need abandon the search for aspects of equality that socialism and democracy have in common. In the social history of medicine, the Revolutionary and imperial period still yields fresh material for research and interpretation, including serious social problems that democratic as well as socialist societies must confront and that our own age has not yet solved.

This book explores numerous aspects of health care for the citizen that should claim the attention of historians and students of modern France, of urban history, and of health policy. It in no way claims originality for the ideas and stratagems of the French Revolutionaries and reformers, who drew on the experience of colleagues in Austria, Italy, and especially Great Britain, and of cities such as Hamburg. Yet they were convinced that given their context—that of a powerful, wealthy, centralized Catholic kingdom living through profound social, intellectual, cultural, religious, economic, and political changes— their experience and experiments with health care for the citizen-patient in Paris were unique.

René Dubos has taught us that health for a whole population is a mirage,[19] and yet, in a democracy, reaching for that mirage remains an inescapable moral imperative. That is not the only paradox we must live with: for while our medical miracles produce increased longevity, they give rise to geriatric illnesses that we cannot cure. We may all become medically indigent, in the sense that few could pay the real cost of heroic surgical interventions or long-term care using advanced technology. Any modern society would bankrupt itself if it offered its citizens "prompt, free, assured, and complete" health care, as the duc de la Rochefoucauld-Liancourt proposed. What the government is compelled to provide on moral and historic grounds, and what medical science is now able to produce, society cannot afford. The burden now falls on the citizen-patients, who will have to establish priorities, given their limited means. A government faces drastic constraints when it attempts to bring good health care within the reach of all citizens, as the French Revolutionaries were the first to discover.

I

TRADITION:

The Grim Reality of the Old Regime

Enlightened Innovation

The state owes every citizen . . . assured subsistence, food, appropriate clothing, and a way of life not injurious to health.

Baron C. L. de S. de Montesquieu, in *The Spirit of the Laws,* 1748

The Humane Legacy of the Enlightenment

In the thirty years between the devastating fire at the Paris Hôtel-Dieu on New Year's Eve of 1773 and the creation of the Public Health Council of the Seine Department in 1802, France laid the foundation for health care in a democracy. This chapter documents the seminal role of the Enlightenment, whose humane legacy encompassed the philosophic convictions and the political theory that established man's right to health care. But the Enlightenment also elaborated model hospitals, well-thought-out plans for medical education and regulations for the practice of medicine, and programs to guide, protect, and police the citizens' personal and public health practices in both civilian and military life. Debates on these issues in pre-Revolutionary years often led to significant action. The spotlight of public attention turned to new ventures such as neighborhood hospitals and nursing homes: we find smallness prized here, and local solidarity, and we identify schemes for self-help and home care. The reformers favored aid that bolstered individual self-reliance and initiative to help the poor safeguard their own health. The Revolution then cleared the stage of long-standing obstructions, permitting reform to proceed. Chapter 2 contrasts this legacy of the Enlightenment with the grim reality of the public hospital on the eve of the Revolution.

Health was not a major theme in the writings of the philosophes, yet many of them took a clear stand on the issue. Thus Montesquieu spelled out fundamental principles in classic terms, asserting that the state owed all citizens "an assured subsistence, food, appropriate clothing, and a way of life *not injurious to health*." He claimed that the worker had a right to a safe environment, protection from disease and a place in the public hospital in case of illness.[1] It is doubtful whether the widely traveled baron ever set foot in a hospital, but the younger generation of philosophes mixed more freely with ordinary people. Denis Diderot (1713–1784), for example, whose empathy for the common man is well known, drew attention to the innate inequality of the handicapped in his *Letters* on the blind and on the deaf.[2] He also pointed to the abject state of the hospitals in his *Encyclopédie* articles "*Infirmier*" and "*Hôtel-Dieu*," describing the Paris Hôtel-Dieu as "the biggest, roomiest, richest and most terrifying of all our hospitals. . . . Imagine . . . every kind of patient, sometimes packed three, four, five, or six into a bed, the living alongside the dead and dying, the air polluted by this mass of sick bodies, passing the pestilential germs of their afflictions from one to the other, and the spectacle of suffering and agony on every hand. That is the Hôtel-Dieu."[3] Even the king's minister A. R. J. Turgot (1727–1781) argued in the *Encyclopédie* that "the poor man has unassailable claims upon the wealth of the rich," and that donors should not control endowments from beyond the grave.[4]

Reformers created a sheaf of projects. Pierre Samuel Dupont de Nemours (1739–1817), for example, devised a plan to assist the ailing poor of Philadelphia,[5] and Claude Piarron de Chamousset (1717–1773) proposed a health insurance scheme.[6] The philosophes generally approved of "medical police," including health measures that the government imposed on the people, such as quarantines that forcibly detained suspected carriers of infection, and cordons sanitaires that prevented such persons from entering healthy places. Under the heading "Police (Jurisprudence)," the *Encyclopédie* specified that "with regard to health, the police must supervise wet-nursing, the cleanliness of air, fountains, wells, and rivers, the quality of food, wine, beer, and other beverages, the distribution of medicines, the incidence of epidemic and contagious disease." The article then detailed precautions regarding food and the urban environment, explaining that "the police regulate the storage of grain . . . the sale of meat . . . fish, butter, cheese, fruit, and vegetables . . . the quality and sale of beverages . . . the control of fires . . . the cleanliness of streets, the maintenance . . . of pavements . . . the use of cabbies . . . mail coaches and rental horses." The *Encyclopédie* even included the teaching and practice of medicine in its definition of health-related "police" and concluded that the government "must aid the deserving poor . . . disperse able-bodied beggars, hospitalize ailing and infirm indigents, and assist both groups with authorized support."[7] The Enlightenment obviously understood the complexities and dangers of ill health.

Nor had the government remained idle. The king had for decades sent "epidemic doctors" (*médecins des épidémies*) to endangered areas and boxes of remedies ranging from specifics, such as cinchona bark, to proprietary mixtures like "purgative febrifuge powder" or "incising dissolving powder."[8] The king also dispatched midwives to the provinces to instruct provincial women. The famous Madame Du Coudray (1715–1794) taught an estimated 5,000 students.[9]

Medical policing fit the mercantilistic strategies and administrative "cameralism" of the major Western states in the seventeenth century,[10] and enlightened despotism in the eighteenth century also filled this role with natural ease. At the end of that century, the classic statement of the subject, Johann Peter Frank's *System einer vollständigen medizinischen Polizei,* appeared.[11] Numerous contemporary doctors, scientists, physiocrats, and reformers shared their governments' outlook and exerted themselves to improve the health-related living and working conditions of the poor. They tested the quality of water and air; toiled to improve foodstuffs; experimented with new seeds, fertilizer, crop rotation, and cross-breeding; introduced drainage and irrigation, new machinery, and schools. Turgot in the Limousin, La Rochefoucauld on his family lands at Liancourt, and scores of less famous men worked tirelessly to improve the diet and skills of their peasants and to instruct them. C. C. Gillispie has abundantly documented their activities.[12]

One outstanding innovator in nutrition, Antoine Augustin Parmentier (1737–1813), devoted his life to developing inexpensive foodstuffs. He was famous, of course, for introducing the potato into France, but alas, Parisian paupers thought potatoes fit food only for horses! Following a career pattern that is typical for a significant number of leaders in health care, Parmentier worked for the old as well as the new regime in professional capacities. He served as Louis XVI's inspector of military pharmacy; inspired the creation of the Central Pharmacy of Paris in 1796; produced the new French pharmacopoeia; and shared in the activities of the Public Health Council of the Seine from 1802 until his death. Under the Consulate, we even find Parmentier and his colleague Antoine Alexis Cadet de Vaux (1743–1828) taste-testing the "economic soup" distributed to the poor.[13]

These pharmacists and others, like Pierre Bayen (1725–1798) and Nicolas Deyeux (1745–1837), did far more than run apothecaries'

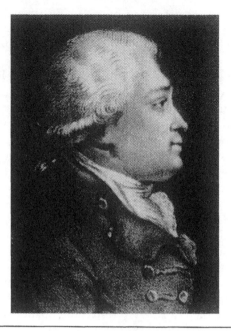

FIGURE 1.1. Félix Vicq d'Azyr (1748–1794). Lithograph from a painting by J. G. Soufflot (1713–1780). Bibliothèque nationale, Paris, Cabinet des estamples.

shops: they functioned as skilled chemists in projects of public usefulness, often using their premises as chemical laboratories. They thus rendered an important public service, for chemistry was not yet an accredited subject of academic study, and few laymen could afford to equip themselves with the expensive apparatus, utensils, furnaces, and materials needed by the pharmacist. Such equipment, however, filled the laboratory of the well-to-do Antoine Laurent Lavoisier (1743–1794), who had already pursued health-related problems in his student days, when he analyzed the quality of a variety of waters during a geological mapping trip.[14] Later he participated in over seventy reports on twenty-three subjects related to medicine and public health. "Of greatest importance were the investigations of prisons and hospitals," write his bibliographers, "they incorporated not only Lavoisier's chemistry, but considerations by him of climate, lighting, water purity and supply, sewage, ventilation and nutrition." His research was cited again and again during the Revolution as the basis of calculations designed to establish how much "respirable air" a hospitalized patient required and therefore what the optimal size of a hospital ward should be.[15]

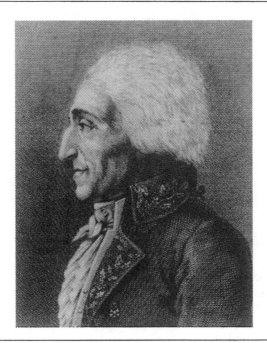

FIGURE 1.2. Antoine Augustín Parmentier (1737–1813). Académie nationale de médecine, Paris.

◆◆◆

Health-related problems concerning air, water, living conditions, and the environment were being discussed with increasing frequency in Parisian academic and social circles in the 1770s and 1780s. The Academy of Sciences had always interpreted "science" to cover medicine. Its membership included physicians, surgeons, pharmacists, and veterinarians, since no academy of medicine existed in France until 1820. The Academy's mandate obligated it to render public judgments on scientific innovations, including those potentially useful or harmful to health. Thus the Academy's decisions ranged from the therapeutic uses of electricity and the validity of Mesmerism to the appropriateness of sign language in teaching the deaf and of raised type to enable the blind to read with their fingertips. The Academy's deliberations and verdicts were published in French, so that all educated persons could understand them. Thus health-related controversy reached the educated public, the salons, the coffeehouses, the press, and, indirectly, the poor.

Reform-oriented doctors met at the Royal Society of Medicine, founded in 1776 by the king's first physician, J. M. F. de Lassone

(1717–1788), and his minister Turgot. This society concerned itself
with nutrition, hygiene, and the purity of food and drugs, as well as
with epidemics, epizootics, the environment, and the control of char-
latanry—in other words, with medical policing.[16] Owing to the active
leadership of its permanent secretary, Félix Vicq d'Azyr (1748–1794),
the society established a network of correspondence among forward-
looking physicians and surgeons throughout the kingdom, and with
provincial colleges, universities, and academies. Vicq d'Azyr publicized the society's prizes for essays on current medical issues.[17] Prize-
winners included some future leaders in health care for the citizen-
patient: the "pediatrician" Jean Abraham Auvity (1754–1821) received
one of four prizes given in 1786 for an essay on a neonatal infection
called *muguet* or *aphthes* (thrush), and the next year his colleague
Charles François Andry (1741–1829) won a gold medal for an article
on sclerema neonatorum, an illness of newborns caused by dehydra-
tion.[18] The military surgeon Pierre François Percy (1754–1825) was
awarded a gold medal worth thirty livres for an essay on artificial feeding of infants.[19] And in 1792 the future "psychiatrist" Philippe Pinel
(1745–1826) won a prize for his answer to the problem: "Indicate the
most effective means for treating patients who have become insane
before reaching old age."[20]

Meanwhile, Vicq d'Azyr was urging provincial physicians to register the daily phenomena determining their local "medical topography." The Royal Society collected these regional records with a view
to publishing a health survey that would be useful to the citizenry.[21]
That project was never completed. In contrast, the Royal Society
spent the major part of its meetings, from 7 August 1789—soon after
the fall of the Bastille—to November 1790, elaborating a New Plan
for French Medicine ("Nouveau plan de constitution pour la médecine
en France"),[22] which Vicq d'Azyr submitted to the Health Committee
of the National Assembly immediately upon completion.[23] This New
Plan directly influenced the curriculum of the new "health schools"
founded in 1794, as well as the legislation to regulate the practice of
medicine, pharmacy, and midwifery promulgated in 1803. It is the
major link between the medical reform ideas of the Enlightenment and
their implementation in the Revolutionary and Napoleonic era. A suc-
cinct analysis of its contents will follow here; its political fortunes are
discussed in Chapter 3.

Part I of the New Plan discussed a reorganized medical school curriculum where anatomy, physiology, and pathology were to be taught
in their relation to the pure or applied basic sciences—then called "ac-
cessory," including natural history, chemistry, and physics.[24] Hygiene

figured prominently. One professor would teach obstetrics as well as women's and children's diseases.

Despite his interest in the advancement of knowledge, Vicq d'Azyr never lost sight of medical care as the chief aim of the enterprise. He realized that clinical medicine requires a totally different approach than research. Doctors must make decisions whether or not they understand the illness they are called to treat. "When one goes from the schoolbench to the sickbed," he wrote, "most theoretical principles no longer apply." The crucial innovation in the plan was the emphasis on clinical medicine, "so important that we felt all the details should be put before the legislature immediately."[25]

In part II of the New Plan, Vicq d'Azyr explained the national health care provisions that the Royal Society proposed. The recent division of France into eighty-three departments was a welcome convenience to the medical reformers. The politicians had devised a pattern that enabled every citizen to reach his departmental administration in one day's travel. The medical reformers used the new national map to assure the citizen-patient equal access to health care: every Frenchman would now be able to reach the best available medical help equally fast. A governing body would gather the physicians of each department into a health council, to plan for the region and keep in touch with Paris.

The following excerpt from the section entitled "The Practice of Medicine in Its Relation to Public Health" illustrates the reformers' arithmetic egalitarianism:

Distribution of Doctors and Surgeons in Countryside and Towns

Doctors and surgeons shall live in the countryside according to the needs of each department. Their assignments are to be established exactly, on the following basis:

since each department measures 18 x 18 leagues [1 league = 2.5 miles], that is, 324 square leagues, has a radius of 9 leagues, and its capital in the center. . . .

each department should be divided into a maximum of 9 districts, each measuring 6 x 6 leagues (or 36 square leagues), each district should be divided into a maximum of 9 cantons of 2 x 2 leagues (or 4 square leagues). That is the basic unit to which doctors should be assigned to watch over the health of the countryside. . . .

Supposing that one person out of 20–40 is sick—which is the proportion prevalent in the army—one canton may contain 50–100 patients on any one day. If the proportion of indigents in France is figured as one-twentieth of the population—as in England—this would mean 3–4 patients a day for the public doctor."[26]

This passage confirms that Vicq d'Azyr was ready to regiment the population for its own good. He was the contemporary of the Utilitarians and, in his health care policy at least, a forerunner of the Utopian Socialists. And he expected that members of the liberal professions would willingly support the national welfare.

In return for a free education and a government salary, an estimated six thousand public doctors would "belong to the departments." Trained at regional teaching hospitals, they learned from government-sponsored textbooks. Graduation qualified them to practice medicine, surgery, obstetrics, pharmacy, veterinary medicine, and inoculations. They supervised foundlings and inspected health conditions in workhouses and jails, because "imprisonment should not exceed deprivation of freedom, it should protect the prisoners' health."[27]

Part III of the New Plan proposed legislation to replace the medical corporations, colleges, and faculties that had clung to outmoded costumes, prerogatives, and the Latin language. They had been sovereign within their boundaries, jealously protective of their own members, imposing costly and discriminatory admissions procedures, dues, rules, and fines. The Royal Society advocated open competition for professorial chairs before public juries. Doctors and pharmacists should be entitled to settle where they pleased, and physicians should not be empowered to dispense drugs.

Vicq d'Azyr saw veterinary medicine as closely allied to its human counterpart (part IV of the New Plan) and emphasized the study of comparative anatomy, his own specialty. But closest to his heart was the encouragement of research (part V of the New Plan). He proposed an academy (the Royal Society, enhanced and enlarged?) as the keystone of the new structure: "It is not enough to establish good medical education; one must also provide for the Advancement of Science [Francis Bacon's phrase, of course]." The new academy should undertake to

> correspond with the best physicians at home and abroad . . . multiply the observations, experiments, and tests that render medical knowledge more precise and of greater use . . . draw up a comprehensive research plan, and submit the details to its collaborators so that they can investigate each aspect. . . . Collect descriptions of all endemic, epidemic, and epizootic diseases and explain their history. . . . publish scientific papers . . . answer inquiries. . . . combat prejudice. . . . stimulate medical symposia in the provinces. . . . in a word, create from among all the citizens of France who love and cultivate Medicine a great body inspired by the same ideals and dedicated to the public weal, reason, and equality.[28]

This plan thus embodies the high hopes and expectations that the medical Enlightenment projected into the new era.

Less prestigious but no less important than the Royal Society of Medicine, the Agricultural Society, founded in 1761, set more modest goals. Targets included the regulation of the sale of remedies and chemical products that could be used to feed animals and fertilize the soil. The veterinary schools at Lyon (founded in 1762) and Alfort near Paris (founded in 1766) were among its concerns, as, of course, was land reform. Communication among the influential members of Parisian learned societies was easy, since a number of men belonged to several of them (Parmentier, Chaptal, Vicq d'Azyr, and Fourcroy, for example, belonged to the Agricultural Society, the Royal Society of Medicine, and the Academy of Sciences). The same learned men thus gathered several times a week to hear papers and discuss questions which frequently touched on the promotion and protection of citizens' health.

We cannot recapture the tone or sparkle of conversations in the Parisian salons where the philosophes and their friends met regularly under the auspices of intelligent and well-read women. But we know the substance of their discussions: these included all the ideas and problems of the day. The salon of the philosophe C. A. Helvétius's widow in Auteuil was of special importance for the citizen-patient. Benjamin Franklin was a regular guest there, as was Pierre Jean Georges Cabanis (1757–1808), the hostess's adoptive son. Michel Augustin Thouret, Condorcet, and the physician Pinel, whom Franklin tried to lure to America, were all visitors.

The citizen's experience as patient also attracted attention, particularly among Ideologue thinkers. As disciples of John Locke, Sir Francis Bacon, and the abbé de Condillac (1715–1780) they promoted a "science of man" rooted in observation, believing that only the inductive method brings results. Among physicians, the leading Ideologue was Cabanis, whose famous lectures on the mind-body problem at the Institut de France in 1796 can be considered the manifesto of contemporary medical science. Cabanis was a materialist, who based his theory of life on the vital properties of matter. "We feel, therefore we are," he proclaimed.[29]

Medical Ideologues rose to positions of importance at the turn of the nineteenth century. Cabanis served in the Council of 500 under the Directory and as a senator during the Consulate; at that time, Jean Louis Moreau de la Sarthe (1771–1826) lectured on the natural history of women at the Lycée républicain;[30] Jean Antoine Chaptal, sympathetic to Ideology, though not one of its leaders, seized unparalleled opportunities during his tenure as minister of internal affairs from 1801 to 1804. Through their newspaper, the *Décade philosophique*,[31] and as members of the Institut de France, the Normal and Central

School faculties, and "free" associations such as the Lycée républicain, the Society of the Observers of Man, and the Philomatic and Natural History Societies, Ideologue thinkers, both medical and lay, refor- mulated French thought about health.

The Ideologues were interventionists in the spirit of "medical po- lice." Seeing women and men as the products of their environment, they planned to revolutionize the setting in which the population lived, whether at home or in the hospital. In "Observations sur les hôpitaux," a widely quoted essay published in the winter of 1789– 1790, Cabanis summarized contemporary ideas. Typically for a Pari- sian, he remarks in the foreword that he will discuss conditions in the capital but speak for all of France. He thinks that the optimal size for a hospital is between 100 and 150 beds. The 120-bed Necker Hospital should serve as a model. Huge hospitals are hotbeds of contagion: "Simple wounds become serious, the serious ones, fatal; and major operations hardly ever succeed." Paris hospitals were overcrowded, stuffy, and wasteful. At the Hôtel-Dieu of Paris, patient care was rou- tine at best: everyone received the identical bouillon—often in exces- sive strength and quantity. "There are days for clysters [enemas], and days without clysters." Administrators should be paid employees, not volunteers, and so should the staff: the rough work is at present "entrusted to people lost to debauchery and debts . . . a mass of bandits who engage in domestic work to elude the police." Doctors must be put in charge of every aspect of patient care, including diet and, of course, drugs. They must take careful histories, keep records, and publish their journals. "The best professors of medicine are the patients."[32]

Cabanis's views on bedside teaching agreed with the international consensus. Among Frenchmen, the most widely quoted essays were those of Chambon de Montaux, C. F. Duchanoy and J. B. Jumelin, and G. C. Würtz;[33] among foreigners, those of S. A. Tissot and J. P. Frank.[34] Cabanis had some original views: physicians and surgeons should collaborate, so that physicians acquired some knowledge of surgery, and surgeons, of medicine. He disagreed with received wis- dom when he argued that surgery was better taught at a small hospi- tal, to avoid "the tumult of an immense practice where the observer has no time to see, where details crowd each other from his memory and leave confused impressions." He emphasized the unorthodox view that practical training in anatomy, surgery, midwifery, and phar- macy should be offered at any hospital throughout the country where the physician or surgeon was able and willing: the students would quickly appraise the quality of the instruction! In what must be the earliest instance of pointing to the United States as a model in medicine, Cabanis remarked approvingly that medical students in North America apprenticed themselves to an apothecary to master the compounding of remedies and learn the signs of illnesses at the bedside.[35]

Yet Cabanis's most original and sensitive proposal concerned the future of hospital nursing. He wrote:

> The National Assembly has raised our hopes that the shackles binding religious women will finally fall. These women now pay with their life-long happiness for a youthful lack of foresight or a momentary illusion. . . . The voluntary association of the Sisters of Charity is unquestionably the best institution for patient care. The government should entrust hospital service to them. . . . The most important source of their dedication may well be that they make only an annual commitment, after which they may reenter the world. . . .
>
> I would wish that any nun who has erred or been misled regarding her vocation might leave the cloister. . . . If a worldly life attracted her strongly, she would stop suffering and cease cursing laws that had immolated her by authorizing the irrevocable alienation of her person and life . . . ; this procedure deserves the approval of religion, reason, and humanity.[36]

This statement takes on poignancy when we learn that Cabanis's sister Francoise, who was two years his junior, and his paternal aunt Jeanne were Ursuline nuns. He may well here have been broadcasting intimate reflections that these two women had shared with him in private conversation.

Cabanis's sometimes original views on nursing, small hospitals, practical medical schools, clinical teaching, and the relation of urban to provincial hospitals earned him appointment to the Paris Hospital Commission in 1792. He thus helped administer the patients and institutions of the capital. This kind of public service based on expertise was precisely the role to which Ideologues aspired.

◆◆◆

Public interest suddenly focused on the hospital when the Hôtel-Dieu of Paris burned in a devastating fire on 30 December 1772. The fire raged for a week. Little wonder that frightened public imagination "raised the number of dead even beyond that of patients in the burning building."[37] The damage was enormous and everyone, from the king to private persons, donated food, blankets, clothes, and money to alleviate the emergency. The murderous overcrowding at the Hôtel-Dieu and the neglect of safety in its layout and storage of inflammable materials became topics of daily discussion.

Hospital-building now provided a fashionable topic of conversation. Books and memoirs on the subject abounded in the 1770s and

1780s. Central to the dispute was the proposal to fragment the enormous and unmanageable congeries of institutions in the middle of Paris into four medium-sized hospitals on the city's periphery. In 1773, Louis XV ordered the demolition of the Hôtel-Dieu. But when his grandson Louis XVI ascended the throne in 1774, he hesitated, preferring to submit a project for its transfer and reconstruction by C. P. Coquéau, with an architectural plan by Bernard Poyet, to the Academy of Sciences for study.[38] The Academy decided to form its own opinion. (Thirteen years had by then elapsed since the fire, and the burnt-down wing of the Hôtel-Dieu had been rebuilt.) To accomplish the task, the Academy chose a distinguished commission chaired by the astronomer Jean Sylvain Bailly (1736–1793), soon to be mayor of Paris and to die under the guillotine. He in turn selected Lavoisier, de Lassone, the renowned surgeon Jacques Tenon (1724–1816), the famous mathematician Pierre Simon de Laplace (1749–1827), the naturalist Louis Jean Marie Daubenton (1716–1800), the chemist Jean Darcet (1725–1801), the physicist Charles Augustin Coulomb (1736–1806), and the agronomist Mathieu Tillet (1714–1791).

The published result of the commission's work, Tenon's *Mémoires sur les hôpitaux de Paris,* remained famous as the most detailed and reliable source of information on French hospital reform for decades after its publication in 1788. Here the would-be reformer could for the first time find precise data about the Hôtel-Dieu's dimensions, layout, staff, and cost. Tenon evidenced an insatiable appetite for quantitative information about everything that impinged on patient welfare: the sizes and uses of wards and beds, staircases, kitchenettes, and toilets; the activities and hierarchies of nurses and servants; the routines of feeding, cleaning, and laundering; the quantities and quality of food, wine, and medicines; of mattresses, straw, sheets, and shirts; of water, wood, candles, and utensils. Tenon documented the staggering amounts of goods consumed, the incredible crowding, pollution, stench, and confusion. He wanted the Hôtel-Dieu replaced with four peripheral hospitals, administered and supplied by a "community center"(*maison commune*) on the Ile de la Cité, which would also house an emergency service.

Tenon provided standards: the minimum for "respirable air" per patient, for the width of staircases so that a stretcher could pass, for the height of a stair so that a convalescent could manage to climb it, for the optimal size of a bed so that a patient could rest, sleep, and turn over. Tenon measured the hospital on the human scale, envisaging an "instrument for recovery" in the hands of surgeons and a place of therapy for the mentally ill.[39] The Academy and Tenon agreed in

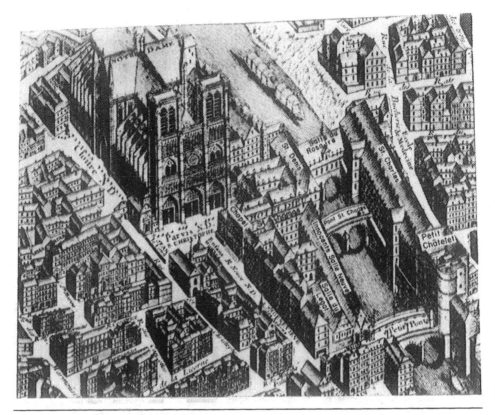

FIGURE 1.3. The Hôtel-Dieu of Paris, from Turgot's plan of Paris, 1739.

advocating the pavilion plan, with wards of about forty patients, as the basic module for future hospitals.[40]

But alas, before 1789, all efforts for reform of the Hôtel-Dieu came to naught, largely because the trustees and the sisters resisted change. They even refused the Academy of Sciences' commissioners access to their registers, while Tenon obtained his data through the good offices of friendly insiders, the head midwife and a doctor named Cochu. Thus, in the microcosm of the Paris Hôtel-Dieu the same struggle took place as on the national stage: the magistrates, financiers, and wealthy burghers who formed the hospital's board of trustees belonged to the same group of notables who, in 1787–1788, refused the government's plea that they tax themselves in order to relieve the national deficit. A stalemate resulted. A noted historian comments that the struggle was "bitter and passionate. . . . The past and the present

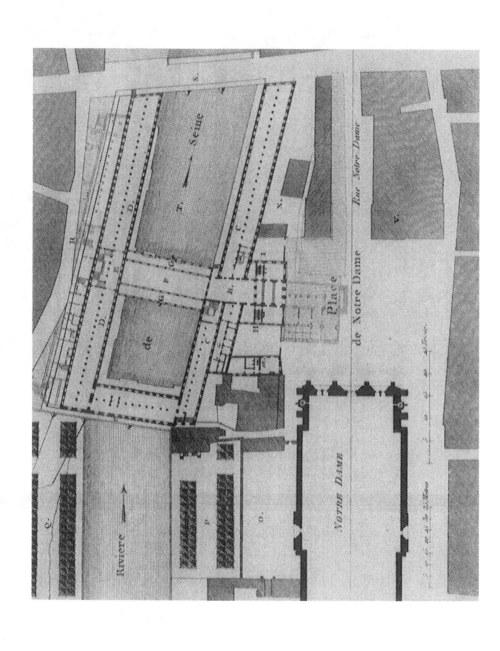

FIGURE 1.4. The Hôtel-Dieu of Paris, from Nicolas Clavareau, *Mémoires sur les hôpitaux civils* (Paris: Prault, 1805). The northwest wing (bottom right) on the Ile de la Cité was destroyed by fire in 1773 but rebuilt before the Revolution.

Location of the Hôtel-Dieu of Paris

A   Covered entrance with staircase to employees' lodgings

B   Hall leading to all sick wards and to the admitting office

CC Women's wards

DD Men's wards; in center

E   Large staircase leading to upper levels

F   Bridge to men's wards

GG Covered promenoirs for each gender

H   Kitchen courtyard

I   Courtyard for wine cellar

L   Dependencies of admitting office below: kitchen, butcher shop, refectory

M Pharmacy, laboratory, etc.

N Courtyard for stables and carriage sheds

O Passage to the archbishopric

P Garden, divided for both genders

Q Proposed male patients' garden

R Rue de la Bûcherie: will be 20 m wide (like rue Tournon) when the double connecting wards are completed

S Châtelet bridge

T River Seine

U Pont aux doubles

V Central Hospital Pharmacy

were locked in a fight. Only the Revolution would solve the conflict by destroying the social order."[41] Yet while tradition prevailed at the Hôtel-Dieu, innovation in hospital building and management elsewhere in Paris was cracking the shell of the past.

The Small Hospital: Public and Private Initiative

Between 1775 and 1785, Ackerknecht has pointed out, as many new hospitals were built in Paris as in the preceding 130 years.[42] Many of them can be viewed as pilot projects, a combination of public and private enterprise. Their distinguishing new features enhanced the importance and comfort of the individual patient and emphasized regular medical supervision and well-trained nursing personnel. The new hospital aimed at the patients' recovery rather than their salvation, and hospitalization sometimes even included a week's stay in a convalescents' section with permission to go out and find work. At the same time, nursing homes of varied sponsorship and clientele appeared. Catholic charity no longer held a monopoly of geriatric custodial care.

Soon after the monumental Academy of Surgery was inaugurated in 1774, the surgeons established a small postgraduate hospital nearby. In this *hospice de perfectionnement,* the "first French university hospital center,"[43] the indigent sick took on the dignified role of medical patients, each occupying a single bed. Ten beds were reserved for women and twelve for men, in meticulously clean, well-aired, and plentifully supplied wards. Admission hinged on the patients having "serious surgical illnesses . . . preferably those that are totally or virtually unknown," wrote Tenon. The members of the College's faculty took charge of the service in turn, but all consulted together when a patient's condition baffled them. Tenon proudly described this hospital as "a unique and invaluable institution" with a mission "to make the art of medicine progress and to help humanity."[44]

Surgery had come a long way since the day when the barber surgeons' guild was the butt of doctors' contempt. A career now beckoned at the hospital, and particularly at the Hôtel-Dieu of Paris, where a prototype of hospital internship already existed. Journeymen surgeons (*compagnons chirurgiens*) assisted residents (*chirurgiens gagnant maîtrise*), who could, in six years, become master surgeons. Externs came for part of the day, to work and to watch. During years of extern- and internship and residency, a surgeon had daily contact with the human body and its ailments. He gained experience and gathered knowledge that contemporary physicians lacked; Toby Gelfand has convincingly argued that the eighteenth-century surgeon knew more medicine than the physician.[45]

Soon the magnificent Academy of Surgery would be transformed into the Revolutionary Health School, absorbing the postgraduate facilities under the new name of "Hôpital des cliniques." It was the reformers' hope, made explicit in Vicq d'Azyr's New Plan, that patients from all over the country who suffered from exceptionally puzzling, complex, or recalcitrant surgical illnesses would be brought here for study and treatment. We cannot assess whether this improbable expectation materialized. The surviving patient records—such as they are—rarely indicate place of birth, and never the date when a provincial may have moved to Paris.

Equally small and specialized, but experimental in purpose, was a hospital that foreshadowed the interest in child health so noticeable in the Revolutionary and Napoleonic era, when strenuous efforts saved babies at risk. A hospital for newborns with venereal disease founded by the Paris police lieutenant Lenoir on rue de Vaugirard in 1780 was coordinated with the Foundlings' Hospice (Enfants trouvés) in 1781.[46] It aimed at salvaging babies infected with syphilis. Their condition was a medical disaster, and it seemed particularly unfair that infants should suffer for the "transgressions" of their parents. Almost all syphilitic babies in public institutions died soon after birth: such was the grim reality. At Vaugirard Hospital, under the supervision of Chief Inspector Jean Colombier (1736–1789) and of René Alexandre Faguer (1740–1785), chief surgeon at Bicêtre, therapy was based on the intriguing theory that mother's milk would transmit curative substances to the infant. The doctors admitted pregnant syphilitic women on the condition that, after delivery, they breast-feed an abandoned infant in addition to their own. The hospital had room for 69 women and 90 babies. Treatment usually began ten to fifteen days after delivery and consisted of "the anti-venereal remedy in appropriate dosages and a mixed method including frictions, baths, mercurial and sudorific medication together with laxatives."[47] Liancourt found "the idea of this treatment both ingenious and humane. . . . It seems that the nurses of these babies are more attached to them, and care better for them, than the nurses of healthy children . . . without them these unlucky infants are sure to die."[48] Treatment normally lasted four months and often led to the women's "cure." The figures indicate that in the decade of the 1780s, 703 women were admitted, and that 47 of them died of causes unrelated to syphilis, diagnosed as puerperal fever, consumption, hydropsy, scurvy, and other infectious or deficiency diseases. The salvaging of the babies, as will be seen, was another matter.

The therapy attempted at Vaugirard Hospital and the bold interventions undertaken at the postgraduate center were exceptional ventures. Other small hospitals had simpler goals—namely, to provide

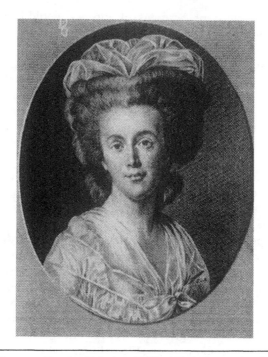

FIGURE 1.5. Suzanne Curchod Necker (1739–1794). Engraving by Blanchard. Bibliothèque interuniversitaire de médecine, Paris.

tures. Other small hospitals had simpler goals—namely, to provide decent accommodations for the sick poor, close to their homes if possible, so that friends and family could visit. By common consent the neighborhood hospital emerged as the favored model.

Exemplary management prevailed at Necker Hospital, officially the "Hospice de la Charité des paroisses de St. Sulpice et du Gros Caillou." Having secured funding from the king, Suzanne Curchod Necker (1739–1794) undertook the administration of this hospital in 1778. She demonstrated that proper medical care and humane treatment could be provided in a financially responsible manner. Her monthly accounts averaged the cost per patient at seventeen sous per day.[49] The Hospital Council named the establishment for her in 1802 and the official report on Paris hospitals characterized her accounts as "models of clarity and exactness, destined to serve forever as guides."[50]

Half of the 24 attendants who cared for the 120 patients were Sisters of Charity; in 1789 they were under the direction of Sister Cassegrain, who was succeeded by Sister Braujon in 1791 and by Sister Clavelot in 1803. They shepherded their hospital through the Revolution. When the Poverty Committee requested accounts in April 1791, Sister Braujon sent them immediately, impressing the duc de la Rochefoucauld-Liancourt with her efficiency.[51] The sisters lived communally and knew how to manage their staff; the servants, the almoner, the gardener, and the porter all took their meals at the hospital.[52] A resident physician, surgeon, and apothecary made rounds twice daily. François Doublet (1751–1795) served as physician from 1780 to 1783; C. Mongenot, later a physician at the Children's Hospital, served at Mme. Necker's institution from 1803 to 1809; and it was here that R. T. H. Laënnec (1781–1826) developed the stethoscope in 1816.

Necker Hospital followed an admissions policy typical of private institutions in all of Western Europe, excluding persons then considered "unclean"—meaning not only those with venereal and other communicable diseases, but pregnant women as well. The mentally ill were not welcome either. Medical discrimination thus prevailed, but there were no religious admission requirements, even though the parish priest officially certified an applicant's poverty and consequent eligibility for free hospitalization.

These policies should have allayed some of the citizenry's fears of entering the hospital. Excluding strangers protected the parish's funds and limited patients to neighbors, with whom one could share sorrows and confidences. Visitors, freely admitted in those days, brought support and distraction. But mortality was 1:7, "too high, considering the good care that patients receive in this hospital," the Poverty Committee commented in 1791.[53] One can only speculate that the poor were so afraid of the hospital, even a good one, that they shunned it until they were very sick and ready to die. The fact that British mortality figures were so much lower than their French counterparts relates to hospital admissions in a different way: British voluntary hospitals selected their patients with an eye to a rate of cure that would please their private patrons and contributors. In contrast, the French charity hospital took in everyone (with the previously stated exceptions).

Madame Necker had adapted a building vacated by the Benedictines of Notre-Dame de Liesse. The parish priest of St. Jacques-du-Haut-Pas, Jean Denis Cochin (1726–1783), built a new hospital at his own expense, in 1780–1782, at the corner of the faubourg St. Jacques and the rue des Capucins. With forty beds—half for women, half for men—and several rooms upstairs for senile or invalid parishioners, scurvy (then thought to be contagious), pregnancy, venereal disease, mental illness, and surgical emergencies. Eight Sisters of Charity, headed by Sister Déthienne, and five servants, cared for the patients, one-fifth of whom paid for their stay (usually 450–500 livres per year). The well-to-do members of the parish expressed their appreciation for this well-run small hospital through generous donations. By 1791 they had paid for the building and even amassed a small surplus.[54] Once nationalized, Cochin was expanded into one of the four general hospitals located on the periphery of Paris.

The indigent patients of Madame Necker's and the abbé Cochin's parishes thus received the best general hospital care available at the time, according to contemporary opinion. These institutions are the most spectacular examples of what was occurring elsewhere on a more modest scale: two Parisian parish priests, Louis Esprit Viennet and Théodore Marie Desbois de Rochefort, for example, founded hospitals at St. Merri and St. André des Arts in the 1780s, and a wealthy financier, Nicolas Beaujon (1718–1786), built a beautiful orphanage, with an annual revenue of 25,000 livres, for twenty-four children. The Revolution transformed Beaujon into a general hospital, temporarily named "hospice du Roule."[55]

St. Merri and St. André des Arts followed the pattern of Cochin Hospital, but in miniature. Established in private houses with the help of wealthy citizens, they had one room with five or six beds for women and another for men, and a separate room for "respectable paupers." St. Merri could even accommodate two contagious patients in a fourth-floor attic. Between six and eight Sisters of Charity administered each establishment, including a school for little girls at St. Merri and a spinning workshop at St. André des Arts. In the course of seven years, only fifty-six of nine hundred patients died there. "No praise is too high for the services and the zeal of the sisters," commented Liancourt, "nor for the prevailing orderliness."[56] The figures for St. Merri indicate that, with an average of twelve patients a month, these neighborhood hospitals were always filled to capacity.

In addition, Tenon's *Mémoires* drew attention to the Protestant Hospital, with six beds, run by the Swedish embassy and predictably clean and efficient.[57] Protestants had their own strong tradition of hospital nursing, developed during the Reformation, and Jews took care of their own patients, in their homes or in their communities.[58]

Thus a groundswell of local philanthropy enlisted the efforts of architects, administrators, doctors and donors to render hospitals more accessible, affordable, and effective for the citizenry. It is hardly surprising that the court did not remain indifferent.

Royal Efforts

Although absorbed in private pleasures, Louis XV occasionally followed the lead of his first physician, de Lassone, and his first surgeon, François Gigot de La Peyronie (1678–1747), and contributed to the health care of his people. In contrast, his grandson Louis XVI's kindly disposition made him eager to intervene wherever the king's authority could prevail over private interests: the inspection of hospitals and of prison and workhouse infirmaries, and the regulation of their medical and nursing services; the modernization of military medicine; the reassignment and renovation of buildings for health care purposes; and the establishment of retirement homes.

To initiate reform, Louis XVI allowed his finance minister, Jacques Necker (1732–1808), to appoint Dr. Jean Colombier as inspector of hospitals and prisons of the kingdom in 1780. Colombier and his colleague Dr. François Doublet set out on inspection tours that resulted in a series of "Observations made in the Department of Civilian Hospitals" published in 1785. One of these concerned Vaugirard Hospital; another decisively influenced the care of the mentally ill in France.[59]

It was undoubtedly at Colombier's behest (although he remained in the background) that plans to install infirmaries in the General Hospital were initiated in 1781. Of particular urgency were those planned for Salpêtrière and Bicêtre Hospices. Undated, printed "Provisional Regulations" provided for two nurses working twelve-hour shifts, responsible for sixteen patients each, a chief pharmacist with the needful number of residents, a physician-in-chief to visit all the patients twice a day, accompanied by the resident surgeon, an apothecary, and the head nurse.[60] These regulations bear a close resemblance to those spelled out in Colombier's treatise on military medicine of 1778.[61] This similarity suggests that, through inspectors such as Colombier, French military medicine influenced its civilian counterpart in significant ways. The influence of Jean Colombier was pervasive, not only because of his untiring, imaginative activity. He also helped shape and orient the careers of his three sons-in-law, all doctors: François Doublet, Michel Augustin Thouret, and N. R. D. Desgenettes, best known as physician-in-chief of the Egyptian expedition.

The armed forces produced several outstanding inspectors other than Jean Colombier: in the army, Jean François Coste (1741–1819); in the navy, Antoine Poissonnier (1723–1795) and his brother Pierre (1720–1798) (who also had army experience);[62] in pharmacy, Parmentier and Pierre Bayen. All of them had served for many years in army or navy medicine; three were members of the Academy of Sciences;[63]

three were to testify before the Health Committee of the National Assembly.[64] These experienced military and naval physicians and pharmacists formed a strong link between the old and the new regime.[65] As one might imagine, military medicine emphasized, not only nursing, but particularly surgery and hygiene. The army pioneered in teaching these skills: surgical demonstrations in anatomical "amphitheaters" became part of military medical instruction as early as the 1770s. In fact, in the ongoing dispute among scholars as to where clinical teaching originated, a close look at military medicine would probably show French army surgeons to have been the real pioneers. The army medical schools at Metz, Toul, and Verdun took the lead; the navy schools at Brest and Toulon followed suit.[66]

Three successive Bourbon kings founded military hospitals in Paris: Louis XIV built the sumptuous Hôtel royal des Invalides in 1674—in fact, a giant veterans' hospital and nursing home. Tenon offers a detailed description of its infirmaries, which had room for five hundred maimed, wounded, or acutely ill patients. They occupied fifteen wards on the ground and first floors, with plenty of space and fresh air, single beds, and wholesome food. Seventeen Sisters of Charity administered patient care.[67]

Louis XIV's successors provided for their soldiers in more modest proportions. Louis XV created the Hospital of the French Guard; when Liancourt described it, the name had changed to Hospital of the Paris National Guard. Whatever its name, the provisions and amenities for sick soldiers were exemplary: single beds, of course; separate wards for surgical, postoperative, contagious, and fever patients; sufficient domestics, nurses and doctors; fresh air; good food; appropriate hospital clothing; gardens to walk in.[68] To meet the expenses, "each soldier gives up his pay; the king provides the remainder."[69] Tenon calls the royal ordinance that had created the military hospitals "a lasting monument of wisdom and humanity that one must consult prior to building and organizing hospitals."[70]

Under Louis XVI's aegis, the reassignment of unused buildings for health-related purposes proceeded apace: in 1781, the endowments of the Enfants rouges enriched the Paris Foundlings' Hospice; in 1783, the king bought the former Capuchin novitiate building on the rue St. Jacques and ordered its transformation into a venereal disease hospital, and he offered the vacant Celestins barracks as a residential school for deaf children.[71] He also proposed to solve the deadlock over dividing up the Hôtel-Dieu by offering to donate the Ecole militaire building for a municipal hospital. But he intervened too late, for the Revolution halted these efforts forever.[72]

When he learned of the inhumane conditions under which the

mentally ill were kept, Louis XVI ordered the architect Charles François Viel (1745–1819) to destroy the humid underground cells for insane women at the Salpêtrière and to build well-aired, sanitary individual cells above ground. (Some of these can still be seen.) At Bicêtre, Viel's main project was a large new sewer, and it was he who built the great amphitheater at the Hôtel-Dieu.[73]

Concerning care for the elderly, a novel concept found hesitant acceptance under the old regime: nursing homes for the middle class. When the Poverty Committee visitors inspected all Paris hospitals and hospices in 1791, they came upon a variety of Catholic nursing homes, often housing the retired senior members of the community that owned the buildings. This world of the small religious establishment was predominantly a world of elderly women. Typically, such a community consisted of ten to twenty-five members with a number of lay sisters, novices, postulants, part-time associates, volunteers, and paying guests. The only men in the establishment were the gardener, sexton, chaplain, and, sometimes, a physician or surgeon. The site visitors inspected four small Augustinian "hospitals," at Place royale, rue de la Roquette, St. Mandé, and rue Mouffetard. They expressed their appreciation of the services these establishments provided. At St. Mandé, they wrote, "the religious take excellent care"; at Mouffetard, "the treatment seemed good." They also took note of the following annual revenues:

Place royale	33,375 livres
La Roquette	45,473 livres
St. Mandé	16,509 livres plus yield of the land
Mouffetard	33,767 livres, but debts of 14,400 livres

Had the inmates of these homes been able to read the reports, they would have worried about their future. At St. Mandé the commissioners noted: "This establishment is vast and beautiful." At La Roquette, "This establishment is remarkable for the spaciousness and beauty of its terrain." At Place royale, their motivation is clearly recorded: "This community can be liquidated to great advantage for the Nation, considering the matter from an economic point of view."[74]

These homes had been the creation of the Church, but the site visitors also inspected a retirement home in which the king had an interest—namely, the Soldiers' Retirement Home (*maison royale de santé*, best known by its nineteenth-century name, Maison de la Rochefoucauld), situated at Montrouge, south of the present Place Denfert-Rochereau. Inaugurated in 1781, it was run by the Brothers of Charity in partnership with the government, which provided retirement for some officers. This home outraged the Revolutionary commissioners because it flaunted lavish buildings and vast gardens while housing only sixteen inmates. It "seemed to exist for the enjoyment of its administrators; . . . [it is] full of abuses and demands radical reform."[75] This retirement home embodied a novel idea with a significant future—namely, public-private partnership for the care of senior citizens. But it can also be taken to symbolize the corruption that rotted the roots of the royal regime.

◆◆◆

In fact, the experience of the old regime proved vital for the plans and achievement of the Revolutionary reformers in every aspect of health care reviewed in this chapter: the reform of medical education and practice, of patient care and hospital management, of public health and custodial care, of research and rehabilitation. Reformers knew that a challenging task loomed before them: to survey the public hospital and then attempt to change its demeaning, futile, and expensive ways. They would have to create a dignified hospital environment with good professional care and to envisage alternatives to hospitalization that provided more initiative for the citizen as patient. But first, as representatives of the nation, they needed to explore the grim reality of the hospital.

The Grim Reality of the Public Hospital

Hospitals are a measure of civilization: as people agglomerate [and] grow more humane and better educated, the hospitals become more appropriate to their needs and better kept.

Jacques Tenon, *Mémoires sur les hôpitaux de Paris,* 1788

The Poverty Committee and Its Task

The events of the summer of 1789 transferred discussion of human rights and social services from the salons, academies, and societies of the Enlightenment to the floor of the National Assembly. These events also transformed the "ailing poor" of the old regime into patients with a right to health care. This group comprised women, men, and children, babies and the aged, the handicapped and the mentally ill, civilians and soldiers: now they were all citizens who could claim their newfound rights.

As reformers and legislators grappled with the concept of entitlement, they soon realized that the different groups of patients had diverse needs, that personnel, funding, and disbursements were unevenly distributed within the kingdom, and that the assembly lacked information on a national scale. The task loomed enormous, yet the guidelines were clear. The first requirement was to gather facts, both general and specific, regarding the health care needs of the indigent, whether they were institutionalized or sick at home, then to provide for these needs in a manner that raised the ill and ailing indigent to the dignified status of citizen-patient. This could be accomplished with decent hospital accommodations, appropriate medical care, training in a skill and inducements to work, education in hygiene and health maintenance at outpatient clinics and dispensaries, in the hospice, the orphanage, the welfare office, and certain schools. The goal was a

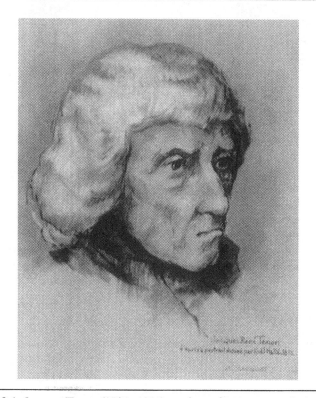

FIGURE 2.1. Jacques Tenon (1724–1816), author of *Mémoires sur les hôpitaux de Paris* (Paris: Pierres, 1788). Drawing by M. Mocquot after a sketch by Jean Noël Hallé at the Académie des sciences. Académie des sciences, Paris.

citizenry conscious of good health as a personal and a public need, a citizenry capable of informed partnership with the physician.

◆◆◆

Soon after the National Assembly settled down to work on a constitution for France, the people of Paris alerted the deputies to the urgent needs of the poor. The assembly responded by creating a Poverty Committee to undertake a variety of tasks—one of them to investigate the health conditions in the nation's hospitals and hospices. The commissioners lacked information for the entire kingdom and therefore focused on the twenty establishments that Jacques Tenon had identified in his *Mémoires sur les hôpitaux de Paris* as medically significant. Strong with the confidence that a political mandate imparts, the commissioners set out personally to investigate the municipal and some religious institutions in the Paris region. They used Tenon's data on the Hôtel-Dieu and scrutinized that hospital and its annexes as well as the hospices, old age homes, and orphanages of the Hôpital général to learn about every detail affecting the institutionalized patient. Thus they prepared the triage of the sick from the destitute that would raise Paris to a model for national health care. This chapter introduces the committee members and their task and follows them on their site visits to the hospitals and hospices of the capital.

The committee had the wisdom to elect a superb chairman. Until 1789, the duc de la Rochefoucauld-Liancourt had spent most of his energies learning how to be a philanthropist, "examining machines, questioning foremen and workers, visiting farms, learning the current methods of husbandry, cultivation and agriculture."[1] His membership in the Philanthropic Society of Paris and in the Royal societies of Medicine and Agriculture gave him easy access to learned colleagues, and his social connections ranged from Jean Sylvain Bailly, now mayor of Paris, to Charles Maurice de Talleyrand-Périgord (1754–1838), in 1790 the president of the National Assembly's Constitution Committee. Liancourt combined urbanity, tact, and determination with an astounding capacity for work.[2]

Like Tenon before him, Liancourt cast his scholarly net wide, consulting the king's library and eliciting testimony from both Frenchmen and foreigners. Though he relied heavily on Tenon's work, he did not coopt him for his committee and gives him scant credit, undoubtedly because of an old feud.[3] Liancourt had trouble gathering information from the provinces. He sent inquiries to the eighty-three departments. Which hospitals were inactive? Which had been merged, transformed into benefices, or transferred to the endowment of a religious community?[4] What were the statistics regarding the poor? What proportion were children? How many were sick, deaf, or blind? What was the cost per patient/day? He requested the same data on 5 and 9 July, and again on 15 October 1790, and even as late as 21 and 27 May 1791, when he was already writing reports.[5] The committee was constantly forced to guess at answers and use Parisian data to draft national legislation.

In contrast to Tenon, who had failed to obtain the registers of the Hôtel-Dieu,[6] Liancourt's commissioners proceeded with "the strength and daring of honest men who are backed by the legislature."[7] On 27 April 1790, they wrote to the trustees of the Hôtel-Dieu: "We have the honor to request that you send us as soon as possible the administrative regulations and the budget of your institution. We would appreciate the most detailed information available."[8] Not only did the administrators comply, but they personally conducted the commissioners during their on-site inspection.

In contrast to Tenon's rather homogeneous committee of academicians, appointed by the chairman, Bailly, from among colleagues, the Poverty Committee's variegated membership reflects the chance results of democratic elections: it included two doctors, four administrators, one engineer, two merchants, one lawyer, and one professional soldier. Half of the nineteen members were aristocrats; one-third, clerics. François Simonnet de Coulmiers (1741–1818), abbé d'Abbécourt; Pierre Louis Prieur de la Marne (1756–1827); and Jean Baptiste Massieu (1743–1818), Liancourt's initial three colleagues, were headed for distinguished participation in the reform of health care.[9]

In addition to elections, the committee enlisted six members by cooptation, and two of these men were outanding experts: Charles de Montlinot (1732–1805), a former cleric, author of the widely read *Essai sur la mendicité* (1786), and inspector of poorhouses at Soissons, and A. L. de la Millière (1746–1803), a lawyer, administrator, and chief of the department of hospitals and poorhouses in the finance ministry.[10]

Liancourt's most valuable colleague, Dr. Michel Augustin Thouret, is a personality central to this book. As a member of the Royal Society of Medicine, he had acquired multifaceted experience in medical and public health issues of continuing importance to the citizenry. He had dealt with epidemics, water pollution, charlatanism, and illicit drugs and spearheaded an extraordinary feat of medical diplomacy, the liquidation of the Holy Innocents Cemetery and the reburial of its contents outside the city limits. Chosen as dean of the new Paris health school in 1794, he implemented the reform of medical teaching in France and, after 1801, served on the Hospital and Public Health Councils of the Seine. Thouret personifies the most important link between Enlightenment ideas on health care and their implementation during the Revolution and Empire.

When it was ten members strong, the committee asked the National Assembly for six more deputies. Three of these turned out to be clergymen soon to emigrate,[11] another joined the constitutional clergy,[12] one was a merchant,[13] and the sixth, Dr. Joseph Ignace Guillotin (1738–1814), was famous at the time for having sponsored a "Petition from the Citizens of Paris" requesting that Louis XVI double the representation of the middle class in the Estates General.[14] To this total of sixteen men should be added two substitutes, one of them the well-known Jacobin Barère de Vieuzac (1755–1841).[15] In addition a deputy from Lyon, Jean André Périsse du Luc (1738–1800), joined the committee by special invitation on 16 July 1790.[16] The urbane and astute chairman treated all members equally in parceling out site-visiting and report-writing assignments.[17] But Liancourt and Thouret worked hardest.

Among the six major and twelve minor Poverty Committee reports issued in 1790–1791, the 120-page Fourth Report deserves our special attention.[18] Here the commissioners surveyed the grim reality of the patients' experience in forty-eight Parisian hospitals and hospices, "with scrupulous care and remarkable insight."[19]

The Poverty Committee's most immediate concern focused on a city with a population of about 660,000 on the eve of the Revolution.[20] Among these, Tenon counted 6,236 acutely ill hospitalized patients, almost 1 percent (0.94 percent) of the population. In addition, he found that Parisians supported 15,000 foundlings in the provinces and 14,105 ailing poor and aged women and men in custodial care.[21] Together, these 35,241 sick and ailing indigents of pre-Revolutionary Paris amounted to about 5 percent (5.35 percent) of the population. The Poverty Committee adopted Tenon's data for a projection of national needs, estimating that 5 percent of the population required institutional care and 1 percent needed medical attention, in or out of a hospital.

The poor feared hospitals as dangerous and degrading places.[22] "Indigent patients are so convinced of the dangers that await them at the Hôtel-Dieu," wrote Tenon, "that they only enter it *in extremis,* after exhausting all their means."[23] Yet despite their reluctance, they filled the city's hospitals and custodial hospices to overflowing.

These facilities now faced their first inspection by critical outsiders, whose reports permit us to accompany them through the hospital wards and courtyards, kitchens, pharmacies, and workrooms. Their horror was at times visceral. Whatever their differences in background and outlook, all the committee members belonged to the upper middle class, the clergy, or the aristocracy. These men lived amidst the comforts and exquisite luxuries of late eighteenth-century interiors—the satins, lacquers, porcelains, wigs, crinolines, and perfumes of the Rococo era. They literally reeled when the smells, grime, and filth that surrounded the hospitalized indigent citizen-patient assailed their senses. "If you lift the covers off these sickbeds," shuddered Tenon, "hot and humid vapors rise as from an abyss. They spread and thicken the air into an atmosphere so tangible that, on a winter morning, it seems to part as one ventures into it; and one cannot penetrate there without an overwhelming feeling of disgust."[24]

The other commissioners lacked Tenon's personal experience and relied to some extent on preconceived ideas and on information collected by others. In fact, the published minutes raise some doubts about the care with which they conducted their investigations. For example, five men took only four hours to inspect the enormous Paris Hôtel-Dieu on the morning of 21 May 1790. Liancourt, possibly alone, gave the municipal hospice of Petites Maisons a quick once-over at 5 P.M., on Saturday, 15 May, and inspected the Pitié Hospice, the maison de Scipion, and Ste. Pélagie with two colleagues on either 10 or 11 May. In the end, though, this skeptical question may not matter because the site visit evidence confirmed recent information collected by the new deputy mayor for hospital affairs, the distinguished botanist Antoine Laurent de Jussieu (1748–1836). He was well acquainted with the appalling conditions, and he had sent a detailed questionnaire to the hospital administrators. Given his doggedly specific questions, they had no alternative but to provide exact information. In some cases the replies arrived before the Poverty Committee inspectors set out on their site visits, and we can safely assume that Jussieu shared useful information with the inspectors.

The committee's initial, daunting task lay in grasping the organization and faults of the so-called Hôpital général, a group of institutions that served thirty thousand indigents whose problems were not strictly medical. The inspectors' chief objective was not a critique of medical care: only two of them were physicians. Their basic aim was to discriminate between hospice and hospital inmates, between permanent and transient occupants. The committee needed to ascertain the health level of this huge mass of confined indigents and to weigh the possibility that, given proper medical care and health support, inmates might be discharged. The visitors were shocked to find that the medical profession tagged hospice inmates as incurable and thereafter ignored them.

It seemed that living conditions in the hospice aggravated, if they did not cause, the inmates' ailments, some of which, such as scabies, were endemic because patients constantly reinfected each other.[25] The visitors intended to find out if contagion could not be checked. They believed that the nation had a solemn obligation to make certain that the permanent inhabitants of Bicêtre, the Salpêtrière, and other old age homes, and the fifteen thousand foundlings and orphans for whose subsistence Paris was responsible were at least living a decent existence.

The visiting teams' specific charge was to make legislative recommendations. Therefore they aimed at gathering facts and figures regarding hospital administration, budget, and personnel, but especially the inmates: their numbers, lodgings, food, clothing, education, religious practices, opportunities for work, leisure activities, and morale; the state of their health, their ailments, and the medical and nursing care they received. The visitors also wished to find out whether each hospitalized indigent was legally entitled to public assistance, or whether some might be excluded; whether each person was housed in the appropriate institution, or whether these huge numbers of indigents should be further subdivided according to medical criteria so that their health needs might be better served.

Site Visits to Hospitals and Hospices

On 21 May 1790, doctors Guillotin and Thouret, the bishop of Rodez, Montlinot, and Lambert undertook their inspection tour of the Hôtel-Dieu.[26] They approached their task knowing that this huge municipal hospital system had been under lay control since the Renaissance, even though the archbishop of Paris headed its board of trustees and Augustinian nurses administered patient care.[27] They faced the inertia and traditionalism of both lay and religious vested interests.[28]

The Hôtel-Dieu and its dependencies covered nearly forty acres, with storehouses for wheat and wine and the Clamart cemetery on the left bank; a farm at Aubervilliers; and a home for retired nuns at Gentilly.[29] The giant hospital occupied a site in the heart of the city that "all good citizens really interested in the fate of the poor" judged inappropriate.[30] Its mortality was the highest in the world. Tenon reports the following figures for the major European hospitals:[31]

Edinburgh	1 of 15 patients admitted
Allgemeines Krankenhaus, Vienna	1 of 13
Hôtel-Dieu, Lyon	1 of 12
Santo Spiritu, Rome	1 of 11
St. Bartholomew, London	1 of 8
Charité, Paris	1 of 7
Hôtel-Dieu, Paris	1 of 4½

The Hôtel-Dieu's main patients' building on the left bank was narrow and high, with only two staircases: in the event of another a fire, it would be a death trap. The inmates endured ubiquitous filth and stench, and the ceaseless clatter of traffic that lumbered over the two bridges and rumbled along the rue de la Bûcherie, where an assistant to the tireless Tenon had, on an October day in 1786, spent one hour counting ninety-two wagons loaded down with wood, stones, and casks of wine.[32] The basements under the wards on both banks of the river held the kitchens, laundries, granaries, slaughtering facilities, tallow shops, furnaces, and storage for wood, coal, oil, and brandy; all of these were sources of odors, noise, and fire hazards.

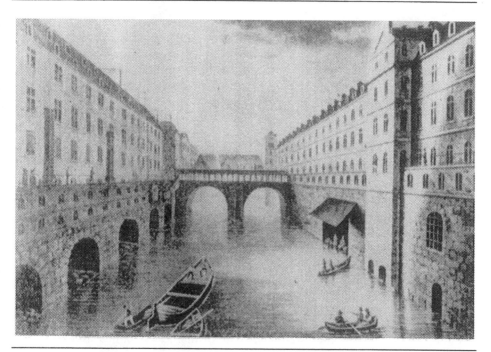

FIGURE 2.2. The Hôtel-Dieu of Paris, view from the Petit Pont eastward toward the Pont St. Charles (a covered passageway between the Ile de la Cité and the left bank of the Seine). Etching, author unknown. Bibliothèque nationale, Paris, Cabinet des estampes.

The overcrowding was murderous, and, even though the commissioners knew what to expect, they were amazed by what they saw. Male patients were grouped in twelve sections and women in thirteen, each amounting to separate hospitals within a common structure. "The St. Charles and St. Antoine wards hold more patients than any of the major hospitals in the kingdom, with the sole exception of Lyon," commented Tenon.[33] Two sick wards, with 202 patients, stood *on* the Pont-au-double above the river; three wards, with 589 patients, occupied a building on the Ile de la Cité; the remaining twenty wards were located on the left bank: these housed over three quarters of all patients, 2,627 on the day Tenon had them counted, out of a total of 3,418.[34]

The administrative structure of the Hôtel-Dieu compounded the confusion. Indeed, twenty-six separate "departments" regulated activities ranging from upholstery, tailor, and candle shops, cleaning operations, and building inspection to the preparation of bread, meat, wine, and medications. But the Hôtel-Dieu was so huge that each

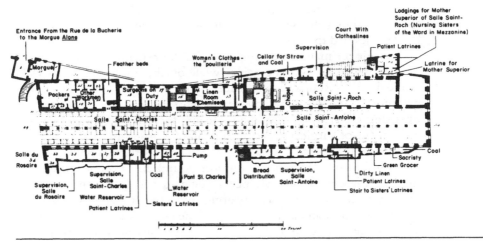

FIGURE 2.3. The Hôtel-Dieu of Paris, left bank, from Jacques Tenon, *Mémoires sur les hôpitaux de Paris* (Paris: Pierres, 1788), pl. 9., as interpreted and Anglicized in John D. Thompson and Grace Goldin, *The Hospital: A Social and Architectural History* (New Haven, Conn.: Yale University Press, 1975), fig. 126. Courtesy Yale University Press.

On Tenon's ground floor plan, two huge wards accommodated male patients with "fevers," the St. Charles ward (A), with room for 413, and the St. Antoine ward (B), with room for 145 men. A smaller ward, St. Roch (C) served 143 children. The peripheral cubicles served for storage, and rooms at the southeast corner to deposit, shroud, and dispose of cadavers.

section (*emploi*) developed its own administration and policies regarding meals, snacks, bouillon and infusions, linen and laundries, medicine cabinets, chapels and sacristies; and innumerable cubicles served for storing small amounts of linen, wood, wine, water, for soiled linen and dishes, and for laundering of small articles other than sheets. Personnel proliferated accordingly.

The location of the wards hindered the patients' comfort and exposed them to infection. The morgue, located on the ground, or first, floor (*rez-de-chaussée*) at the southeast corner of the left bank building, opened onto the St. Charles fever ward, subjecting 413 men who shared large beds there to "fetid smells." The location of the main surgical ward on the second floor (*premier étage*) directly above the morgue could hardly have reassured the patients, who were, moreover, in earshot of the St. Joseph maternity ward on the third floor (*second étage*), with its 182 places. Above all this, yet another floor, St. Landry, housed 374 women fever patients. It was here that the great surgeon Pierre Joseph Desault had his apartment and his dissection room. A stinking gutter served to remove blood and offal. The toilets overhung the Seine: five seats served hundreds of patients; the head nurses had their own.

Outside the main wards on the second floor, damp sheets curtained off side windows over the Seine, while on the inside the south wall blocked off the stairwell and offices. In the corner of one ward stood bathtubs for the hydrotherapy treatment of the insane. The St. Jerome operating room was, according to Tenon, the place where "the greatest number of surgical procedures in all of Europe are performed."[35] The new amphitheater, replacing the St. Yves ward, was built in 1788. One can imagine the noise, commotion, and dust occasioned by the masons, carpenters, and plumbers going to and fro in the St. Paul ward, which also served as a waiting room for outpatients seeking a free consultation and as passageway to the chapel and to the St. Louis ward on the Pont-au-double, where forty-two insane men noisily protested being strapped to their beds.

Surgeons, male nurses, and apprentice midwives used between sixteen and twenty-one alcoves and closets in each ward as bedrooms. The best accommodations, in some cases four- or five-room apartments, located at the periphery of the wards, and thus able to catch some sunshine, a breeze, and a view of Notre-Dame cathedral, were reserved for the Augustinian nurses. The head midwife occupied a two-room apartment on the second floor. The privileged accommodations of the nuns reflected their heavy responsibilities: yet they occupied these only during the day, retiring to their convent at night.[36]

A footnote in Tenon's book allows us a glimpse of some very French housekeeping in those numerous kitchenettes, which were needed because the food arrived cold, having been carried along multiple passageways and staircases. The head nurse would recook the broth that was the mainstay of patients on a liquid diet. This was called *raccommoder le bouillon.* "She could not possibly afford to do this," commented Tenon, "but for the patients' earrings, watches, jewelry, and coins, which are locked away and registered by the head nurse of each section. If the patients recover, everything is scrupulously returned. If they die, these objects go to finance the snacks."[37]

The nurses struggled against the doctors' intrusion into the realm of nutrition. "Formerly the food distribution was decorous, clean, and almost majestic," protested the superior, Sister de la Croix, to the trustees. "First, a sister apportioned the bread, soup, and wine; then followed the head nurse with the meat, the very image of Providence endowing her children; her gifts were gratefully received." Then the superior came to the point and argued that "a doctor who sees two hundred patients an hour" could not possibly allot portions correctly.

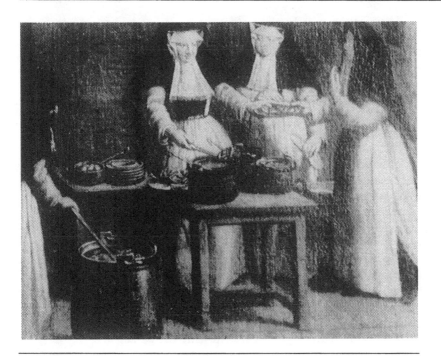

FIGURE 2.4. Nursing sisters at food distribution. Detail from an oil painting by Jan Beerblock of a ward in the Sint Jans Hospital, Bruges (1788). Memling-Musuem, Bruges. Photograph, Grace Golding. Reproduced by kind permission of the Institut royal du patrimoine artistique, Belgium.

The head nurse alone knew the patient, being "at the bedside from four o'clock in the morning until nine at night; she talks to him, comforts and watches him, apportions the food and can judge how it agrees with him."[38] Despite the nurses' valiant struggle, Revolutionary reforms established the physician's overriding authority in matters of diet. An equally fierce battle raged over the adoption of single beds.

The varied shapes and sizes of the beds made it impossible to align them and thus difficult to follow the instructions on the rudimentary tags and charts. "The number of beds in the Hôtel-Dieu is 1,219," Tenon informs us; "733 are large, or 4½ feet wide, and 486 are small, or 3 feet wide; they stand in two, three, or four rows, the small mixed with the large, some facing the windows, others adjoining the walls. These arrangements are bad for the service, the patients, and medical practice." Elsewhere in the book he continues: "When each bed contains four to six patients, a single tag does not tell who should get the medicines or the food, nor in what quantities. . . . Thus, orderly expenditures and exact distribution are impossible."[39]

The well-known battle over the benefits of arranging identical, single beds in an orderly manner is typical of the conflict between old and new. The advantage of single beds was obvious to anyone mainly concerned with rest, cleanliness, and privacy for the patient, and with preventing confusion in the distribution of diets and medicines. The king kept endowing single beds, and, in the smaller hospitals where medical care, not poor relief, determined hospital policy, all beds were single; the large beds were gone from all hospitals by 1815.[40]

But why large beds in the first place?

The indignant modern historian should perhaps be reminded that large beds—the size of our "king" and "queen" size ones—were then in common use among peasants and poorer folk. More important, the nursing orders were concerned with their obligation to shelter *all* the poor. It is in this context that one must read the prioress's lament that recent introduction of single beds made her "lose 922 places."[41]

The lack of decent patient accommodations was partly caused by those convalescents whom the Augustinians employed to sweep floors, change beds, pull food carts, and wash patients, dishes, and linens. Tenon identified 287 persons in this category, but no sleeping space for them is discernible on his diagrams. The nuns rewarded these workers with single beds, displacing the patients.[42]

The site visitors seemed unimpressed by recent government efforts to rebuild the burnt-down sections of the Hôtel-Dieu and bring about improvements through architectural renovation: "All that was done are some additions to the buildings on the north bank and a few improvements on the south bank of the Seine," they commented.[43] The architect Clavareau, writing in 1803, also minimized the pre-1789 changes in comparison to later ones (his own).[44] The earlier improvements were the result of ceaseless prodding by the inspector general, Jean Colombier. Trying to please both the conservatives and the innovators, he not only "accommodated the Augustinian nuns in rebuilding their chapel, infirmary, dormitories, and novitiate" (which took up a significant portion of the new building on the place du Parvis Notre-Dame), but he also "designed and supervised construction of wards, laundries, kitchens, fixtures, beds, transferred various services between wings, planned a new obstetrics service, and promulgated regulations for their operation." The trustees were right to emphasize recent progress: the number of those objectionable large beds had diminished in the huge fever and lying-in wards. These now boasted 144 additional single beds (most of them undoubtedly freed by dislodged employees), and 53 new "double beds," the compromise solution.[45]

The significance of these improvements remains slight when it is contrasted with the irreconcilable perceptions that result from a comparison of the *Délibérations* of the Hôtel-Dieu trustees with the accounts of the Poverty Commissioners. Whereas the trustees reported that their visitors "found the meat of superior quality, the bread and wine very good and above reproach, and that they seemed rather satisfied with the way the wards were run, and found the air, on the whole, pure and odorless,"[46] the commissioners described "a narrow locale, disgusting because of the immense number of inmates."[47] When the visitors searched the ledgers for an exact patient census, the *Délibérations* reported that "the commissioners . . . made some observations about the fact that the departure of convalescents was not registered." The response was that, "once cured, patients had no interest in announcing their departure and they often left without being noticed, since they could not be identified . . . and that, as long as the names of all patients were listed, and of all who died, it was certain that all who were not dead and were no longer present, had left."[48]

This know-nothing attitude could only stiffen the commissioners' conviction that nothing short of a drastic reform of the Hôtel-Dieu would create conditions favorable to the emergence of citizen-patients. First a deep cut in the patient census must curtail overcrowding so that indigent citizens could receive good care. Then the segregation of patients with communicable diseases must lower the danger of contagion. Single beds for all would result from a speedy discharge of convalescents. Rigorous accounting must prevail, and nurses must be subordinated to the doctors in the matter of patient care. In other words, the site visitors demanded a total reform of the Hôtel-Dieu of Paris.

Yet the Hôtel-Dieu was neither to be subdivided nor moved farther than one city block. As the modern visitor gazes from the square René Viviani northward across the Seine and the place du Parvis Notre-Dame, there looms the present-day Hôtel-Dieu, built in the 1860s, massive and forbidding, with its ten three-storey pavilions, claiming its thousand-year-old privileged place on the Ile de la Cité, next to the cathedral.

◆◆◆

In addition to the Hôtel-Dieu properly so called, three other hospitals depended upon the same administration. St. Louis, the seventeenth-century plague house built by Henri IV, was located on the northern outskirts of the city. It is a striking structure, not a transformed monastery like several other Revolutionary hospitals; rather, its unique architectural design totally isolated the patients. Two concentric squares of buildings, surrounded by walls and separated by

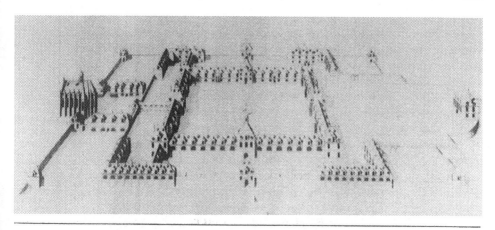

FIGURE 2.5. St. Louis Hospital. Engraving from Jacques Tenon, *Mémoires sur les hôpitaux de Paris* (Paris: Pierres, 1788), pl. 3.

gardens, communicated only through a gallery, with a turntable that linked the kitchens to the wards. Thus the patients, a source of contamination, were locked into the inner structure. The outer buildings housed the surgeons, nurses, and priests. St. Louis had room for about 700 patients, but in the eighteenth century, when plague was no longer a threat, this hospital served mainly to house the overflow from the Hôtel-Dieu in emergencies and epidemics. During the era under discussion, it reverted to its origins and specialized in the treatment of skin diseases. In the nineteenth century, St. Louis reached fame in dermatology.[49]

Another dependency of the Hôtel-Dieu was Ste. Anne, also known as "La santé." Begun under Henri IV and endowed by Queen Anne of Austria, it was dilapidated on the eve of the Revolution. Advocates of gardening and farm labor for hospice inmates and mental patients sporadically proposed Ste. Anne for such occupational therapy. Rebuilt under Baron Haussmann in 1861, it is now the chief psychiatric center in Paris.[50]

The third structure subordinated to the Hôtel-Dieu administration was the Hospice for Incurables located on rue de Sèvres, now the Hôpital Laënnec, specializing in tuberculosis and radiology.[51] In 1790, it housed 446 chronic patients with paralyses, persistent tremors, cancers, gout, hydropsy, asthma, ulcers, and enormous tumors. Many of. the patients were "in a state midway between health and sickness";[52] some were ill, some old, but hale; "all of them malcontent."[53]

These observations strike one as strange, because the Incurables consisted of vast, salubrious buildings and large gardens. The modern visitor can still discern the original cross-shaped wards, one each for women and men, with mansards that document the buildings' seventeenth-century origins. Only the chapel is now in disarray. On Tenon's plan one can locate the large orangery to the north that later isolated children with contagious diseases; one is surprised to find a prison used for uncooperative inmates; one can identify several peripheral lodgings and gardens that were rented out. Perhaps the inmates were malcontent because they were daily witnesses of these outsiders' exclusive use of several large gardens.

At the Incurables, all beds were endowed, and the ratio of servants to patients was 1:5.[54] So the chronic resentment of the patients may simply have been the anger that old age often entails. The Incurables must have been a rather disorderly establishment, for the hospital administrator, Camus, later reported that male patients who were transferred elsewhere took with them the habit of selling their portions of food, drinking in the cabarets, and begging for alms when their funds ran out.[55] The Poverty Committee drew the conclusion that the hospice should be sold, and that the inmates should return to their families and receive pensions. Up to 1,500 ailing citizen-patients could live on the proceeds from such a sale, calculated Liancourt.[56] But the establishment has remained a chronic diseases hospital.

The site visitors were astonished to find acres of orchards and vegetable plots at St. Louis, Ste. Anne, and the Hospice for Incurables, with chicken coops, cowsheds and pigsties, indicating hidden wealth and potential self-sufficiency. Such vital strength was typical of many confiscated institutions: the Necker and Children's hospitals also fed their patients vegetables and fruit grown on their lands, and so did the Salpêtrière and Bicêtre. That was how they survived the Revolution. The site visitors came away convinced that only national ownership and central management would allow an equitable allotment of resources.

The General Hospital for Adults and Children

The confusing title of "Hôpital général" was applied to the institutions housing elderly indigents, undesirables, and even criminals who were not acutely ill but ailing or incurable. Many of them would have benefited from medical attention, but medical care for incurables was considered a waste of money, time, and effort. The logic of this argument led to an arrangement whereby one physician and one surgeon, with four assistants each, were responsible for the whole Hôpital général—that is, about 15,000 women, men, and children.

La Rochefoucauld-Liancourt himself undertook the inspection

of the Hôpital général, with Massieu, de Crétot, Montlinot, and Thouret.[57] In preparation for the site visits, which began on 5 May 1790, the Poverty Committee may have been able to study the hospital administrators' replies to Jussieu's detailed questionnaires, particularly those by Regnard for Scipion, Hagnon for Bicêtre, Doumey for the Salpêtrière, and an unsigned response for the Pitié.[58]

The duke, with Massieu and de Crétot, inspected the maison de Scipion, an elegant, rambling building that remained the Paris hospital bakery and a supply center for all Paris hospitals until 1978. Here the visitors for the first time faced the staggering quantities pertaining to their task. At the time of the Revolution, Scipion's seventy-four employees provisioned the Parisian hospitals with bread, meat, wine, and candles. Every day, twenty-four bakers produced about 22,000 pounds of bread. Every year, the patients of Paris consumed some 1,800 heads of cattle, 800 calves, and 6,000 sheep. Some of the cattle were slaughtered at Scipion, and the tallow yielded the 90,000 pounds of candles needed annually to light Paris's hospitals and hospices.[59] The purchase of most other supplies had been contracted out (á la régie), on the assumption of considerable savings. But the commissioners grew quite convinced that the supply system for Paris hospitals needed the firm hand of a central administration.

In the two giant custodial institutions of the Hôpital général, the Bicêtre and Salpêtrière hospices, the commissioners faced the nadir of traditional medical charity. At Bicêtre, according to Hagnon, seven "governors" administered services subdivided into fifty-two dormitories and infirmaries, while sixty sisters supervised the wards and staffed the kitchens and laundry.[60] Liancourt perceived no such distinctions: he saw only a shocking mass of suffering men. "Bicêtre houses paupers, and four categories of paying patients," he wrote.

> There are epileptics; scrofulous and paralytic men and boys; mental patients; prisoners jailed by order of king or *parlement,* with or without a pension; boys picked up by the police or condemned for theft and other offenses; children, neither corrupt nor ill, housed free of charge; and finally, syphilitic men and women. The institution thus serves as hospice, hôtel-Dieu, boarding house, hospital, prison, and correctional institution. The total number of inmates on 5 May [1790] was 3,874, of whom 769 were servants, among whom figure 435 male paupers, who receive additional food and four livres a month pocket money.[61]

Patients with some money could buy all sorts of daily comforts such as illegally sold liquor, a single bed, or extra food.[62] Inmates entitled to supplementary rations ate at the common table, causing all the others daily moments of envy; "a humiliating and distasteful experience," commented Liancourt.[63]

The administrators perceived most of the inmates as physically fit. For the acutely ill, five new infirmaries had recently been set aside in obedience to the royal decree of 1781. These were no more than separate rooms: *infirmary* did not yet imply medical attention. The St. Martin and St. Roch infirmaries, with patients from the reformatory and prison sections, seemed to Liancourt to be "a school for vice and crime," where children met hardened criminals.[64] St. Joseph infirmary housed the terminally ill, epileptics, imbeciles, and the incontinent, pell-mell with children suffering from scrofula or ringworm. St. Henry infirmary was reserved for employees, servants, and the deserving poor. An effort had thus been made to segregate the patients by status and afflictions—at least that is what the report claimed. Yet Liancourt flatly states that Bicêtre had "no facilities to care for patients. . . . As soon as a poor man falls ill, he is taken to the Hôtel-Dieu."[65]

An unexpected experience awaited the site visitors in the St. Prix ward, where about two hundred insane men were incarcerated under the governorship of a former inmate, Jean Baptiste Pussin (1745–1811). "The insane housed at Bicêtre . . . seem generally to be treated with kindness," reads Liancourt's report.

> Their accommodations consist of 178 cells and a two-storey pavilion where they sleep in single beds with the exception of three double beds. . . . an administrator and thirteen employees work in this division. The madmen are locked into their rooms or dormitories every night, but during the whole day they are free in the courtyards, as long as they are not violent. The number of these is small and varies with the seasons: only ten out of 270 were chained the day of our visit.[66]

While no one in Paris seems to have known about the humane treatment of the mentally ill at Bicêtre in the 1780s, the venereal disease clinic at this hospice was notorious as the only treatment center for syphilis in the capital. It had room for 54 women and 56 men at a time, in the Saint Eustache and Miséricorde wards respectively. The treatment took six weeks, under the supervision of Chief Surgeon Michel Jean Cullerier (1758–1827).[67] A waiting room with 20–25 beds often accommodated 200 men and women applicants, lying on beds and floors, too ill, weak, and dejected to move, "like a cargo of negroes in an African vessel," wrote the comte de Mirabeau, who knew the place.[68] Cullerier gives horrifying details:

In the waiting room, half of the patients went to bed from 8 P.M. to 1 A.M., the other half till 7 in the morning: thus all had half the night to rest, maybe to sleep. The room was dark and the walls covered with all kinds of filth. The windows, nailed shut, never let in any air. They would have broken in an attempt to open them. Many were walled in, thus transforming the sick ward into a dungeon. Garbage covered the tiled floors; the straw in the mattresses had not been renewed for years; sheets and blankets were tattered and their cloth impregnated with excrements and pus; pillows lacked covers, so that the patients' heads lay on ticking soiled with the putrid emanations of successive occupants. These 200 to 250 candidates for treatment received little attention. Their external sores were perfunctorily dressed. And so they waited, six months, nine months, sometimes a year. The illness worsened; new symptoms developed; the genital organs degenerated, and many of the patients died.[69]

The remaining two-thirds of the "expectants" finally reached therapy. They were bled once, purged twice, and took nine baths and fourteen treatments with sudorific mercury unguents. In a ten-year period, 3,400 men and 3,000 women had been treated, of whom 442 and 440 respectively had died, whereas about 3,000 men and 2,500 women were "cured."[70] We have no way of knowing what "cured" means; there was no follow-up of patients. They may have felt better temporarily, or the symptoms may really have disappeared, or they may have applied for renewed treatment. La Rochefoucauld-Liancourt, shocked by the sight, found it "very urgent that Bicêtre be relieved of this [venereal disease] service, which has existed there for about fifty years . . . and occupies space that could well serve as an infirmary.[71] In fact, royal orders had long been given to transfer this clinic to the new Venereal Diseases Hospital at the Capuchins. It is significant that Liancourt was evidently unaware of these plans, and nothing at Bicêtre seems to have alerted the site visitors to impending changes.

As for the general health of the inmate population, Liancourt concluded that "all kinds of diseases spread throughout the hospice, and everyone ends up suffering from all of them."[72] Scabies and ringworm remained endemic despite a clinic set up in 1787 that treated between 100 and 160 patients daily.[73] Liancourt encountered some boys who, cured of scabies, had evidently been forgotten.[74] It was mainly the employees who received medical attention and Liancourt found invidious distinctions and preferment wherever he went.

One question foremost on the commissioners' minds was the availability of remunerated work for the inmates whose idleness they all considered as an evil, the very antithesis of a citizen-patient's way of life. The administrator of Bicêtre, Hagnon, answered Jussieu's questionnaire of 12 April 1791 as follows:

Question: What is the proportion, among the total of poor men, of individuals capable of doing some work?

Answer: At least half.

Question: Is any kind of work required of those who are able to perform it?

Answer: No.

Question: Are not a certain number of poor employed working for the establishment? What is their number, what is their work, and how are they treated?

Answer: There are sixteen deserving poor at the head of various employments and shops, and they are considered masters or foremen. Their subordinates are:

Assistant masters, overseers, and aides	4
Poor employed as journeymen	11
Shop apprentices	19
Assistant gardeners	19
Assistant launderers	27
Masons and carpenters	14
Mattress workers	8
Latrine cleaners	4

In addition to the listed total of 122 deserving poor, 74 paid volunteers regularly raised water at the big well, 40 or 50 more deserving poor were employed as weavers and worked on looms set up in a basement, 60 or 70 of them carded and spun wool for the upholsterer, and an unspecified number of men polished mirrors in a workshop leased out to a manufacturer in town. It is safe to conclude that no more than 10 percent of the inmates were gainfully employed. Or, to put this another way, about 3,000 men spent the whole day idling.[75] Here was an opportunity to provide work and create training programs from which citizen-patients might emerge in considerable numbers.

At the Salpêtrière, which was almost twice the size of Bicêtre, lived 6,704 destitute women in 1790, the majority aged and infirm. In close proximity, at the same institution, 1,600 abandoned girls, from toddlers to teenagers, and some one hundred prostitutes, jailed as public nuisances, wasted their lives away. A special seventeenth-century endowment by Cardinal Mazarin provided for 108 indigent married couples (both partners had to be over sixty years old); they lived in a special "Householders' Section" (*ménages*).[76] Tenon, the site visitors knew, had described the Salpêtrière as

> the largest hospital in Paris, perhaps in Europe. It serves as a women's hospital and as a prison and shelters pregnant women and girls, wet nurses

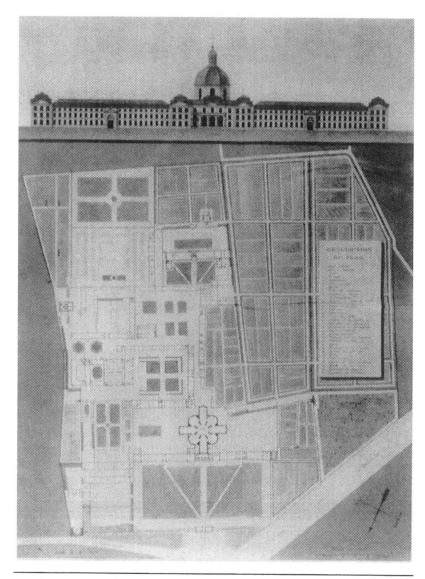

FIGURE 2.6. Salpêtrière Hospice. Ground plan. Note the eglise St. Louis, with eight chapels, and the vast fields and orchards. From A. Malo and N. M. Maire, *Atlas administratif de la Ville de Paris* (Paris: Lottin de St. Germain, 1821).

with their nurslings, male children from seven or eight months to four or five years of age, girls of all ages, elderly women and couples, agitated madwomen, imbeciles, epileptics, paralytics, the blind, cripples, patients with ringworm, all kinds of incurables, children with scrofula, and so on and so forth.[77]

In the center of this hospital stood the prison, divided into four sections: the common jail for the most dissolute inmates; the reformatory for less serious offenders; a lock-up for women detained by *lettre de cachet*; the maximum security cells for branded criminals. One can imagine Doumey, the administrator, squirm as he answered de Jussieu's detailed and probing questions: his answers could not hide the total neglect.[78]

At the Salpêtrière, as at Bicêtre, money could procure advantages: here sixty-six women paid for single beds, private rooms, better food.[79] The most galling daily experience for all these confined women must have been the sight of how well the administrative staff lived,[80] particularly the thirty-two head nurses, known as *soeurs officières*, who formed a quasi-feudal, hierarchical, authoritarian clan. They chose the servants and even the teachers and priests employed at the hospice. Clad in a costume resembling that of the Sisters of Charity, they lived in comfortable quarters, ate well and entertained guests, in particular the fifteen ecclesiastics on the staff. Everyone held them in awe, and the anticlerical Revolutionary legislation left them untouched because they were a lay group. [81] They derived income from a boarding school for little girls established within the Salpêtrière complex and recruited their successors from groomed and favored orphans, publicly derided as "jewels." On 24 November 1790, the Poverty Committee demanded the expulsion of these "privileged children. . . . [who] eat the portion of the poor and are a subject of scandal, envy and depredation." At the same time, Liancourt recommended that priests be refused the right to have women in their households at the hospice.[82]

The presence of prostitutes provided another target of the visitors' criticism. If pregnant, they were sent to the Hôtel-Dieu to give birth, but expelled as soon as manageable after their return. Pregnant prisoners, on the other hand, gave birth in the hospice. While most of these women abandoned their newborns, twenty to thirty each year breastfed their infants, hence the presence of little boys as well as girls. Some years later, Parent-Duchâtelet, in his humane treatise on prostitution in Paris, remarked how eager these women were to care for their babies, even taking them along to prison.[83]

Some accommodations were unbelievably primitive. One group of girls lived above the pigsty and the dissection room. Many of the

550 mentally ill women were chained: their new cells, built by Viel, were "a little larger, airier and less conducive to infection" than the notorious dungeons that the king had ordered replaced; but conditions for the insane were "much less adequate than at Bicêtre" with its good water supply and fresh breezes.[84] The Salpêtrière is located in a low-lying area near the Seine and is subject to periodic flooding and, two hundred years ago at least, to a consequent invasion of rats. The surrounding stagnant water, open sewers, garbage dumps, and the river Bièvre, which carried down industrial waste from the Gobelins manufactory, all stank and spread "putrid fevers." Liancourt lamented that "fresh air, water and cleanliness are totally unknown."[85]

The inmates' provision of clothing, renewed every two years, consisted of a skirt and cloak for the women (or pants and a jacket for the men at Bicêtre) made of gray homespun (*bure grise*) or linsey-woolsey (*tiretaine sur fil*). The regulations stipulated that everyone receive a new pair of stockings once a year, clean sheets every month, a clean kerchief, shirt, and cap per week, and wooden clogs when needed. The commissioners had no way of finding out whether these conditions were fulfilled.[86]

As for work, little girls carded wool, "a murderous regimen," because they inhaled dust and lint all day.[87] Only about 400 adults earned some pocket money by spinning, knitting, sewing, embroidery, or lace-making. Yet Doumey falsely claimed that "all able-bodied women and children work daily . . . and only the paralytics, infirm and insane do not."[88] As usual, wide discrepancies separate the administrators' claims from the commissioners' findings. Invidious petty or punitive distinctions compounded the prevalent misery. For example, prostitutes received the usual 1½ lbs. of bread per day, but if they were syphilitic the ration was cut by ¼ lb. Whereas women in advanced pregnancy were expected to do unremunerated needlework, a few young ones and those incarcerated at the behest of their families could receive an allowance "to make life more pleasant."[89]

How this could be done becomes apparent when one learns that inmates could visit a market within the hospice where merchants peddled their wares daily. The published Salpêtrière budgets reveal revenue of 6,355 francs in 1789 from the sale of wine and 9,214 francs from the sale of brandy: business in liquor and tobacco was brisk in this hospice for women.[90] Second to brandy ranked pig feed, indicating the large number of animals raised, either for food or for sale. Business was so good and rental fees so high that the Salpêtrière earned 27,000 francs in 1811, and 30,000 in 1812.[91]

This traffic furnished additional proof to the site visitors that the

TABLE 2.1. Revenues from Shops at the Salpêtrière Hospice, 1811 (in francs)

Name of merchant	Trade	One year's rent
Aubry	wine	3,000
Morand	brandy	1,500
Destacets	tobacco	1,205
Deshayes	pig feed	2,000
Brunet	dry goods	400
Mme Daniau	lemonade	350
Mlle Coré	grocer	350
Mlle Sorel	grocer	300
Mme Dijard	fruit	150
Femme Gonneau	fruit	150
Mlle Hauteplain	fruit	100
Femme Coré	fruit	100
Femme Violet	fruit	100
Leclerc	sausages	150
Gaultron	laundress	200
Widow Varingue	rolls	25
Lemaire	laundress	200

SOURCE: A figure for "revenue" from these shops appears regularly, beginning with Year XI (1802–1803) in Seine, CGAHHCP, *Comptes généraux des hôpitaux et hospices civils . . . Recettes, dépenses, population* (Paris: Imprimerie des hospices, 1805–1813). It is here supplemented with details taken from the manuscript version of the report for 1811, found by the author under the eaves of the Chapelle St. Louis at the Salpêtrière in 1982.

General Hospital's administrators had not focused their attention on the ailing indigents. The commissioners objected in particular to the punishment of unruly patients by food deprivation, demotion from single to large beds, or incarceration among the mentally ill, and to the cruel practice of putting mental patients on public view for pay, "showing them to visitors, like wild beasts."[92] Liancourt believed that many quiet patients became violent owing to the provocations that they had to endure. The commissioners concluded:

> At Bicêtre, the despotism of minor officials is more insidious and smooth; men command here. At the Salpêtrière, where women reign, their despotism is more active, vexatious, and harsh. Laziness, vice, and villainy prevail at Bicêtre, bitterness, envy, and corruption permeate the Salpêtrière. Idleness debilitates the men at Bicêtre, forced labor kills the children at the Salpêtrière. Cleanliness is lacking everywhere, but for the women's health this is particularly dangerous; Bicêtre looks more horrible, the Salpêtrière more disgusting.[93]

At both institutions a degrading environment and deficient health care perpetuated these abject conditions. The cold wind plagued the men at Bicêtre, while lack of space and fresh air exhausted the women at the Salpêtrière. Overcrowding precluded privacy and meant a daily sharing of bitter memories and a demeaning existence. This sapped the inmates' strength and impaired their resistance to acute illnesses. They suffered from the chronic ailments of old age—pulmonary catarrh, ulcers, tumors, paralyses, and blindness. Dysentery was endemic and poorly understood "fevers" were rampant. Pervasive senility, dementia, and incontinence further troubled these women's declining lives.

Perhaps the most discouraging aspect of the Hôpital général was that it seemed to be a self-perpetuating institution: an endless influx of men and women sought admission to its adult wards, while a steady stream of newborns flooded its Foundlings' Hospice, and older children filled its Pitié and St. Antoine orphanages to capacity.

The Foundlings' Hospice and Orphanages

Almost one-half (about 43 percent) of the human beings who depended on the city of Paris for support were young children whose lives were at risk: upon entering the Foundlings' Hospice, the Poverty Commissioners came face to face with a problem that was disastrous for the city of Paris, and they learned that it was acute all over France. Between 5,000 and 6,000 unwanted babies were abandoned annually in the capital. As far as could be ascertained, 10 to 20 percent of them originated in the provinces. About 60 percent died within the first few months, another 30 percent before reaching the age of five. This left Parisian charity with the obligation to support the cumulative remnant, about 15,000 children, who lived with foster parents in the provinces or in Parisian orphanages.[94] We shall examine the health of older needy Parisian children in Chapter 7, turning our immediate attention to the survival of infants.

By legal definition, foundlings, abandoned children and orphans belonged to three different categories. Foundlings were children of unknown parents found somewhere by someone, often in entranceways and at church doors. By the eighteenth century such exposure by unknown hands had become rare, in part because turntables at foundlings' hospices made the abandonment of infants a safe procedure.[95] The law assigned responsibility for foundlings to the nobleman on whose domain an infant was discovered: he was its legal guardian. We shall see that under the Republic and Empire, guardianship de-

TABLE 2.2. Orphanages in Paris on the Eve of the Revolution

	Boys	Girls	Total
Orphanages			
Foundlings' Hospice			80
Vaugirard Hospice			90
Pitié Hospice	1,400		1,400
Maison St. Antoine		800	800
Trinité Hospice, rue St. Denis	100	36	136
St. Esprit Hospice, place de Grève			100
Hôpital de la miséricorde, ou des 100 filles[a]		100	100
Maison des orphelines de la mère de Dieu	6	38	44
Filles de la Providence, rue de l'arbalète			?
St. Enfant Jésus et de la mère de la Pureté, cul de sac des vignes		15	15
Hospice Beaujon[b]	12	12	24
Maison de l'enfant Jésus, rue de Sèvres[c]		28	28
Filles séculières de Ste. Agnes			60–200
Schools			
Ecole d'orphelins[d]	200		200
Charity offices[e]			
Day-care centers at charity offices and workshops			
Filature de la paroisse St. Sulpice		16	16
Maison de la dentelle noire, rue St. Placide		56	56

SOURCES: Adapted from Jacques Tenon, *Mémoires sur les hôpitaux de Paris* (Paris: Pierres, 1788); A. Tuetey, ed., *L'Assistance publique à Paris pendant la révolution* (Paris: Imprimerie nationale, 1895–1897), vol. 1, 721–783; and AN, Série S, 7051.
[a] Legitimate and doubly orphaned.
[b] Beaujon became a hospital in 1794.
[c] The maison de l'enfant Jésus served as the national orphanage for girls for seven years (1795–1802) and then became the Children's Hospital.
[d] The Ecole d'orphelins, sponsored by the comte de Pawlet, was for the sons of officers and invalid veterans.
[e] Charity offices throughout Paris taught, fed, and sometimes housed varying numbers of children, many of them orphaned.

volved upon the department and its hospital council. Both the law and Catholic ethics enjoined the finder to bring an exposed infant to the nearest hospice immediately. But while speed was of the essence for the baby's survival, secrecy motivated the guilt-ridden parent, and this often caused delays. Such delay surely accounts for numerous infants discovered dying or dead from exposure to the elements or from starvation.

While exposure of infants declined in the eighteenth century, the abandonment of newborns rose to monstrous proportions. Thousands of parents, single or married, gave up their babies to the Foundlings' Hospice, either because of gnawing poverty, or in expectation of good care for a sick child, or even to save burial fees. Freestanding babies' hospitals did not yet exist. Close to half of the annual number of newborns were carried to the Foundlings' Hospice from the maternity ward of the Hôtel-Dieu immediately after their birth because their mothers decided to abandon them. For provincials, faraway Paris offered the best chance of anonymity, and the number of unwanted babies transported to the capital and deposited at the Foundlings' Hospice rose to alarming proportions, from about thirty per year in Louis XIV's day to over 1,700 by the turn of the seventeenth century, 4,000 by midcentury, and an all-time high of 7,676 in 1772.[96] The hospital administrator Camus tells us that a total of 55,106 babies were brought to the Foundlings' Hospice between 1790 and 1803, an average of 4,158 per year.[97]

The literature repeatedly asserts that most of these abandoned children were illegitimate.[98] But a baby's legitimacy cannot be determined from the Foundlings' Hospice registers, because the authorities were only interested in recording three details: the infant's name, the date of baptism, and the identity of at least one parent—someone responsible for the child's upkeep.

It is a mistake to assume that none of the parents wanted to reclaim their children when they could afford to do so, or when the child could start working. They sometimes attached identification to their infants: nametags, trinkets, a message saying the baby had been baptized, an intricately cut paper—half of it affixed to the child, the other half kept to provide convincing evidence at some future time. These foundlings and abandoned children were legally distinct from orphans whose known parents were dead.

One could hardly gather a favorable impression of this widespread rejection of newborns. And yet the well-known German dramatist August F. F. von Kotzebue (1761–1819), who visited Paris in 1790, drew a tender and romantic portrait of Sister Claudine Guillot, head nurse of the Foundlings' Hospice:

> This sister is surely among the happiest human beings, not only in Paris but in the whole world. . . . She pointed to a pretty little girl and asked

that we question her where she had been found. "In the snow," answered the poor little creature. . . .

This good Sister of Charity told us that she had never been infected, even though she had for thirty-five years been in daily contact with children who suffered from venereal disease, scabies, and leprosy. She washes and cleans them, and rubs them with unguents, using no other preservative on herself but pure water.[99]

The commissioners did not share this sentimental point of view.

Liancourt thought deeply about the fate of orphaned and abandoned children and made a number of suggestions, which led nowhere in the short run but resurfaced later, because he raised the fundamental issues. He perceived that the crucial first need for an infant's survival was a wet nurse. Such women were available to middle-class households for good pay through a wet nurses' referral service (bureau des recommendaresses), leaving only poorer women, who lived farther away and commanded low pay, as wet nurses for the foundlings.[100] Liancourt deplored the insufficient number of these women, their advanced age, and their poor health. He recommended that they be taught artificial feeding methods so as to eliminate dependence on their lactation. The doctors at the Port-Royal Foundlings' Hospice were to explore alternative infant-feeding methods at the turn of the century, but no efficacious substitute for mother's milk existed at that time. As the ultimate remedy, Liancourt urged adoption, hoping that the bond between nurse and infant might gradually encompass the woman's family. He advocated the idea in a speech to the National Assembly in December 1790, but without success.[101]

Facing the national tragedy of child abandonment, the commissioners questioned the wisdom of rendering public care attractive: this might encourage the poor, and especially unwed mothers, to give up even more children. That argument was to be typical of nineteenth-century Economic Liberalism and remained a preoccupation in France and abroad.[102] Liancourt persistently tried to introduce Anglo-Saxon voluntarism into the French welfare system, particularly the care for foundlings. He failed. Most Parisian orphans spent their early years with foster parents, impoverished peasants who welcomed the minimal monthly payments. The reformers deluded themselves into believing that the natural kindness of the peasant would make up for the callousness of city folk toward their babies. In fact, the city fathers had long turned a deaf ear to the peasants' argument that these children were much more expensive than lucrative to raise. Might one devise a means of inducing peasants to keep foster children longer? The sad fact was that, when the salary stopped on the child's seventh birthday, most peasants shipped the youngster back to Paris, where the girls were assigned to St. Antoine orphanage and the boys to the Pitié hospice.

The Poverty Commissioners learned, partly from Tenon's survey, partly from their own research, that some 3,000 children lived in Paris institutions: the Hospice de la Pitié, the maison St. Antoine, and a variety of religious establishments here and there in the capital. The Pitié was home to 1,400 boys—foundlings, abandoned youngsters, and orphans aged four to twelve, including the young sons of indigent Parisians, who had developed the habit of temporarily abandoning their boys to this surrogate home, only to reclaim them when they were grown and useful—a habit the Poverty Committee sharply condemned.[103]

The boys lived in huge dormitories. They were separated into groups, below and above the age of eight, and slept in ingeniously constructed but unhygienic bunkbeds (*lits à tiroir*), closed up during the day.[104] Liancourt disliked everything about this establishment, beginning with its location near the Salpêtrière instead of in the countryside. "Fresh air and movement are the primary needs at this age," he argued.[105] The commissioners took great pains to investigate the food, apportioned and used to dole out favors and to control behavior in a way that would require a Balzac or a Dickens to describe. The boys received four ounces of meat, weighed raw (that is, two ounces cooked), on Sundays, Tuesdays, and Thursdays. The daily soup for fourteen hundred children contained one bushel of legumes and twenty-eight pounds of butter; for the servants' soup, the cook doubled the fat. Everyone received 1¼ pounds of bread daily, 1½ ounces of rice with a speck of butter (one-fifth of an ounce per portion), and five ounces of prunes a week.[106]

Wine was allotted in "double portions, half-double [sic], ¾, ¾ plus ⅛, and ⅜, and these bizarre measurements compounded the complex administrative details."[107] A different rationing system prevailed in the infirmaries: ailing orphans rated one pound of white bread per day, male employees and choirboys received one pound of meat, other boys and female employees, ¾ pound. As for wine, men employed in the infirmary were granted ½ liter, women and choirboys ¼ liter, but ordinary boys only ⅛ liter. The infirmary "sometimes served fruit compote, preserves, and milk," reserved for the privileged few.[108]

The vitamin deficiencies in this diet, obvious to the modern investigator, are confirmed by the prevalent scurvy. If one counts calories, as Jean Paul Aron did for early-nineteenth-century Paris, one arrives at a sufficient ration.[109] But can one assume that these boys ate all they

were offered? At the Salpêtrière, the commissioners asked for food
and tasted it, trying to disregard complaints. "We found it of poor
quality, unappetizing, poorly cooked, tasteless. The proof is unan-
swerable: most of the children discard the soup and refuse to eat it."[110]
The reformers concluded that living conditions and food for these
public wards did not strengthen their health or their resistance to illness. The children faced adult life disadvantaged by their upbringing.

Distress in the Hospice: Sickly Orphans and Ailing Adults

The few small orphanages under Catholic auspices that the
commissioners visited seemed comparatively well run and the children relatively lucky: short of adoption, life in such a charitable institution represented the optimal chance for reasonably adequate care. At
the St. Esprit Hospice for 120 doubly orphaned Parisian children, the
administrators apprenticed their wards at sixteen and paid out a small
dowry at marriage or at age twenty-five. They thus raised a privileged
minority, well cared-for by eighteenth-century standards. Yet Liancourt found that St. Esprit produced "only ordinary workers who
were often bad and sometimes dangerous."[111] Their education seemed
to him defective, their health and manual training neglected.[112] Strict
regulation prevailed, and constant supervision, without attention to
the youngsters' need for fresh air, exercise, and play.

The children's education included "a little drawing and plainsong,"
and the youngest boys spent most of their mornings assisting and
singing at masses. "Of the five priests who belong to this house, only
one teaches them to read, write, and figure, another the catechism,
and the other three take these children to funeral processions." This
"disgusting and vagabond practice" of playacting grief for pay infuri-
ated the committee.[113] "It seems to us," commented the duke, "that
young men thus accustomed to mimic near corpses and at the saddest
religious ceremonies must form a habit of hardness and immorality
dangerous for the rest of their lives."[114] Habitual begging was not
much preferable, and yet, at the Foundlings' Hospice, about eighty
children were used for this task: "Chosen from the best-looking boys
and girls, they live at the hospice until they are apprenticed; since their
upbringing is more regular, their education succeeds better than at
St. Antoine. A greater proportion turn out well."[115] By no means,
however, did Liancourt approve of turning little children into professional beggars. The youngsters might have enjoyed mastering some
useful skills, Liancourt mused, such as carpentry, leatherwork, print-

ing, or gardening. He found that the young boys at St. Antoine knitted socks and caps, while the girls learned how to sew or embroider. We shall see later that the headmasters of the deaf and the blind children used more imagination in educating and training their wards.

Age twelve was considered the appropriate time to apprentice the boys to Parisian artisans, the girls to householders or shopkeepers. But these employers found only "a very small number . . . of good workers and loyal citizens," Liancourt reported.[116] "The gentlemen of the administration admitted that, to their great sorrow, more than three-fourths of these children ran away," and swelled the gangs of beggars and prostitutes—only to end up on the venereal wards of Bicêtre or at the Salpêtrière, or in jail . . . a vicious circle. . . . They turn out badly because they are badly raised," concluded the duke.[117]

In theory, these boys and girls in the orphanage were healthy, since a triage at admission weeded out "epileptics, or those with other physical defects, like deaf-mutes, the incontinent, and . . . children with herpes, scrofula, or cold humors." As for the acutely ill, "the traditional usage has been to send . . . [them] to the Hôtel-Dieu, except choirboys, professional mourners, and all surgical cases." [118] And yet, despite this triage, Tenon had found 301 boys at the Pitié to be seriously ill in 1786. A projected infirmary had not been begun, but four small rooms—so-called infirmaries—were set aside for female employees (eighteen beds), male employees (fourteen beds), domestics (five beds), choirboys and professional mourners (eighteen beds).

What ailed Parisian children at the turn of the nineteenth century? We are fortunate to have authoritative information on the medical history of the boys at the Pitié, recorded by their surgeon, Anne Brun, who lived there from 1770 to 1802, when the infirmary closed because the new Children's Hospital opened its doors. Trying to care for the boys, he performed surgical interventions at the Pitié, even though there was no special locale for such operations. The children dreaded being sent to the Hôtel-Dieu with its disgusting and frightening sights and dangerous contagious diseases. We do not know how many were transferred, because separate data were not kept for patients under twelve years of age. Not even the death of a child at the Pitié rated undue notice. "No special records are kept of children who die here, nor of their illnesses: they are included in the number of poor who die in this establishment." [119]

Brun wrote the following report for Antoine Laurent de Jussieu, the hospital commissioner of Paris, in the spring of 1790:

Each kind of illness has its season. Spring is the time for pleurisies, pneumonias, nervous and inflammatory complaints; summer, for high, eruptive, and malignant fevers; fall, for bilious, putrid, verminous fevers and dysenteries; winter, for many colds, catarrhs, and pneumonias. All year round, apathy and consumptive fevers abound, the result of boredom, a poor constitution, and long deprivation.[120]

This mixture of humoral pathology and observation led Brun to favor a conservative therapy, because "gentle means are most successful"; he withheld bleeding, emetics, and purgatives. When "antiseptics" were indicated, he preferred vegetable to mineral "acids"; he used cinchona sparingly, because "it has often been observed in intermittent fevers that [cinchona] caused stomach pain, heat flushes, colic, diarrhoea." He prevented whooping cough as a complication of scarlet fever by administering diaphoretic liquids and refraining from purgatives.

No therapy seemed effective against "cold humors" or scrofula, although Brun tried soapy remedies, diaphoretics, absorptives, tonics, bitters, diuretics, antiscorbutics, resinous purgatives with mercury, and even "an opiate with extracts of monkshood, rue, figwort [Scrophularia], soap, quinine, calcinated oyster shells, diagrede, and mineral oethiops."[121] Brun treated ulcers with unguents and swollen glands with plasters. He mentions jaundice and frostbite but no relevant therapy. He called for more vegetables and sauerkraut to combat scurvy but sent serious cases, as well as cases of violent toothaches, persistent scabies, and ringworm, to be treated at St. Louis. At the same time, he kept some 100 boys with scabies and 136 with ringworm in special isolated wards. When bone decay (probably following an infection) spread in a joint, he dared undertake amputations and other "triumphs of surgery."

Thus Brun usually avoided heroic measures but tried new remedies. He dealt with a chronically ailing population of children, suffering from deficiency diseases, malnutrition, and probably chronic anemia. If one adds lice, fleas, and bedbugs, one can imagine the constant itching and scratching, the coughing, sneezing, and spitting. Given the deficient sanitary facilities and the confining environment, the Pitié was a demeaning and "miasmatic" institution, with a poor prognosis for raising healthy children. In describing them, Brun seems to refer most significantly to "apathy," "a poor constitution," and "long deprivation."

◆◆◆

Despite Brun's efforts to be a good doctor for 1,400 boys, these orphans suffered mainly from neglect. The other adult inmates of the Hôpital général, and some of the children, had been classified as incurable patients, and medical attention was supposed to be useless for them. In fact, the medical staff of the Paris hospices had little to be proud of. They lived in the constant presence of these unfortunates, whose health was decaying, and they managed to ignore them. They condoned and profited from inveterate abuses that a doctor should not allow: they cared for the sisters, priests, and staff, not the inmates; permitted children to be hospitalized pell-mell with adults; tolerated filth and squalor and poor food. Nor did they care for the acutely ill: children and adult patients were carried to the Hôtel-Dieu, regardless of their condition, the long distance, or the weather, "on open stretchers, lying on plain canvas, and entrusted to aged employees whose lack of strength made them stop constantly during a walk of about one league. Many patients died on the way."[122]

The Hôpital général thus neglected its inmates and harmed their chances of emerging as citizen-patients, the Poverty Committee concluded, and the Hôtel-Dieu served them badly. Hospitals and hospices needed total reform: that conclusion was unanimous and clear. Buildings must be renovated, staffs secularized and streamlined, supplies produced more efficiently, daily care improved. At stake was the creation of a medical space where the ordinary poor citizen could be ill without worry, in decent surroundings and attended by well-trained personnel. Many illnesses would then be of limited duration, so that the citizen-patient, restored to health, could resume a productive life. How the new National Constituent Assembly would now implement the right to health care, find the funds and harness the medical manpower to maintain and guard the people's health—that was as fundamental a medical, economic, and moral challenge as any elected national legislature has ever faced.

II

CONFRONTATION:

Reform and Resistance

CHAPTER THREE

The Rights and Duties of Citizen-Patients and Citizen-Doctors

Long-neglected major improvements emerged from the Revolutionary shock.

Paris Hospital Commission, 1801

Noble utopias . . . the grandiose plans of powdered and sincere reformers.

Jacques Léonard, *La médecine entre les pouvoirs et les savoirs,* 1981

The issues were clear by the fall of 1790, and the citizen-patient's health needs urgent. But how would they fare in the political arena before deputies who, if we believe Edmund Burke, "could not be expected to bear with moderation, or to conduct with discretion, a power, which they themselves, more than any others, must be surprised to find in their hand?"[1] That is the question pursued in Part 2 of this study.

Desiderata for the Hospitals

As the Poverty Committee site visitors gathered to share their impressions, their sense of outrage and urgency mounted. They found Paris hospitals and hospices in desperate need of reform, a need they knew to be nationwide. Also, they worked under increasing pressure, because their time might run out: the National Assembly was scheduled to disband as soon as it completed a constitution.

The Poverty Committee's list of desiderata is of great interest to the historian because it echoes the consensus of the Enlightenment, while establishing future guidelines for the citizen-patient's hospital admission and care. Providing considerable authority for the doctor, it also envisaged municipal hospital administrations under national supervision.

A major unforeseen stumbling block loomed for the Poverty Committee, whose members never wondered (at least not in print) whether the medical profession would willingly participate in its projected program. Yet doctors turned out to be so hostile to social medicine as to found their own Health Committee (*Comité de salubrité*), which succeeded in claiming medical education, buildings, and care as their province. With ample support from Paris experts, powerful help from the Royal Society of Medicine, and especially the "New Plan for the Reform of French Medicine" submitted by Félix Vicq d'Azyr, the Health Committee elaborated the basis for the medical curriculum issued in December 1794 and for the law regulating the practice of medicine promulgated in 1803.

Health care for the poor was left in limbo, although not for long. True, projects of national scope remained beyond the reformers' reach, but in 1796, after the high tide of Revolutionary violence subsided, municipal governments resumed an active involvement in health care for the poor, under the direction of the ministry of internal affairs. In Paris especially, municipal initiative produced innovation, which also influenced the provinces. The imprint of the Poverty Committee's thought on these changes was pervasive and long-lasting.

Historians have judged the committee harshly because little came of its recommendations. This critique is justified only if one takes the short view. If, on the other hand, one compares the draft laws of 1791 with the regulations of 1803, it becomes evident that the Revolutionary decade forms only a hiatus. Liancourt and his committee in fact wrote the rules of health care for the citizen-patient in modern France, which were basic to the Assistance publique established in 1849 and developed thereafter.

In judging the historic role of the Poverty and Health Committees, the scope adopted for this study becomes crucial. Viewed within the confines of 1789–1815, the bridge between the early Revolution and the Consulate emerges as a central reality. The commissioners' list of desiderata closely resembles that of the armchair reformers and Ideologues of the 1780s—Charles de Montlinot and A. L. de la Millière being such reformers and M. A. Thouret such an Ideologue. During the Enlightenment, they had often reasoned in the abstract; now, as the nation's political representatives, they came armed with their eyewitness documentation. Under the Consulate, Thouret, Cabanis, Parmentier, Hallé, Cadet de Gassicourt, and others, already vocal critics on the eve of the Revolution, staffed the Paris Health School as well as the Hospital and Public Health Councils, seizing the chance to transform earlier plans into reality. Discussions in the late Enlightenment and investigations in the early days of the Revolution, based largely on Paris conditions, gave rise to legislation for all of France.

◆◆◆

The year 1791 was the time to write the guidelines for achieving two initial goals: selective admission and secular efficiency. As a priority, the Poverty Committee sought a procedure to sift the enormous mass of ailing indigents in the capital so as to reserve the hospital for medical patients only. We shall see in Chapter 5 how a careful triage of applicants curbed the flow of admissions, while a refurbished admitting office and streamlined administration eased the doctor's task. But initially the government had to establish criteria to identify medical need, to decide on the legally valid domicile where a citizen could claim health support (*domicile de secours*), and to set the goals of home care (*secours á domicile*). Also, the tasks of the country doctor, pharmacist, and midwife needed definition, as did the safest procedure for dispensing drugs.

The goal of selective admission presented the doctor with serious dilemmas. Should he hospitalize a patient only if he knew that specific therapy was available, as in the case of syphilis, dropsy, malaria, mental illness, kidney stones, and surgery of the head or limbs? Should he admit a person who "felt ill," even if the physician could find "nothing wrong"—that is, if he could identify no lesion, disease, or disturbance of function? In trying to assess the criteria of a late-eighteenth-century physician, the modern historian is constantly reminded of how relative and changing our notions of "health" and "illness" are. Many more diseases can, of course, be identified today, and modern doctors would therefore have designated an even larger number of applicants as bona fide patients. They would have considered syndromes such as advanced malnutrition, anemia, alcoholism, and depression as illnesses. But they would know how to treat these, whereas their eighteenth-century colleagues did not. A further dilemma was whether or not to admit and swell the ranks of hospitalized patients, knowing that the overcrowded hospital, with its endemic communicable diseases, was dangerous to health. Many applicants had no home or caregiver: they were in fact aspiring to hospital admission to secure food and shelter. They cried out for medical charity as formerly dispensed by the Church.

This charity was precisely what the Poverty Committee wanted to stop. The committee shared the widespread public irritation at the religious nurses' practice of hospitalizing an excessive number of paupers and then retaining them as convalescents to do menial work in return for food, shelter, and a single bed. The Poverty Committee argued that to stem the overcrowding, doctors must reject applicants they perceived as malingerers and admit only according to exclusively medical criteria. But we shall see that the committee underestimated the difficulty of this task, performed hitherto by an ill-trained surgeon or sister.[2]

To achieve an optimal distribution of patients, the Poverty Committee advised that one central admitting office should assign the sick to the various city hospitals. No one asked whether ailing individuals could be expected to walk or be transported all the way to the center of town in order to seek hospital admission, or whether the doctors had sufficient time for thorough intake interviews and examinations. We shall see these problems surface after 1801, when triage was practiced under the auspices of the new Paris Hospital Council.

Hospitals should be located in healthful parts of town, Tenon had argued, adding: "We need not follow the old custom of placing hospitals near cathedrals; this tradition is not based on principles of health, and the reasons for this proximity no longer exist."[3] He also believed hospitals should be of manageable size. The Poverty Committee agreed, and expressed a special preference for neighborhood hospitals, because they had the local inhabitants' support and could be run at reasonable cost: Madame Necker's establishment was a much-cited example, and so were the parish hospitals of St. André des Arts, St. Merri, and Cochin. This trend continued with the transformation of Beaujon into a hospital and the creation of a district hospital adjoining the St. Antoine orphanage.

The trend favored small, specialized institutions. Two of these had long been in operation inside the Hôtel-Dieu—a fact not obvious to the casual observer. The maternity service occupied inadequate, cramped quarters, dangerous for parturient and postpartum women, their newborns, and the midwives. Similarly, the accommodations and treatment facilities for mental patients lay in harmful proximity to the surgical and fever wards. Both services needed to be moved to the outskirts of town, into more appropriate buildings and a healthier environment. By focusing attention on these hospitals-within-the-hospital for lying-in and mental illness, Tenon's *Memoirs* and the Poverty Committee's reports stirred up much publicity in favor of reform, thus furthering the citizen-patient's cause.

Nor could this vital evolution be implemented, argued the committee, unless the nurse yielded command to the physician and the requirements of religion were subordinated to those of medicine. While the commissioners never directly discussed the function of religion in the hospital, their point of view transpires in a variety of statements. One example is their condemnation of the requirement by the Brothers of Charity that patients confess their sins before receiving hospital services, "as if charitable help should not be proffered to all," wrote Liancourt. "We do not believe that any valid reason can be adduced to justify this practice."[4] Just as priests were too large an item in hospital budgets, the committee argued, so altars occupied too much space in wards. The primacy of religion over medicine was as patent in the architecture as in the hierarchy of hospital personnel.

It was this primacy that the Poverty Committee wished to disestablish, and the secularization of the hospital stood out as a crucial goal in its deliberations. The "internal warfare" carried on against innovative physicians must stop. "Depredation and waste will continue to plague [the Hôtel-Dieu] until the doctor's orders become the only rule for the distribution of medicines and food . . . as in the military hospitals," wrote Liancourt.[5]

Secular efficiency would also improve the flow of supplies on which the hospitalized citizens' daily well-being depended and curtail waste, argued the committee. It recommended scrutiny of the production and distribution of food and other goods, including wine, surgical dressings, and medicines. Perhaps middlemen should be engaged; the processing and storage of food and supplies must be removed from the cellars of the Hôtel-Dieu, where they created fire hazards and compounded the traffic congestion. One central pharmacy, located outside the Hôtel-Dieu, should provision all the hospitals. An inventory of hospital furnishings should be undertaken, as should the total elimination of those notorious large beds. A survey of all personnel was needed, because the hospices were overstaffed with servants for the sisters and priests. Money could buy a shockingly varied array of favors and goods: "In these houses of charity, charity is always for sale," the committee tartly concluded.[6]

To improve patient morale and hospice finances, Liancourt advocated work for the inmates. He pilloried idleness as "the most striking vice of the system." Work relieved monotony and put a little money in the pockets of the invalids. They might produce candlewicks, plain furniture, and cloth. "The manufacture of all the articles of clothing for the 15,000 inmates of the Hôpital général would provide useful and guaranteed work for many paupers. But a principle of total idleness seems to have been adopted by the administration. This system would appear to be the vicious result of hoary habit. The administrators themselves told us it was the result of careful deliberation. It is difficult to admit this as true," the committee argued.[7] "It would be easy," concluded Liancourt "for the administration to mend its ways."[8] Absent its willingness to do so, Revolutionary legislation would attempt to compel change.

Legislative Proposals

Even while they were visiting hospitals, hospices, and orphanages, the members of the Poverty Committee held their meetings and drafted their proposals. Between 2 February 1790, when they began, and 25 September 1791, when they disbanded, they met seventy times—often three times a week. Their Fourth Report, "On Assistance to Paupers at Different Ages and in Diverse Circumstances of Life," was read to the National Assembly on 31 January 1791. It is the object of our special attention, and we shall focus on titles I–III, proposing aid to patients, children, the aged, and the infirm (for the text of the report, see Appendix A). This document was an ambitious attempt to spell out nationwide health care for the poor. In the committee's view, indigent patients were coming of age as citizens, so that their duties formed the logical counterpart to their rights as responsible adults. As for these rights, the committee addressed them under three main headings: eligibility, a legal domicile, and home care.

The legislators adopted the philosophic tenet that "every man has a right to his subsistence," otherwise liberty and equality would be denied. It followed that "society must provide for the subsistence of all those in need."[9] And "need" encompassed the citizen's legitimate claim in case of illness or disability. It had thus taken two generations for Montesquieu's idea to find its way into a bill. The local government would decide who was "indigent," and each community would publish an annual list of citizens for the guidance of doctors and midwives. Similar criteria applied to children who were public wards and to indigents over sixty years of age. This proposal broke new ground, the committee argued, for "no state has ever included the poor in its constitution. Many have concerned themselves with relief . . . but never . . . [with] the claims of the poor man upon society. . . . Here is the great task that the French constitution will accomplish."[10]

Once eligibility was established, the committee wrestled with the notion of a "legal domicile" as the place where citizens were entitled to aid and where they must return to receive it.[11] If they fell ill away from home, they would be cared for in the local hospital until they felt well enough to go home. This measure would have relieved the welfare budgets of major cities, where ailing indigents tended to seek refuge. But this rule was impossible to enforce, and it discriminated against the homeless, who claimed their share of public aid wherever they happened to be. Two years later, the Jacobins passed more generous legislation, making aged patients eligible for aid after one year's residence, but they had little time to put their egalitarian principles to the practical test.[12]

It was in the poor man's home that health support would be most effective: the Enlightenment had long advocated this strategy. The members of a patient's family are his natural nurses, Bernardin de St. Pierre had recently written, and to be ill at home is less frightening than to be hospitalized.[13] The poor needed to learn that home care could be dispensed without religious overtones; indiscriminate outdoor relief would be abolished. Liancourt commented that, if home care were to prevail, "that system would present many advantages: it would spread benefits to the whole family, let the indigent patient remain in cherished surroundings, use public assistance to strengthen natural bonds and affection." He firmly believed that timely and personal assistance with food, fuel, and medications would nurture individual natural virtues.

Liancourt further argued that home care would "result in considerable economy since it costs half of hospital care or less. Eight out of eleven thousand indigents could be aided in this way."[14] Among these, children and the elderly were foremost on the commissioners' minds. They had by then seen rooms full of abandoned babies, dormitories and courtyards teeming with unwanted youngsters, wards and infirmaries warehousing rejected old folk. They wished to discourage child abandonment by generously supporting poor parents who raised their children at home.

Elderly ailing citizens would also be most content in a family setting, and the committee emphasized its preference for home care in Title III, on aid to the aged and infirm, which stated that "support in public asylums shall be available only to individuals unable to receive it at home, either because they have no family, or because their serious infirmities require special care, or for similar reasons." But even unattached or unloved old people might find families to take them in, the committee suggested, particularly if the elderly performed some remunerated work.

Medically ill and indigent citizens were thus seen by the Poverty Committee as patients entitled to public aid, and this aid should reach them at home. This policy attempted cleverly to undercut the role of the Catholic Church both as dispenser of aid and of nursing care. As for hospices and hospitals, the Poverty Committee envisaged them only for communities of over four thousand inhabitants. Their number and size would increase proportionately with population. But no institution should exceed five hundred patients.

Health needs differed in town and country, it was widely believed, and Matthew Ramsey has recently explored that distinction. To settle that issue, the Poverty Committee made two sweeping assumptions at the outset of its Fourth Report, where it asserted that "indigent patients shall be treated free of charge in their homes, by surgeons or doctors established in the countryside." This implied the availability of citizen-doctors in the provinces and their willingness to make housecalls. The committee then further embellished its image of the country doctor by deciding that, as a familiar visitor in the peasant's home, the doctor could examine any foster children in that house and "render a monthly account of their condition." That overly solicitous schedule conveys the committee's suspicions that babies were at risk and that foster fees might be being illegally collected for children who had died. The public doctors should also inspect the wet nurses, it was decided: the legislators feared syphilis transmitted by the Parisian foundlings. And the doctors should inoculate against smallpox (ten years later vaccination was substituted).

Another public service that the citizen-doctors could perform pertained to the medical topography so dear to the Royal Society of Medicine, "an annual report containing their comments on the climate and soil of their canton, on epidemic diseases and their treatment, and a comparative overview of births, marriages, and deaths." This was precisely what Vicq d'Azyr had encouraged local doctors to do voluntarily for almost fifteen years. The Poverty Committee thus supported the Royal Society's determination to complete, and periodically to update, a statistical overview of the nation's health.

In emergencies, particularly in epidemic outbreaks, the doctors would alert the district relief agencies. Doctors could always refer their problems to consultants, hospital physicians or professors who would keep an eye on the performance of their young colleagues: young, because it is difficult to imagine that anyone but a beginner would assume the obligations of a citizen-doctor for a salary of 500 livres per year, when, in a community of 4,000, he might be responsible for as many as 120 patients. Moreover, the position was not only underpaid but insecure, for he could be dismissed if the majority of cantonal municipalities complained about his "bad conduct, negligence, or incapacity."

Midwives also figured in the draft legislation, which required their certification by the departmental health agency. The public midwife was to assist the women on the poor list and deliver them in their homes, free of charge. After 1802, as we shall see, quite a few departments offered scholarships for midwifery training in Paris. A special provision in the Fourth Report confirmed the traditional precaution that physicians "shall not be in charge of dispensing drugs; in each canton a centrally located depository shall be established." It is not clear who was to be entrusted with the task—perhaps the Sisters of Charity, for the document states cryptically: "The preparation and distribution of medications and of free food and soup shall be the task of persons chosen for this work by the communities." It is interesting to note that this bill mentions access to specialized hospitals for "contagious and venereal diseases, curable mental illness, major surgical operations, and deliveries." We hardly needed to be reminded that Paris served as a model for the commissioners. They encouraged provincial communities to segregate patients with these illnesses and to avail themselves of the specific remedies and treatments available in the capital.

Problems of Implementation

Whatever the difficulties in his path, Liancourt held to his conviction that "public welfare . . . owes the ailing poor assistance that is prompt, free, assured, and complete." [15] The problems were staggering, particularly as regards the sources of funding, the budget, and, unexpectedly, the supply of physicians.

The cost of a national medical welfare program would predictably be enormous. But in September 1790, when Liancourt read his Fifth Report on "Estimated Funds Needed for Public Assistance," the committee still believed that the hospitals themselves would contribute a major portion of the moneys needed to run them. True, they had lost their traditional tax exemptions and their considerable revenues from the Paris tolls and amusement tax and were now expected to pay certain levies. But they still retained the rest of their property, particularly real estate. Whether this was to be sold at auction remained to be decided.

The problem of endowments (*fondations*) preoccupied the committee. These funds were often earmarked for masses, for designated beneficiaries, or for expenditures of which the committee disapproved, but it hesitated to tamper with this tradition for fear of risking its obliteration. In the end, the committee recommended that donors be free to determine the use of their funds for their own lifetimes and up to fifty years after death. The Jacobins abolished this principle in 1793, but the Consulate reestablished it on 29 September 1802 (7 Vendémiaire, Year XI). This pattern of return to traditional practices frequently prevailed.

Not only hospital property should pay for indigent patients, the committee argued, but also confiscated Church property. The rationale underlying this argument was that all funds donated for charitable purposes belonged to the poor. Therefore France's abbeys, monasteries, cathedrals, bishoprics, and parishes now belonged to the nation and should help pay for poor relief and medical aid. It was from the national treasury that aid would be "disbursed to the departments, the districts, the municipalities."[16] Thus:

> Assistance to disadvantaged citizens is a national obligation, just like the payment of public servants, the cost of public worship, or any other national expenditure.
>
> The citizen pays his taxes without differentiating between the portions that will relieve poverty, maintain the highways, or pay the army. Thus the state alone provides for the poor.[17]

A "new legislative system of public assistance" was being born, comments Jean Imbert, the expert on Revolutionary hospital law.[18]

To establish such a system, the number of indigents in need of medical welfare aid had to be ascertained. No national survey had ever been undertaken. Thouret submitted two long memoranda, on 11 and 14 June 1790. He based his calculations in part on English statistics and the English poor tax, in part on reports from various French cities, such as Soissons, Lille, Le Mans, Rouen, and Paris, and in very large part on guesswork. Estimates of the number of needy poor in France varied widely: Thouret settled for about one twenty-fifth of the population—that is, one million. Half of these he assumed to be in good health and able to work, the other 500,000 were invalids, aged persons in need of lifelong assistance, and homeless children who must be nurtured till adulthood. The English supported their poor too lavishly, Thouret argued, spending about £140 per head annually. In France, one might "relieve misery at small expense without, like in England, encouraging indolence and laziness."[19] In France, it should cost no more than six sous a day—or 100 livres per year—to support each of the 500,000 invalids. This calculation provided the convenient figure of 50 million livres per year as the cost of general welfare support.[20]

The committee estimated there to be 50,000 medical patients among the 500,000 dependent paupers. This proportion of 10 percent, borrowed from the army, was subject to debate: should one compare the health needs of soldiers to those of a population of undernourished paupers, including infants and the aged? In fact, the data resulted from so many imponderables and variables that disagreement is not surprising. Thouret calculated the expense for a medical welfare patient as 18 sous a day. This was based on the experience of the model Necker Hospital in Paris and was therefore, he argued, a lavish basis for calculation if applied to all of France, where costs were lower. A hospitalized welfare patient would thus cost the nation 300 livres per year, and, if there were 50,000 of them nationwide, the expense would be 15 million livres. Liancourt reduced this estimate by 20 percent and asked the National Assembly for 12 million livres annually for medical aid.[21]

Liancourt and Thouret must have heaved a sigh of relief when these calculations were accepted. Surely they believed that the questions of funding and apportionment were the worst they had to wrestle with. Little did they suspect that the insuperable obstacle to national health care would be the medical profession.

Reluctant Physicians

While listening to the grand projects of La Rochefoucauld-Liancourt and Thouret, one medical member of the Poverty Committee felt a growing restlessness. What role were doctors meant to play in the committee's schemes? he mused. Were they to be employed by the state? ordered to the provinces or slums? paid a small salary? Would they practice as the associates of local pharmacists and midwives? as cogs in a nationwide administrative machine? as mere civil servants? This concerned physician was Joseph Ignace Guillotin.

Guillotin was civic-minded and had espoused public causes. Under the old regime, he had helped write reports for the Paris Faculty of Medicine on rabies and the drainage of swamps. He had served with Benjamin Franklin on a major committee that discredited Mesmerism, and made himself useful to the National Assembly by providing its Paris meeting hall with lightning rods, with benches that had backrests and cushions, windows that opened to permit ventilation, and toilet facilities. And of course he participated in the discussion of the death penalty in October 1789, arguing for the egalitarian beheading of aristocrats and commoners alike by a "simple mechanical device."[22]

Guillotin was typical of members of his profession in that, despite all his public service, he did not wish to neglect his private practice. After 1789, and in agreement with many medical leaders, he felt that their most urgent concern should be the reform of education and of the rules for practice. When it came to serving the poor, the physician should continue to be guided only by his conscience. He would enter public service only if he chose.

Organized medicine has always resisted socialization. Economic reasons are an obvious factor in this reluctance, since the discrepancies of remuneration between private and public practice are substantial. But a fundamental professional criterion also requires consideration.

The practice of medicine is traditionally based on the relationship between one physician and one patient, and the diagnosis and therapy of
the sick individual form the crux of the doctor's task. In contrast,
social medicine, public health, and preventive medicine require a different approach. Here the physician takes precautionary measures for
unseen multitudes before they fall ill. The individual doctor-patient
relationship does not exist. The doctor often serves as part of a team,
where the tasks of sanitation and inspection can be performed by para-
medical personnel. This also explains why the promoters of public
health and social medicine have often been laymen. Medical legislators of 1790 understood the widely differing ways of doing medicine,
coping with illness, and curbing diseases: they knew the phenomenon
of contagion even though they did not understand its etiology; they
practiced prevention through inoculation and were familiar with quarantines, isolation hospitals, and certain life-saving techniques. French
legislative debates were revealing the contrasting approaches of therapeutic and preventive medicine to the public when, in September
1790, a completely unexpected development—the creation by the National Assembly of a separate Health Committee—focused that body's
entire attention on the politics of health.

◆◆◆

Perhaps Liancourt's overpowering chairmanship indirectly provoked the eruption of the dispute between advocates of medical welfare and defenders of doctors' privileges on the national rostrum. In
August and September, Thouret read several draft proposals, which
were adopted. At the meeting on September 3d, a reorganization of
subcommittees took place: Thouret and Guillotin collaborated closely,
since their two subcommittees had only four members. According to
the printed record, nothing unusual occurred during fifteen meetings.

Then, on September 12th, Guillotin took a sudden initiative. He
proposed and secured the creation of a Health Committee composed
of all the seventeen doctor deputies and as many lay experts. The bill
authorizing its creation stipulated that the new committee should
"concern itself with all matters pertaining to the teaching and practice
of medicine, with public establishments in towns and the countryside
such as schools, hospitals, nursing homes, etc., and, generally speaking, with all matters pertaining to public health." The committee was
to report to the National Assembly.[23]

Guillotin had acted without consulting his own chairman and had
chosen to speak on a Sunday, when Liancourt was absent. Two days
later the duke complained to the National Assembly: "The Poverty
Committee was distressed to learn that the National Assembly as-

signed to a new committee . . . the work it had already earmarked for the Poverty Committee." Growing as outraged and explicit as an eighteenth-century nobleman could permit himself to be, he continued:

> We were most surprised to learn that one of our own members had, without informing any of us . . . secured the decree that deprives our committee of one of its most interesting tasks. That part of our work has been completed, and this member knows it well, even if his own affairs often deprive us of his presence. But he gave his personal approval, and his action is thus all the more surprising. . . .
>
> M. Guillotin knew very well that your Poverty Committee had decided to submit this part of its work to the most reputable physicians of Paris . . . doubtless a tenacious loyalty to his profession motivated a step that took all of us by surprise.

In a passage full of irony, the duke questioned the eminence, and by implication, the competence, of the physician-deputies, and expressed his preference for consulting "the most experienced physicians in Paris, the members of the Royal Society of Medicine [to which Liancourt and Thouret belonged and Guillotin did not], whose useful work is known throughout Europe, and certain members of the Academy of Sciences who specialize in these matters." Liancourt even resorted to questioning the legality of the new committee, since all physician-deputies were to be members, without an election.

But it was too late. The Health Committee had been voted into existence the previous Sunday. All that Liancourt obtained was this lame decree of September 14th: "The National Assembly declares that, by its decree of the 12th of this month it did not mean to attribute to the Health Committee any of the functions previously assigned to the Poverty Committee.[24]

Underlying this struggle for the control of health care reform lay a problem crucial to this book and still of acute interest to modern medicine. Thouret wanted to help create a national health service, while Guillotin had no intention of becoming a civil servant. Their views were bound to clash, and not just because the two were rivals (Thouret was a founding member of the Royal Society of Medicine ; Guillotin was a professor of anatomy, physiology, and pathology at the old Paris Faculty of Medicine who shared that antiquated body's contemptuous attitude toward the innovative Royal Society and therefore helped hamper its activities). Thouret now planned to involve the medical profession in national health care; Guillotin would guide his Health Committee toward a reform of the medical profession.

But Guillotin's battle was not yet won. Even though he might have outmaneuvered Liancourt, he had not checkmated him yet. Liancourt realized, of course, that his own plans for health care depended on adequate medical staff, and that Guillotin's committee now controlled plans for the education of the nation's doctors. But why not constrain Guillotin in turn? It seems evident that Liancourt discussed Guillotin's outrageous parliamentary ploy with his aristocratic colleague Charles-Maurice de Talleyrand-Périgord, president of the Constitution Committee. The two had ample opportunity to meet in the fall of 1790: both belonged to the Society of 1789, both moved in select circles and entertained lavishly, and they may well have dined regularly at each other's townhouses.[25] It can hardly be a coincidence that, on 13 October 1790, just a month after Guillotin's power grab, Talleyrand asked the National Assembly to reaffirm his Constitution Committee's jurisdiction over educational reform, requesting that all educational proposals be initially processed by his committee. He referred explicitly to Guillotin, explaining wryly:

> A member of this assembly, who is ever eager to serve you, recently took it upon himself to propose and secure a decree that created a Health Committee, specially responsible for the teaching and practice of medicine. A few days later, this assembly also accepted the protests of another committee that feared itself deprived of an essential task and unable to do all the good for which it was intended.

This admonition led the Assembly to declare that "it would not discuss any aspect of public education until the Constitution Committee, which had general jurisdiction over these matters, had submitted a report."[26] The reform of medical education would now be a part of general educational reform, while health care for the poor was demoted to secondary importance.

Personal animosities thus dealt a severe blow to the citizen-patient's interests. Two aristocratic gentlemen, bent on reform, here joined ranks against a commoner, two laymen against a physician, two liberals against a conservative. At the same time, the conservative physician successfully undercut a public welfare plan. These maneuvers severed two interdependent and fundamental parts of national health care and separated the power to create a network of facilities from the authority to train the appropriate professional personnel. The government could set up the network, but only the medical profession could bring it to life. The situation may have seemed hopeless, and it threatened to cause lengthy delays, but neither the problem nor the moral imperative to solve it would ever go away.

The historian can, at this point in the parliamentary debates, discern the complexities and paradoxes that make the "politics of health" so intractable and persistent a problem. The Poverty Committee's reports—well-informed, thoughtful, humane, and farsighted—dealt with a national system of health care for the poor in the abstract. The training of adequate staff—doctors, pharmacists, and midwives—would be discussed in the Health Committee, but from the point of view of the professions, not that of the needs of the poor. General requirements for medical education would then have to gain approval from the Constitution Committee and fit into the overall national plans for educational reform. Budget questions had to be submitted to the Finance Committee. And how, in the end, the National Assembly would react to huge outlays for the poor remained a matter for conjecture.

Guillotin's bill is more specific than Vicq's regarding doctors' qualifications and their duty to report infractions of the law, but by and large Guillotin adopted the Royal Society of Medicine's recommendations. Title X carries a footnote stating that the principles underlying this report had been endorsed by the Poverty Committee. Indeed, Title X of Guillotin's bill consolidates the relevant articles of Liancourt's Titles I, II, and III (see Appendix A).

Planning the Future of Medicine

The Health Committee had barely begun its work when an event occurred that was even more surprising than the unorthodox circumstances attendant upon its creation.[27] On 25 November 1790, six weeks after the first meeting, each committee member received a printed document of 170 pages, namely, the "New Plan for the Reform of French Medicine" ("Nouveau plan de constitution pour la médecine en France"), the work of the Royal Society of Medicine, under the leadership of its permanent secretary, Félix Vicq d'Azyr.

The evidence suggests that Vicq d'Azyr projected as early as May 1789 to use the doctor-deputies in the National Assembly as agents of reform. We gain some insight from the correspondence of one of those doctors, Jean Gabriel Gallot (1744–1794), a practitioner from the small town of Saint Maurice-le-Girard in lower Poitou, soon to be elected secretary of the Health Committee.[28] Gallot was delighted to receive an invitation to dine at Vicq d'Azyr's house on 20 May, soon after his arrival at Versailles as deputy. Weekly dinners for the seventeen doctor-deputies were being planned.[29] (Actually, only three of them materialized, presumably because Vicq d'Azyr, the personal physician of Marie Antoinette, was kept busy at court.)

Several short pieces from Vicq d'Azyr's pen convey his purpose with striking brevity. The first, dated 1787, is the article "Abuse, History of Medicine" in the *Encyclopédie méthodique . . . Médecine,* of which he was the editor. It reads:

> Sickness and death can teach important lessons in the hospitals. Does anyone study there? Is anyone writing the history of the diseases that claim so many victims? Are autopsies done to discover the seat of the illnesses and the causes of death? Are accounts of the various diseases being written? Are the numerous, interesting new occurrences being recorded? Are the arts of observation and therapy taught? Are there chairs of clinical medicine? Only in our day have able men begun to correct the numerous *abuses* widespread in our hospitals.[30]

Vicq charged that students mainly memorized Latin texts and had minimal exposure to patients, and he wrote a scathing critique of French medical education in the preface to the New Plan:

> The Royal Society of Medicine realizes that . . . medical teaching is almost everywhere corrupt or nonexistent, that the degree-granting institutions are too numerous to remain strong, that the competitive examinations for professorial chairs and for graduate degrees in our schools favor mediocrity if not ignorance, that useless traditions and formalities hamper our students, that the most essential parts of medical learning are forgotten, and that none of our hospitals offer facilities for medical teaching or progress.
>
> The Society finds that almost all midwives lack indispensable knowledge, that doctors have all but abandoned our peasantry to ignorance and empiricism, that medicine is subjected to local rules and exclusive privileges contrary to the spirit of the French Constitution, that the drugs most popular in the provinces are badly compounded and mixed, that, despite much legislation, charlatans continue to spread dangerous poisons, that legal medicine needs reform, and mortality statistics need improvement. All these subjects are dealt with in the present proposal.[31]

Given his eagerness for reform, it is likely that Vicq d'Azyr grew impatient, in the fall of 1790, as he watched the Poverty Committee cast its reformers' net so wide, and as he saw Liancourt submerge urgent medical reform in the morass of social welfare problems. Vicq feared lest health care reform be lost in the surging tide of the Revolutionary upheaval. He therefore decided to act. Not being a deputy, he took the indirect route. He exercised caution, because his close association with the royal family might render him suspect to some.

The creation of a separate Health Committee in the Constituent Assembly, in rivalry with the Poverty Committee, thus takes on new meaning. So does the fact that, at the third meeting, it was decided to invite a large number of learned distinguished outsiders to enlighten the Health Committee. "The speed of this measure," comments a historian, "shows clearly that it was prearranged."[32] The strategy also suggests that someone realized how ordinary a group of citizens the seventeen provincial doctor-deputies turned out to be. True, the nonmedical members of the Health Committee included the abbé Grégoire, Talleyrand, and a duc de la Rochefoucauld, cousin of the Poverty Committee's chairman. But these laymen seem to have taken little part in the deliberations.[33] The selection of the subservient Gallot as secretary and of the pompous Guillotin as chairman fit Vicq d'Azyr's design well.[34] Even in the absence of conclusive proof, one may surmise that he masterminded these choices.

Indeed, fourteen years of correspondence with Gallot had convinced Vicq d'Azyr of his provincial colleague's qualifications for the secretarial job: he was hard-working, punctual, respectful, honest, discreet—and, moreover, devoid of original ideas, ambition, oratorical talent, and love of intrigue. Gallot seemed typecast for the post of secretary,[35] and Ingrand exaggerates this doctor's importance when he writes that Gallot's "Vues générales . . . provided the guidelines for the committee's work."[36]

As for Guillotin, he turned out to be more effective in fostering his own priorities than Vicq d'Azyr had anticipated. He accepted a suggestion that the Health Committee use Vicq's d'Azyr's New Plan as a working draft for its report. This obvious course of least resistance led to fifty meetings in which the committee discussed the plan point by point.[37] But Guillotin also shunted committee debates toward the traditional interests of the medical profession, to the detriment of public care. Not all historians agree with this interpretation. Jean Noël Biraben, for example, reverses the roles of the two committees: "The good intentions of the [Health] Committee," he comments, "were unfortunately counteracted by other entrenched organisms, particularly the Poverty Committee, and personal quarrels finally ruined the major part of its projects."[38] One can also argue that the Health Committee's "good intentions" toward the citizen-patient in town and country were thwarted by the medical profession's special interests.

In the winter of 1790–1791, Health Committee members still believed that a broad range of reforms were close at hand, and they set to work eagerly. The committee's mandate extended, it will be remembered, from the teaching and practice of medicine to schools and hospitals—in short, to "all matters pertaining to public health." By March of 1791, the Health Committee had arrived at considerable consensus regarding prospective legislation.

But then three specialists from the armed forces presented their views. Pierre Isaac Poissonnier (1720–1798), a physician and chemist, medical inspector of the navy and colonies, attended eight meetings, and initiated discussions about naval health regulations, including the diet of seamen. Expert witnesses for the army were Jacques de Horne, a consulting physician who had for seven years been the editor of the *Journal de médecine militaire,*[39] and Jean François Coste (1741–1819), first physician of the armed forces, who had served as chief medical officer with the French expeditionary corps in the American Revolutionary Wars, where he won the friendship of Benjamin Franklin and George Washington. Coste had recently written a book criticizing the cutbacks of 1788 that subordinated military doctors to a health council. In Guillotin's bill, "secondary medical schools" for the army and navy, with teaching services in the major military and naval hospitals, appeared as article 3 of Title I.[40]

The pharmacists had their say during ten committee meetings, from May to June 1791, through their representatives from the College of Pharmacy, Pierre Bayen and Becqueret. On 5 May 1791, Bayen read a proposal on hospital pharmacy. In Guillotin's bill, plans for the study, teaching, and practice of pharmacy took a prominent place among the provisions for health care.[41]

Following the pharmacists, a steady stream of famous medical men appeared before the committee: the surgeons Bernard Peyrilhe (1737–1804) and Philippe Jean Pelletan (1747–1829), Jean Louis Baudelocque (1747–1810), and Antoine Louis (1723–1791), all of them members of the Academy of Surgery; the dean of the medical faculty, Edmé Claude Bourru (1737–1823); the two most knowledgeable medical reformers in France, Vicq d'Azyr and Tenon, and four other members of the Academy of Sciences, Jean Baptiste Leroy (1720–1800), Antoine Laurent de Jussieu, Bailly, and Lavoisier.[42] How flattered the provincial doctor-deputies must have been to attract the attention of so many famous Parisian personalities! And how easy for brilliant professors and academicians to overawe their listeners! Given this list of experts, one no longer wonders why medical education absorbed so much of the committee's time nor why the poor got short shrift.

The Health Committee's bill, reported out of Guillotin's committee in September 1791, essentially followed Vicq's New Plan where medical education was concerned. Ninety-one articles dealt with the establishment of new medical schools, and forty-five regulated the choice of professors. The bill discussed salaries, including that of the concierge, fixed at four-fifths of three-quarters of the professors' pay! In contrast to medical education, health maintenance and home care rated only twenty-six articles in Guillotin's bill. He adopted some of Liancourt's provisions, but his committee's purview of public health remained narrow.

The Health Committee's discussion about country doctors, for example, was often sidetracked to military and naval medicine, and this happened for a good reason. The planners perceived the military doctors as country doctors in uniform who dealt, in fact, with peasants-in-arms. The experts argued that, in the army as on the farm, the enlisted men's primary needs had to do with hygiene, food, and salubrious accommodations. The Health Committee as well as the Royal Society judged country people to be more vulnerable to epidemic disease than city dwellers because of their constant exposure to animals, the weather, and "miasmata" carried by both. Enlistment did not alter this vulnerability, since on military campaigns the peasant-soldier returned to his normal rural environment. The reformers therefore argued that country doctors, like army doctors, needed primarily to understand the dangers of contagion and contamination, and to master preventive precautions, first aid, sanitation, and surgery. It is not by chance that the Health Committee usually referred to army and country doctors as "surgeons." This reveals their traditional prejudice: physicians who served soldiers and peasants were, in the minds of Parisian experts, those very barber-surgeons whom the medical profession had long despised.

To equate the tasks of army and country doctors was to draw a fallacious analogy, however. An army doctor's task consisted in repairing injuries to the soldier's body and readying him for a return to war. He dealt with cuts, gunshot wounds, fractures, infections, and fevers. Naval surgeons concerned themselves primarily with hygiene, nutrition, and exotic infectious diseases. Thus military and naval needs could be equated with a peasant's problems caused primarily by the environment. But one major difference invalidates the comparison: the armed services consisted of men, most of them young and presumably sturdy. In contrast, the peasantry included men and women, infants and old people. Yet the planners in the Health Committee compared the army to the peasantry, particularly in considering cost. It may well be that a desire to economize motivated this illogical assumption.

Eventually, in May 1791, the training of public doctors appeared on the Health Committee's agenda. Like their colleagues on the Poverty Committee, the doctors decided that these young men should study for one or two years in provincial hospitals or clinical schools, taking courses offered at military, naval, or civilian hospitals.[43] The same professor should teach theoretical and practical medicine and adapt his instruction to local conditions of morbidity, epidemiology, and extraordinary pathologic occurrences. At times he might present an overall report on his patient population, emphasizing for his listeners the relationship of morbidity to the seasons, the weather, and regional health problems. At other times he should lecture on illnesses with similar characteristics but varied physical lesions, or else on the varieties of a disease according to patients' temperaments, ages, professions, and the circumstances surrounding the onset of illness. There should be separate wards for occupational diseases, recent admissions that presented a confusing picture, for convalescents, and, of course, for postoperative cases, contagious illnesses, and women in childbed.[44]

It is instructive to compare the New Plan's provisions for clinical schools with Cabanis's reflections in "Observations on Hospitals" of 1790. Cabanis was more willing than the Royal Society to trust provincial experience and initiative. "The form [of these schools] does not strike me as an important question," he wrote. "Here, as in many other things, the best idea is to regulate least. Everything would fall into the optimal pattern if one merely established the qualifications that young students must acquire for admission to all the medical schools, by attending a clinical school for two or three years. . . . It would be proper to leave the method of instruction to the choice and talent of the professors."[45] So permissive an approach did not find favor with the majority of medical reformers.

Under the New Plan, government doctors were to be elected by their constituents.[46] The Health Committee agreed to a "health council" for each department to provide emergency aid in epidemics; to supervise food, drugs, and the qualifications of midwives; and to control the sanitary condition of public establishments such as hospitals, prisons, and cemeteries. The details are spelled out in Title IX of the bill, "Relief and Health Agency." For, indeed, the Health Committee recommended an amalgamation of provincial public health agencies with the relief agencies already planned for all departments by the Poverty Committee. The discussion of relief led to the topic of medical home care, which did not fascinate the Health Committee members: they adopted the Poverty Committee's plans.

But the proposal for abbreviated basic training for government doctors encountered formidable opposition from Talleyrand, the chairman of the Constitution Committee, which controlled educational legislation. Talleyrand was then preparing his Report on Education for presentation to the National Assembly on 10 September 1791.[47] "To do justice to this vast undertaking," he wrote in his *Memoirs,* "I consulted the best-educated men and the most remarkable scientists of the time, men such a M. de Lagrange, M. de Lavoisier, M. de Laplace, M. Monge, M. de Condorcet, M. Vicq d'Azyr, M. de la Harpe. They all helped me. The reputation that this work of mine has since acquired obligated me to name them."[48] There was no such thing as "big medicine" and "little medicine," Talleyrand argued. "In teaching, one must above all avoid mediocrity. Mediocre professors teach nothing, or teach badly and fail to inspire students with the eagerness and creative enthusiasm that only great talent can arouse."[49] He carried the day, and the training centers of country doctors temporarily receded from the national agenda. Talleyrand incorporated the main proposals concerning medical education into his influential report. He assigned the exclusive power for medical accreditation to four medical schools (the fourth, at Bordeaux, would later be dropped). Provincial hospitals could offer courses: freedom of teaching would thus be respected. But only fully trained and licensed physicians would have the right to practice.

Talleyrand thus adopted the major part of Vicq d'Azyr's plan and thus of Guillotin's bill. The proposals contained in the clauses of this bill in turn shaped the Revolutionary "Health Schools" established in 1794 in Paris, Montpellier, and Strasbourg. And these two committees' debates informed the Law of 1803 that regulated the practice of medicine, pharmacy, and midwifery.

But Talleyrand removed Titles IX and X from Guillotin's bill, thereby causing a serious setback to health care for the citizen-patient. His was a reactionary move: it re-separated national health care from medical education. By implication this meant that the health of the poor need not concern young doctors: a welfare program would suffice. The citizen-patient would not be able to rely on a national health network, but would have to resort, as in the past, to individual local practitioners. Talleyrand's reactionary move undoubtedly reflected the consensus of the National Assembly. No one protested.[50]

The fact remains that the Poverty Committee's recommendations and the two related titles of the Health Committee's bill that Talleyrand eliminated from his report constituted a comprehensive plan for national health care in France. Although political events temporarily swept them aside, they soon resurfaced; in 1796 the disarray in the nation's hospitals led the Directory to reform hospital administration; the need for sanitary and public health regulation resulted in the creation of the influential Public Health Council of Paris in 1802; and the damage done by unlicensed practitioners hastened elaboration of the law of 1803 that regulated, not only the practice of physicians, but also that of health officers, pharmacists, and midwives throughout the nineteenth century.

The Next Assignment: The Delivery of Health Care

Liancourt and Vicq d'Azyr "failed" to create a national health service, but they set the goal and spelled out the rules. Their views were complementary, inasmuch as Vicq d'Azyr dealt with the desiderata of national health care from the physician's point of view and the duke sought to address the health needs of patients, the handicapped, children, and the aged. These two leaders, products of the Enlightenment, idealistic, energetic, and determined men in their early forties, each prestigious in his own way, had produced reform projects well adapted to the French academic and professional traditions, responsive to the needs of the poor and mindful of the new constitution. Had the Revolution not gotten out of hand, would the legislature have appropriated the needed funds? Would the medical profession have agreed to train public doctors? We do not know.

In retrospect, it seems remarkable that provisions for social medicine should have been included in a reform program of 1791. This occurred partly because both the national constitution and medicine needed reform in 1789. The social needs of the country were therefore on the mind of every citizen, including every doctor, and seventeen of these doctors were deputies and thus members of Guillotin's committee. Second, the fact that Liancourt's Poverty Committee had formulated detailed plans for social medicine before the Health Committee was even founded meant that Guillotin had to harmonize his proposals with Liancourt's and Thouret's. This was done, at what cost to the two doctors' pride only their personal papers could reveal. Third, and most important, a distinguished reform-minded group of physicians, the Royal Society of Medicine, came forward at the crucial moment with a thoughtful, scientific, and progressive new plan, thereby exerting a decisive influence on medical thought. Finally, Poverty Committee members emphasized sickness among the etiologic factors of indigence from the start, thus directing their attention to health care personnel and institutions, and to the needs of the citizen as patient. This lends their work significance far ahead of its time.

◆◆◆

In the fall of 1791, the Constituent Assembly was drawing to a close, its main task achieved: France now had a constitutional monarchy, an elected legislature, a Civil Constitution of the Clergy, a new administrative pattern. But there was troublesome unfinished business and ominous dissent. The country's finances were in disarray, and the new currency was losing value; the pope had refused to sanction a national French church, thus splitting French Catholics into two irreconcilable factions; the king had attempted to flee to his bellicose brother-in-law, the Austrian emperor, thus hopelessly discrediting the monarchy. The hereditary rulers of Prussia, Austria, Russia, and England felt threatened by the progress of equality in France. A general war seemed likely. Under those circumstances the legislature had more pressing problems than the citizens' health.

But while the deputies and doctors of France were the most important professional groups involved in planning for the patient of the future, it was the caring professions—nurses, pharmacists, professional midwives, and medical students—that were most immediately and pressingly affected by the Revolutionary developments. We shall see in the next chapter how they related to the patient population. The nurse was closest to the acutely ill, as well as to the ailing citizen. The nursing orders differed sharply in tradition and behavior. Some nurses, like the Augustinians, continued to practice patient care as a religious calling; others, like the Sisters of Charity, shed their religious habits and stayed close to their patients out of a feeling of professional responsibility. Nursing survived because it was essential, but the nurse found her activities curtailed. The male pharmacist stepped into the place of the sister apothecary. Women had no access to training in the medical or pharmacological sciences, and their practices thus became increasingly obsolete. We shall see the pharmacist acquire a fine scientific education and Parmentier's pharmacopoeia for home use meet with great demand. The professional midwife experienced a period of high regard and prominence, but this was brief. And, finally, we meet the medical student of this era, a newcomer to the hospital ward. These young men became conduits of the new attitude of the Revolution toward the citizen-patient—a special fraternity that flowered on military campaigns and the battlefield, as we shall see at the end of this book.

Liancourt sensed the temper of the National Assembly and knew that his projects for health care reform were now untimely. In the hope of provoking at least some action, he submitted a "Report on the Distribution of Aid for the Department of Paris," on 26 September 1791.[51] But the next morning the Assembly merely passed this lame decree: "The National Assembly is pained to admit that its enormous workload in this session has prevented the elaboration of aid that the Assembly itself had ordered in the constitution. It leaves to the subsequent legislature the honorable task of fulfilling this important duty."[52]

That "honorable task" would take many years. But the adaptations of the caring professions to the new, Revolutionary needs of the citizen-patient were already proceeding apace.

The Caring Professions

This decree does not concern women.
> Civilian Committee, section faubourg du Nord, 1792

Public patient care under the old regime satisfied no one and the agenda for change in the new era was long, burdensome, and contradictory. The reformers' most difficult long-range project would be to alter the indigent patients' traditional concept of what a hospital could do for them, lower their expectations, and instill a motivation to return home as soon as they were physically well enough. But the reformers' immediate tasks concerned readjustments in the complex relationships among hospitalized patients and the caring professions: the nursing orders, pharmacists, midwives, and medical students.

The events of the Revolutionary decade affected these four groups in diverse ways. Despite persecution of the religious orders, nurses remained at the patients' side, struggling to maintain their professional role and their ties to the Catholic Church. Both nursing and hospital pharmacy suffered from problems related to gender, as well as from internecine rivalries. The sister apothecary experienced a curtailment and eventual abolition of her job, while the male pharmacist emerged with a scientific education and helped instruct the citizen-patient in compounding home remedies that were effective and safe. Midwives succeeded owing to government support, but competing obstetricians and tradition-bound women colleagues and customers hampered their advancement. A group of young men, rarely admitted to the hospital in large numbers under the old regime, now beleaguered the patient on the sick wards: the medical students. They came to look and to learn; as residents and interns, they examined, admitted, treated, and counseled the citizen-patient. Before long they would meet him as a wounded soldier. The Revolution thus changed the patients' hospital experience in many ways.

Nursing: Vocation or Profession?

Two hundred years ago, most poor people did not consult a doctor when they were ill; in Catholic countries they depended on the nursing sisters and brothers in hospital wards, in pharmacies, in dispensaries, and in their homes, and on midwives to deliver their babies. The nurses responded to the pain, hunger, homelessness, and helplessness of a petitioner rather than to specific medical needs as a physician would. They responded with charity, for their mission was to comfort, feed, and shelter, but also to convince and convert. The indigent patient had been their silent partner in this relationship for a thousand years.

The nursing orders perpetuated the spirit of hospitality of many centuries toward pilgrims, who had gratefully accepted ablutions, food, rest, and the large variety of unguents, plasters, lotions, and potions that the religious created over the years. Active ingredients derived mainly from their medicinal herb garden. Eventually the monastery added hospital wards, and the religious turned to nursing. Their cloistered existence provided the daily pattern and their home the framework for the patients in the hospitals they administered. Nursing was originally organized by men, the rules for the chief French orders being Augustinian, as adopted by the Knights of the Hospital of St. John of Jerusalem around 1100.[1] They admitted women from the start, and separate communities for women proliferated and mastered hospital administration as well. Nursing was already a well-managed and lavishly financed profession when the first modern medical schools were just being established.

In Paris at the time of the Revolution, eighty religious communities for women comprised 2,523 members, and close to half of these women were nurses.[2] While the women far outnumbered men in the nursing profession, we shall soon see that the men were the innovators. All religious nurses lived a communal life of poverty, chastity, and obedience to their superiors; the vows of some orders (such as the Augustinian Religious of the Hôtel-Dieu of Paris and the Brothers of St. John of God, or Brothers of Charity) required a strictly cloistered life. Other vows (like those of the Ladies of St. Thomas de Villeneuve, and especially of the Sisters of Charity and the Sisters of St. Martha) left religious free to live in the world and pursue their calling.

The Revolutionaries abolished all religious orders: they grudgingly tolerated individual female nurses, but effectively dispersed the men, who did not resume their work until the Restoration. The history of nursing during the Revolutionary and imperial period is thus a history of women.[3] A brief look at these nursing orders active in France at the beginning of the Revolution will permit us to assess their varying attitudes toward religion, politics, and medicine, and thus toward the patient.

The Augustinians of the Paris Hôtel-Dieu assembled patients under their own roof and nursed them according to long-established practices.[4] They referred to the French Revolution as a storm, "*la tourmente révolutionnaire*," with a nice play on words that associates a hurricane with passing torment. They faced the Revolutionaries with incredulous and stubborn resistance, opposing their own absolute ideal of Christian service to the ideal of liberty proffered by the politicians and to the scientific medicine proposed by the doctors. About three dozen Augustinians and over two thousand patients somehow survived at the Hôtel-Dieu during the Revolutionary decade. The nurses complied with the decree of 18 August 1793 that simultaneously commanded them to disperse and to remain at their posts as lay individuals.[5] Their own records provide the most reliable illustration of their monastic existence. Hours for prayer regulated their day, service to patients represented care for Christ. They perceived their working environment at the Hôtel-Dieu—the overcrowding and confusion, the foul smells, and filth—as tribulations set by God to test their piety. In this emotional context, they equated advocacy of change with heresy. Had anyone presented them with the notion of the citizen-patient, a patient with rights and duties, they would have stared in disbelief.[6]

The prioress, Sister de la Croix, warned the National Assembly in July 1790 against abrogating the novitiate. She predicted that without the commitment of holy vows, women would lack the strength to follow the exhausting schedule. But the Revolutionaries abolished the novitiates, and as a result the thirty-eight Augustinian nurses remaining at the Hôtel-Dieu in 1800 included only eleven under fifty years old and nine in their seventies. Their activities during the Revolutionary decade focused of necessity on finding enough food to keep their patients alive and 400 to 800 servants content enough to continue working.

Somehow they succeeded, but it is almost impossible to imagine how women who had not set foot outside the Hôtel-Dieu for fifty or sixty years experienced the French Revolution. Daily life for the patients inside that hospital still followed the regulations of the old regime. The nurses' daybooks and registers indicate that Augustinians and Revolutionaries lived in different worlds.

◆◆◆

By the eighteenth century, the Brothers of Charity, founded two hundred years earlier by Saint John of God, had grown into a power-

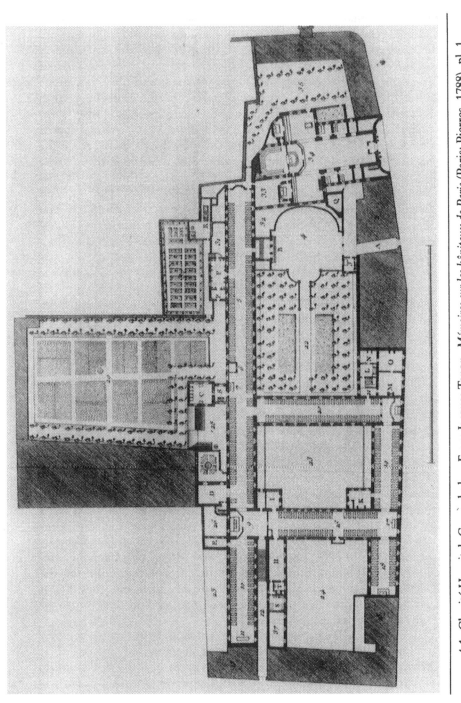

FIGURE 4.1. Charité Hospital. Ground plan. From Jacques Tenon, *Mémoires sur les hôpitaux de Paris* (Paris: Pierres, 1788), pl. 1.

ful international corporation: their mother house in Paris staffed and supervised thirty-seven *charités* in France and her colonies, and the brothers developed into skilled specialists in pharmacy, surgery, and nursing. In Tenon's day, the Charité hospital in Paris boasted 216 single beds in six clean, well-aired wards. It excluded contagious and incurable patients and women. Tenon considered this hospital as an architectural model because all wards were of moderate size; fever, surgical, and convalescent patients had separate wards; five courtyards provided plenty of air and light; and three gardens were reserved for patients, medicinal herbs, and vegetable plots. At the Paris Charité, the brothers usually employed two surgeons and three physicians, among these Louis Desbois de Rochefort (1750–1786), Pierre Joseph Desault (1744–1795), and Jean Nicolas Corvisart (1755–1821). The Charité became so famous for surgery that, the authoritative Fosse-yeux tells us, lay apprentices joined the order so as to gain thorough training and attain expertise.[7] The brothers admitted only paying patients or those sponsored by donors. Because the Paris Charité was the order's only novitiate, the ratio of servants to patients was 1:2, assuring excellent care. The brothers also ran a busy outpatient service and their pharmacy on the rue Jacob served as a dispensary.[8] A home on rue du Bac sheltered convalescents for eight days while they looked for work.[9] The patients, all of them Catholic men, here experienced medical charity at its best.

One little-known expertise of the brothers was psychiatric nursing, a branch of health care that literally emerged from medieval horrors at the time of the Revolution. At the Charité de Charenton, in a Paris suburb, as at *charités* throughout France, the brothers cared for wealthy, mentally ill Frenchmen confined by *lettre de cachet*. The patients lived under strict but thoughtful supervision, ate well, and were treated by knowledgeable physicians (if we are to believe the brothers' advocates). Charenton later became a model public psychiatric institution under the supervision of the Seine Department. The links to its charitable past were many: the grounds, facilities, and amenities remained exceptional, as the vast asylum still suggests. Its first administrator, de Coulmiers, was a former Premonstrant priest and member of the Poverty Committee.[10] Had not the Revolution dispersed the brothers out of fear of their powerful sponsor in Rome, they might have become invaluable teachers of nursing care and thus improved the patient's hospital experience.

In contrast to contacts with Augustinians and Brothers of Charity in cloistered hospitals, the French poor encountered the Sisters of Charity and the multiple variants of their order in many walks of life, in their own homes, and even in dangerous and filthy places such as prisons and galleys. In Paris, 182 out of a total of 590 of these sisters worked in the hospitals on the eve of the Revolution.[11] The Sisters of Charity constituted by far the largest group of religious nurses, and they served wherever they were needed. One might consider them the forerunners of the modern public health nurse, the visiting nurse, or the social worker who brought support to the citizen-patient. The order's founder, Saint Vincent de Paul (1576–1660), always stressed service to the poor and directed the sisters to "say little and do much." They made only an annual commitment to their communities instead of taking vows for life: this intelligent innovation by Vincent de Paul attracted numerous women to this order and accounts for its vitality ever since its inception.

After the dissolution of the nursing orders, the government kept the former sisters under close surveillance. We can tell from a document in the Archives nationales, dated "Year IX," that 458 "former religious women" lived together in Paris. Their addresses indicate that many were neighbors (for example, at 205, 212, and 214 "rue Jacques" and 10 and 13 rue des Postes). Several groups found lodgings near the very doors of their former hospitals.[12]

In this context, entirely new significance accrues to a decision taken in 1798 by François de Neufchâteau, the minister of internal affairs, to use contractors (*entrepreneurs*) to supply the hospitals. These private entrepreneurs furnished supplies, food, and nursing personnel. No one asked them about the background of the nurses they hired. It is surely not farfetched to suggest that the five contractors employed these religious-in-hiding, dispersed because they would not deny their faith, but eager to nurse their patients and earn a livelihood, however meager. This collusion explains why the hospitalized patients continued to be cared for by the same persons, regardless of the political regime in power.

For the patients bedded down in the hospital, the one reassuring person was the nurse. The "sister" came from their social milieu and spoke their language. She relied, as they did, on traditional remedies and food. She took orders from the doctor, as they did. Commanded to deny her faith, she may have shed her habit and bit her tongue, but who knows whether she did not whisper reassuring prayers to the patient in pain or near death?

These sisters also played a prominent role in the "charity" or "welfare" offices in the inner city and the slums (*bureaux de charité*; then *bureaux de bienfaisance*). In 1791 in Paris, they staffed twenty-two of these, but had been expelled from five. Their efforts aimed particularly at children and the elderly, at persons not ill enough to require hospitalization but too unwell to work. They functioned as administrators, nurses, counselors, teachers, cooks, and pharmacists. They visited the bedridden, bringing food, clothing, fuel, and medicines. At the welfare office, they taught orphaned and poor children the 3 Rs (here to be interpreted as reading, writing, and religion), and simple skills such as rope-making, sewing, and embroidery. They served the children a good meal, particularly if the office included a soup kitchen. They were instrumental in helping to keep the citizen-patient out of the hospital. (We shall meet them again in the next chapter in connection with the "outpatient.")[13]

Ailing indigents thus encountered hundreds of women whose services they had experienced since childhood, women dressed in religious or para-religious costumes, serving huge quantities of food and dispensing simple drugs. They provided nutrition and medication all at once, for there was no clear dividing line between the restorative action of drugs, the medicinal quality of food, and the soothing comfort of religion. And who will say that the best therapeutic medication may not consist in food of the right quality, served in appropriate quantity at the opportune time, attractively, and with soothing words by a trusted and gentle woman endowed with motherly feelings? It may well be that expert cooking and traditional trust were indeed, as the sisters claimed, an irreplaceable treasure.

A particularly forlorn group of women, those imprisoned by *lettres de cachet* as incorrigible or mentally ill, or in homes for repentant prostitutes, were nursed by the Ladies of St. Thomas de Villeneuve, an order that stood halfway between the Augustinians of the Hôtel-Dieu and the Sisters of Charity in terms of orthodoxy. Recruited mainly in Brittany, this order consisted of two traditional groups: ladies, often aristocratic and wealthy, who held voting rights in the order, and sisters who performed the rough work. All underwent a seven-year novitiate, but they took simple vows. They owned seven houses in Paris and fifty in the provinces, predominantly in Brittany, Normandy, and Picardy. In 1791, forty-two members of the order lived in their mother house in Paris, known as the "Enfant Jésus," subsequently the world's first children's hospital.[14]

From among the numerous other orders similar to the Sisters of Charity, it seems important to single out the Sisters of St. Martha, who were Jansenists. They relied on the protection of powerful families like the Joly de Fleury and of outstanding philanthropic ecclesiastics like the abbé Cochin and the abbé de l'Epée. A secretly administered fund, familiarly known as "la boîte à Perrette," helped them subsist.[15] Napoleon relied on this order, no doubt because it had suffered persecution under the old regime and might therefore be loyal to a Bonapartist government. In fact, all regimes at the turn of the nineteenth century treated women's nursing orders as a minor pawn.

◆◆◆

When the Revolutionaries nationalized the Catholic Church in November 1789, no one could have been further from their minds than the nurse. Their motive was to confiscate Church lands and to control the nomination of ecclesiastic officials. These measures concerned power and men, and *men* subsumed women in eighteenth-century thinking. The government intended gradually to extinguish monasticism: men's orders were suspect as subversive because of their international ramifications, converging at a high command in Rome, the center of counterrevolution. Women's monasticism suggested "wasted" human lives: women should live in the world, marry, and produce numerous little republicans.

The Jacobin legislators may well have believed that they were bestowing the natural right of "liberty" upon hitherto subjugated women. In reality, liberty opened nothing but frightening perspectives to the many nurses who were aged and depended on the hospital community as their only home. They not only found their corporate existence challenged, but their homes and their means of subsistence nationalized. The Revolutionaries had not immediately connected the abolition of monasticism with the staffing of hospitals and schools. They proceeded gradually: the decree of 3 November 1789 suspended new vows, and that of 19 February 1790 forbade them altogether. After the fall of the monarchy, the Revolutionary leaders grew impatient and abolished "all regular and secular congregations" on 18 August 1792. Finally realizing that most of the nation's schoolteachers and nurses belonged to these associations, the assembly added: "Nevertheless, in hospitals and charitable institutions, the same persons as before shall continue individually to serve the poor and the sick, *under the supervision of the municipal administrators*" (emphasis added). The police commissioner, or the section leader, thus became the judge of a nurse's loyalty to the nation.[16]

Many religious went underground or fled into exile when their new republican masters insisted on a loyalty oath to the secular state. The women's opposition stemmed partly from their dependence on the priest for the sacraments of confession and mass: these ceremonies were essential to their faith and required the services of an ordained man. The nurses shielded priests who refused to take the oath of allegiance to the Civil Constitution of the Clergy, providing a safe haven in the hospitals, where these men secretly officiated.[17] It was this association with priests that rendered nurses suspect.

Yet in the minds of some it was questionable whether women were meant to take any oath at all, and F. S. Bézard, deputy from Oise, asked the Convention to clarify the issue, arguing that the law concerned civil servants and teaching congregations, not nurses. As proof he cited the following certificate:

> We, members of the civilian committee, section faubourg du Nord, certify that, at the time the oath of 18 August 1792 was decreed, the citizenesses Marie Bernard and Marie Claudine Ponard, former Sisters of Charity, presented themselves to take the said oath, *but the city government, consulted about this, replied that this decree does not concern women.*[18]

The Convention, convinced that it must compensate for past oversight, ordered all nurses to take the oath within one month. From time to time the political authorities made a clean sweep of all the nurses who refused to comply: they dismissed a total of forty-three Sisters of Charity—from the Hospice for Incurables at the end of June 1791, from the orphanage in the faubourg St. Antoine in September 1792, and from the infirmary of the Hôtel des Invalides at the end of 1793.[19]

Although the Revolutionary lawmakers, and later Napoleon, threatened cavalierly to fire all unsubmissive women and replace them, it was well-nigh impossible to find suitable laywomen for nursing work. The only ones for hire were usually untrained, undisciplined, and unreliable.[20] The hospitals, in the meantime, were "in a disastrous state": while Revolutionaries and Catholics fought an ideologic battle, thousands of patients starved, deprived of physical comfort and medical aid.[21] How did the hospitalized patients survive—particularly after their ranks were swelled by the influx of sick and wounded veterans from the Italian, German, and Dutch campaigns? We lack specific data about Paris hospital inmates during this era,[22] but one imagines that they helped each other as best they could on the wards, that their families brought food, and that the large hospital gardens yielded produce and sustained cows, pigs, rabbits, and chickens. None of the major Paris institutions closed their doors in the 1790s—evidence of survival, at least.

That the nursing orders emerged from hiding and anonymity at the beginning of the Consulate, and quite suddenly, was owing to the intervention of a man in a uniquely powerful position: the minister of internal affairs, Jean Antoine Chaptal (1756–1832).[23] From 1801 to 1804, this Ideologue physician played a pivotal role in health care for the citizen-patient, particularly in Paris: his reforms began with the recall of the nurses and the creation of the midwifery school at Port-Royal; it culminated in the work of two model administrative councils supervising hospitals and public health. Even before he as-

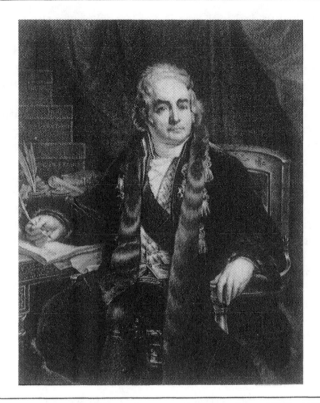

FIGURE 4.2. Jean Antoine Chaptal, comte de Chanteloup (1756–1832), minister of internal affairs, 1801–1804. Bibliothèque nationale, Paris, Cabinet des estampes.

sumed his new duties as minister of internal affairs on 21 January 1801, Chaptal undertook an inspection tour of the Paris Hôtel-Dieu. He came away appalled by the conditions under which the patients lived. Within ten days he invited several nursing orders to resume their activities immediately and begin training novices.[24] The government would eventually legalize nursing orders one by one, after thorough investigations.

The attempt of Revolutionaries and of Napoleon to create a lay national nursing profession was reasonable enough, since there is no necessary logical relation between nursing and religion. But they failed to appreciate the essential motivation of these women. Only a layperson's calling to nursing as a profession might have rivaled a believer's vocation. But that concept of modern nursing would only be imported into France a century later by Protestant English "nightingales."[25] In the meantime, the French Revolutionaries, and after them

Napoleon, had to deal with nursing orders whose loyalty to the new government was untested.

Once they faced the sisters in political negotiations, after the Concordat of 1801, the men realized that they were dealing with stout antagonists, women with power, experience, tradition, and faith. These nurses were professional women who had chosen their work in response to a religious conviction and made a lifelong commitment to their patients and to their God. Centuries of experience had turned them into knowledgeable hospital administrators, who trained their own successors in a tough apprenticeship system. Their religious communities, established in hospitals, participated in the activities of these institutions, derived financial support from the endowments, and regulated the lives of the patients in harmony with monastic rules. The experienced leaders of these nursing orders dealt firmly with their subordinates and with their male supervisors, the municipality on the one hand, the Church hierarchy on the other. They opposed revolutionary change as a matter of principle. If Revolutionaries, medical reformers, and Napoleon's ministers had given serious attention to the nursing orders, they might have foreseen that it would be easier to confiscate their property, proscribe their uniforms, and dismiss and disperse them than to replace them. Nursing services turned out to be essential to the nation, particularly a nation at war, and the image of the "good sister" remained etched into the patient population's consciousness.

For Napoleon, the revival of the nursing orders was, like everything else, a political question, though compounded by his prejudice against women. He was convinced that he could bully mere nurses into forming a single national group, which he would finance and control. He also wanted to bring the nursing orders into line with the Civil Code, under which citizens could neither take religious vows nor renounce their right to own property. Napoleon called together representatives of all the nursing orders on 4–8 December 1807, at a congress under the aegis of his mother, Laetitia, whom he named "General Protectress of Imperial Establishments of Welfare and Charity." The maneuver failed. In the end, the emperor agreed to all the nurses' requests for buildings and funds, and an annual subsidy of 130,000 francs.[26]

A secret "Table of Religious Houses or Groups in Paris" dating from the end of Napoleon's reign indicates that the imperial government continued to keep the nursing orders under careful surveillance.[27] It indicates that the Augustinian nurses of the Hôtel-Dieu numbered thirty-four, with ten novices, and "favor the Pope a little, but mainly their own establishment and His Majesty; very useful";

that the Ladies of St. Thomas de Villeneuve, eighteen strong, with twenty-one novices, were "encrusted with old prejudices, strongly ultramontanist, and in touch with all elements opposed to the government. This establishment is to be closed"; that the Sisters of Charity numbered two hundred and eight in all, and were "precious for humanity and reasonably Papist"; that twenty-five Sisters of St. Martha "are Papists, devoted to the abbé Dastroc, but very useful . . . not to be feared."

Napoleon's spies thus reached conclusions with which the modern historian can agree: they saw the remaining Augustinians as busy and isolated in their cocoon at the Hôtel-Dieu, and the Sisters of Charity and Saint Martha as the most valuable nurses in a modern lay state. Napoleon called them to Cochin Hospital in 1810, to the infirmary of the Collège Louis-le-Grand in 1811, St. Antoine Hospital in 1812, and Beaujon Hospital in 1813. In 1834 they replaced the Sisters of St. Thomas de Villeneuve at the Pitié hospital, and in 1840 they took over nursing at the Quinze-Vingts Hospice.

Successive legislatures never raised the possibility of training professional nurses, even though they elaborated curricula in medicine and pharmacy and created a school for midwives. Politicians and doctors assumed that these women would adapt, comply, keep quiet, and continue to work hard. In repetitive, perfunctory phrases, they praised the dutiful, dedicated, selfless, kindly "girls" (usually the word is the half-condescending, half-derogatory *filles*). But the archives yield no evidence that they considered the sisters as partners. Not until the Consulate, and then only by necessity, did the government negotiate seriously with the nursing orders and only the Third Republic created secular scientific nursing.

Thus the French government, beginning with Napoleon, had to bow to reality: on the hospital ward the Catholic nurse was irreplaceable, and she unquestionably maintained the patients' bond to their religion. In contrast, the hospital pharmacist would be drawn into the lay world owing to a scientific education. His attitude toward the citizen-patient meanwhile underwent significant change.

The Hospital Pharmacist

In the late eighteenth century, hospitalized patients witnessed the gradual eclipse of the sister apothecary, while the male pharmacist rose in importance; the continuing feuds between lay and monastic pharmacists, and between pharmacists and doctors; and the destruction of all traditional corporations and the rise of modern scientific pharmacy. Each set of developments deserves attention.[28]

The poor in France under the old regime relied heavily on medicines distributed by religious establishments. Monasteries and convents grew their own herbs, compounded their own remedies, and had the legal right to dispense substances with mild medicinal qualities, known as "simples." Hospital pharmacies not only furnished medications for the wards, but sold large quantities to the public. Furthermore, they opened an avenue for professional specialization.

The poor were used to the services of women as well as men apothecaries. At the maison de l'Enfant Jésus, the dames de St. Thomas de Villeneuve had a "well-equipped laboratory and a room for drying balsamic herbs picked in their garden, which measured seven acres and adjoined their buildings." The nuns of the rue Mouffetard "compounded medications in their pharmacy, used these for their own patients, and sold them to the local residents at a low price." The nuns at the Miramiones convent manufactured remedies and "ran a veritable clinic."[29] A sister kept the register of deposits and withdrawals of drugs at the Salpêtrière, as well as the keys to the attic where medicinal plants were being dried. The same applied at St. Louis Hospital. The nuns' work as pharmacists was not limited to administering infusions, syrups, unguents, and balms: they knew how to apply plasters, poultices, and bandages, and some of them were experts at bloodletting.[30]

It was reluctantly that brother apothecaries and lay pharmacists acknowledged nuns as skilled and responsible practitioners. How seriously should we take the accusation that the Augustinians at the Hôtel-Dieu pampered their own sweet tooth and were forever preparing syrups and preserves, thus consuming too much sugar? The nuns countered with the charge that the pharmacists practiced sloppy bookkeeping (and they may have been alluding to the chronic shortage of brandy at the Charité). Yet these were but family feuds compared to the more serious attacks on all religious pharmacists by their lay competitors.

For indeed the world of the monastery and convent pharmacy was increasingly at risk. Since the sixteenth century at least, lawsuits had challenged the right of the religious to dispense drugs, and in the eighteenth century litigation grew angrier and more frequent. The brothers readily admitted that the guilds protected the quality of drugs by setting standards of purity and measurement, and trained their apprentices according to strict regulations. But they criticized the pharmacists' monopolies and price-fixing practices. Lay pharmacists, on the other hand, charged their religious rivals with deficient training and incompetence: they often directed their criticisms at the sisters.

An even more serious professional challenge to the pharmacists came from the medical profession. Doctors had long complained that pharmacists overstepped legal bounds: only doctors should control medically active substances, otherwise empirics and charlatans would harm and swindle the public. But the public relied on prescriptions from doctors and quacks alike,[31] and the distinctions between simple and active ingredients were by no means clear. What is more, physicians themselves engaged in quackery—as, for example, in 1746, when the physicians at the Hôtel-Dieu received legal permission to experiment with "universal purgative," "oil of life," and "liquid gold." They used enormous quantities of theriaca, or Venice treacle, made with over seventy ingredients, including the flesh of vipers. At the same time doctors bowed before the patients' praise for "Mother Thecla's unguent," and the restorative virtues of the hospital bouillon and quince jelly.[32] But they attempted to draw a line between over-the-counter drugs and prescription medicines.

Pharmacy eventually emerged as a lay scientific profession: in fact, the Revolution came at an optimal time for this specialty because chemistry had changed radically and pharmacy needed to adjust to the new terms and measures.[33] The most important aspect of this evolution for the citizen-patient was without doubt the modernization of the pharmacopoeia. The new formulas took shape once the kilogram and the meter were enthroned in Meudon in platinum purity in 1799, but how to transfer these measures into the popular traditions of self-medication puzzled even the professors: the old *livre* now equaled almost two *livres*—that is, the new kilogram; the apothecary's traditional grains, scruples, and drams were difficult to render in decimal terms. On the other hand, measures expressed in tablespoons, teaspoons, or drops were "not rigorously exact but convenient and can be used by all kinds of persons," Professors Deyeux, Chaussier, and Pinel resignedly concluded in their report.[34] Citizen-patients would have to be educated slowly, in their own language. Editions of Parmentier's pharmacopoeia now followed one another at a fast pace: from the beginning, he included a note listing the new weights and measures, and the corresponding traditional ones; thirty-eight simple and composite remedies for use in the citizen-patient's home and ninety-three for prisons and workhouses. Parmentier wanted to enable the citizenry to compound approved remedies in the home, community center, school, and factory, and even in prison, and he hoped they would abandon the tradition- and superstition-bound almanac in favor of his pharmacopoeia.[35]

Another aspect of the modernization of pharmacy important for the patient was the creation in 1796 of a central hospital pharmacy for all of Paris that would guarantee the uniformity and purity of medications.[36] This required large sums of money for architectural changes to house well-equipped laboratories. The idea of a central pharmacy for Paris derived from important precedents: the Hôtel-Dieu and the Salpêtrière had long supplied the medicines needed in their dependencies. The government decided in 1795 to form one central pharmacy for Paris at the Hôtel-Dieu.[37] Etienne Guiraudet (1754–1839), its chief,[38] had already succeeded in creating what an eyewitness described as "one of the largest, most efficiently organized and most plentifully supplied, most elegantly appointed—in a word, the most complete and orderly—pharmacies in the republic."[39] Its transfer across the street to the premises of the former Foundlings' Hospice, vacated by the creation of the new maternity hospice at Port-Royal, began a year and a half later on 12 November 1796. For several years, the architect Clavareau adapted, rebuilt, and perfected laboratories with intricate installations, and as usual he seems to have been well-pleased with the result. He describes "vast and beautiful lofts serving to store and dry simples, both herbs and flowers, others holding powders, mineral substances and liquids, both alcoholic and plain. In a word, this central pharmacy contains all that is needed to serve the hospitals of Paris."[40] As of 1803, its staff included a chief pharmacist, two chiefs of service for supplies and the laboratory, two assistants, a bookkeeper, a shipping clerk, and seven other employees.[41]

But this happy state was not to last, for Napoleon decided quite suddenly, it seems, that the central pharmacy building was needed for other purposes. All the costly installations were to be moved elsewhere, and quickly. The imperial decree of 10 February 1810, proclaimed for reasons to which no one was privy, caught the pharmacists by surprise.[42] Their objections proved futile. The Hospital Council thereupon found a new locale at the corner of the rue de la Bûcherie and the rue du Fouarre—the medieval site of the University of Paris. This may well have been a stalling maneuver, for these buildings were inadequate, and the council pleaded with the prefect of Paris to preserve the laboratories and other facilities at its previous locale. Finally an appropriate building was found, the Hôtel des Miramiones, and by 1813 the central pharmacy moved into magnificent new quarters.

The central pharmacy could now finally provision all the health care facilities of Paris, and to some extent the provinces. This was the dream of the chief promoter of the whole enterprise, Parmentier. He, and the pharmacist-in-chief of this era, Noël Etienne Henry (1769–1832),[43] now prodded the Hospital Council to confiscate all utensils and substances remaining in hospital pharmacies. This effort would hasten what the expert historian Maurice Bouvet calls the "in-

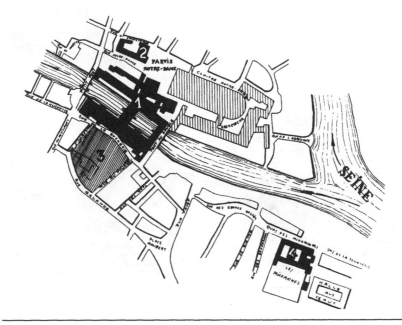

FIGURE 4.3. The four locations of the Pharmacie Centrale des Hôpitaux during the Revolution and under the Empire. From M. Bouvet, *La pharmacy hospitalière à Paris de 1789 à 1815* (Paris: Société d'histoire de la pharmacie, 1943), 32. Between 1789 and 1815, the central hospital pharmacy was relocated three times. The Hôtel-Dieu fire in 1773 warned Parisians that it must be moved from the basements of the Hôtel-Dieu (1); in the mid 1790s, an elaborate site was ready at the former Foundlings' Hospice (2); Napoleon dislodged the Pharmacie to inadequate temporary quarters on the left bank (3); finally, it moved into the former Miramiones Convent, today the Musée de l'Assistance publique.

dustrialization" of pharmacy. Sisters and brothers were now expelled, except from institutions such as the Salpêtrière, where the "*soeurs officières*" obstructed change to the best of their abilities.

War, in this case, hastened modernization. The centralization of manufacture and distribution of pharmaceuticals became a necessity, as did research to find substitutes for tropical substances such as cane sugar, opium, castor oil, and cinchona bark, not to mention lemons, tea, and coffee: the British blockade had cut off supplies. French chemists developed beet sugar, and chicory for coffee, and eventually isolated strychnine (1818), quinine (1820), caffeine (1821), and codeine (1832). Ackerknecht comments that "a new era of therapeutics, domi-

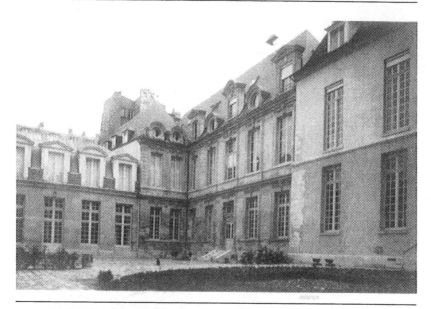

FIGURE 4.4 Hôtel des Miramiones, Pharmacie centrale hospitalière. Now the Musée de l'Assistance publique. On permanent display are the huge kettles, elaborate vials, and elegant pottery of the Pharmacie centrale, as well as a turntable from the Foundlings' Hospice.

nated by the newly created experimental pharmacology, began: in this movement, the old opposition between "rational" and "empirical" treatment disappeared.[44]

The patient in the ward or at the dispensary now invariably encountered the lay professional pharmacists whose requirements of eligibility were definitively established by the decree of 22 February 1802. Trained according to a basic science curriculum similar to that of the doctors, the pharmacist could now aspire to an internship after three years' experience with an apothecary or in the army, followed by two years at the central pharmacy or four years in a hospital. A six-year hospital internship qualified him for the residency if he passed examinations in botany, chemistry, and theoretical and practical pharmacy. It was from these residents that the chiefs of service were chosen, two for the central pharmacy, one for each major hospital. A pharmacist-in-chief, who was also a member of the Paris College of Pharmacy, was the official head of the profession. The quarters where sister and brother apothecaries had officiated gradually disappeared: that of the Maternity Hospice, for example, ceased operations owing to a decree of 4 May 1802, and henceforth Madame Boivin, supervisor of the neonate infirmary, obtained the bulk of her supplies from the central pharmacy and special medication from the nearby Venereal Diseases Hospital.[45] Women pharmacists faced special restrictions, such as the guidelines issued by Dean Thouret and the pharmacist Nicolas Deyeux under the Consulate directing doctors periodically to verify that the sisters kept exact accounts, used only proper ingredients, and did not sell these to the poor. If a salaried pharmacist was present in the establishment, the nurses "should in no way participate in the preparation of medicines."[46]

As nuns yielded influence to physicians and pharmacists, patients experienced a gradual shift of attention from food to medication. The personal and domestic details of patient comfort—the delicate daily adjustment of food intake to strength, medication to pain, therapy to morale and recovery—tended now to be superseded by scientific pharmacy, particularly, as we shall see, in the teaching wards. Progress was indubitably made in protecting the citizen-patient from poorly compounded drugs. Chemical analysis and precise measurement gradually enabled the legislator, the health authorities, and the police to target an increasing variety of dangerous substances and harmful foodstuffs, control proprietary medicines, protect patents, ferret out nostrums and quackery and punish offenders.[47] Toxicology and forensic medicine could not have emerged without the modernization of pharmacy. Protective government control of the medications consumed by the public thus paralleled the rise of scientific pharmacy and the demise of the traditional apothecary. We shall now see how the medical revolution affected a special kind of citizen, the indigent pregnant woman, and attempted to bring about her evolution into a citizen-patient.

Midwives for a Safe Delivery

Indigent women who entered the lying-in section of the Paris Hôtel-Dieu when the time for the birth of their child approached had long received the attention of an excellent midwife. But immediately after birth, mother and child were returned to the polluted, overcrowded general wards, where five out of every nine patients died. The Revolutionary decade brought dramatic improvements in this situation for the midwife, the Hôtel-Dieu, mother and child.[48]

Poor women trusted the midwife, the "*sage-femme*" and her traditional practical wisdom, and the head midwife at the Hôtel-Dieu of Paris held an honored position, handed down from one generation to another within the same family. Marie Louise Lachapelle (1769–1821), the incumbent during our era, followed her mother and grandmother in that post.[49] She trained four apprentices at a time. Usually

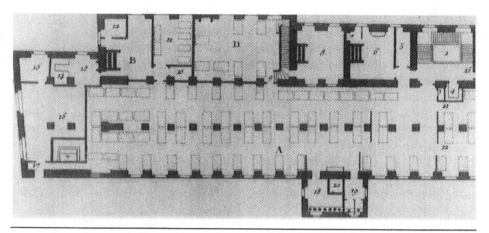

FIGURE 4.5. The lying-in service at the Hôtel-Dieu, left bank, second floor, southeast corner. A: ward for pregnant and postpartum women. B: delivery room. D: ward for nursing mothers. 1: staircase. 6, 8, 15: head nurses' offices. 11: apprentice midwives' dormitory. 12: apprentice midwives' dining room. 13–14: head midwife's apartment. 16: chapel and sacristy, for baptism, 18, 19: toilets. From Jacques Tenon, *Mémoires sur les hôpitaux de Paris* (Paris: Pierres, 1788), pl. 9.

they came from the provinces and stayed a short three or four months. Sharing a small dormitory next to the delivery room, they ate in a small special dining room overlooking the rue de la Bûcherie. Training was intensive; they watched their teacher perform an average of six deliveries a day. Eventually they were allowed to assist, then to attempt complex maneuvers such as podalic versions to correct the position of the child in the womb under the eye of their tutor.

The debate over the relative competence of midwives and surgeons to deliver babies barely touched the poor, who may not even have known that the medical profession scorned midwives as ignorant, stubborn, and inclined to call the surgeon when it was too late. Some critics, on the other hand, accused surgeons of unjustified eagerness to perform risky interventions such as cesarean sections, which usually proved fatal. According to Tenon, seventy-nine such procedures had been performed successfully at the Paris Hôtel-Dieu since 1500 (by this he apparently means that the baby was saved).[50] The available data suggest that only the hospitalized poor were subjected to this "heroic" measure. On the other hand, the forceps was evidently popular among wealthier women.[51] Surgeons argued that midwives had no right to use this instrument. Madame Lachapelle used it rarely and, when she did, always showed it to the woman and explained its use and her manipulations.[52]

Parturient women lay at the center of controversy between accoucheurs and midwives with regard not only to surgical interventions but to the important issue of student training. Madame Lachapelle argued for the continued exclusion of young doctors from the labor room, and even from the whole maternity service, so as to ensure decency. Helping Minister of Internal Affairs Chaptal write the ground rules for the new midwifery school of Port-Royal in 1802, she argued that a school for both midwives and young accoucheurs would be too large; it would not be proper to instruct men and women together, especially in view of the subject matter; it was unlikely that young surgeons would settle in the countryside, where care for women in childbirth was most needed; women would do so, and be content with the low pay; women apprentices needed the government scholarships available at the new school, whereas young doctors did not. Chaptal surrendered.

The private practices of surgeons were thus the scant remaining source of instruction for would-be obstetricians,[53] but medical students found a legal way of gaining obstetrical experience by paying indigent women to give birth in private anatomy "amphitheaters." The Hospital Council disliked this practice but lacked means of stopping it. Camus wrote in 1803: "These births in the amphitheaters deserve the government's attention. Under the supervision of a skillful and prudent master, the women's lives and decency are doubtless respected; but are we equally guaranteed such precautions in all the amphitheaters of Paris?"[54] For the moment, attendance at the births in the Hôtel-Dieu remained the midwife's world, a world that was transformed, at least in Paris, by the transfer of the lying-in section of the Hôtel-Dieu to a large and healthful establishment on the southern edge of the capital. By the end of the Revolutionary decade, poor parturient patients would receive the best care available at the time, which meant a better chance for the survival of mother and child.

The first attempted transfer, in the summer of 1795, was a fumble. It aimed at the transformation of the Val-de-Grâce monastery into a lying-in hospital.[55] Eventually the newborns, wet nurses, pregnant women, and midwives moved instead to the nearby Oratory and Port-Royal monasteries.[56] The latter—it had previously been a prison under the Revolutionary name of "Port-libre"—was gradually adapted to its new purpose as foundlings' hospice (hospice d'allaitement).[57] Yet a disgruntled employee described "a labyrinth of small, dark, and stuffy rooms, the largest of which were to house six wet nurses and twelve infants in a miasmatic atmosphere. In the infirmary the largest room held five beds. The pregnant women's dormitory, in

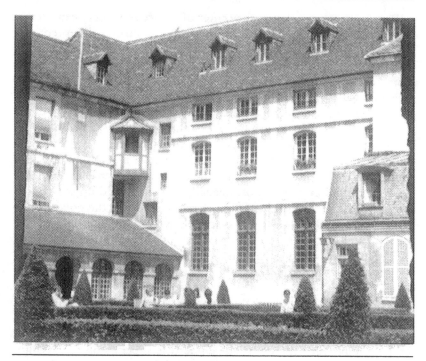

FIGURE 4.6. The maternity hospice of Port-Royal, old cloister and chapter house. Photograph by the author.

the former chapter hall on the ground floor, contained forty beds: it was somber and dank." [58]

In contrast, the transformation of the Oratory into a lying-in hospital (*hospice d'accouchement*) is one of the most impressive changes studied in this book. The twenty-eight-year-old Madame Lachapelle guided Viel, the architect, in providing the Oratory with dormitories for women before and after delivery, for midwifery students, and for domestics; a lecture hall; a well-appointed delivery room with a slightly tilted, tiled floor to facilitate cleaning and a large stove; several infirmaries; apartments for the head midwife and for the administrator. A visitor can still see that Viel added a floor supported by "a new type of girder" to divide the lofty structure horizontally, creating a refectory and amphitheater downstairs and an infirmary upstairs. [59]

"In comparison with the old maternity wards at the Hôtel-Dieu, the Oratory was a palace," writes Dupoux. [60] The innovators undertook "the purposeful demolition of old structures, amassed without order, neither solid nor in good taste, and harmful to the hospital service." [61] The renovations were accomplished between 1 August

1796 and 9 December 1797, no mean feat if one remembers the disorganized state of the Directory's politics and finances. But even in the new surroundings, Madame Lachapelle was guided by her mother: "The rules of the old Hôtel-Dieu regulated the new maternity services: the only difference were the new accommodations."[62]

As he watched the lying-in hospital prosper, Minister of Internal Affairs Chaptal was planning the next step: a national midwifery school to provide poor citizens in the provinces with skills honed in Paris.[63] The school opened its doors in 1802 at the Oratory, providing for a six-month course of study,[64] which included not only the theory and practice of deliveries, phlebotomy, and vaccination, but the study of anatomy, physiology, obstetrics, and medicinal plants. The professor of obstetrics, Jean Louis Baudelocque (1746–1810), and his successor Antoine Dubois (1756–1837) volunteered their services twice a week. For Baudelocque, who had even written a special textbook for his women students, this course was the continuation of many years of teaching obstetrics.[65] To facilitate learning, particularly for peasant women, "nothing can replace mannequins," he commented. "Some people may have praised these with too much enthusiasm, but they are neither well enough known nor sufficiently appreciated."[66] Madame Lachapelle always used them in the classroom.

The midwives' teachers also included Charles Francois Andry (1741–1829), who had joined the staff of the Foundlings' Hospice in 1785 and taught midwives at the medical faculty since 1788. In 1804 he was replaced by François Chaussier (1746–1828), who used some two hundred plants, most of them grown in the Oratory's herb garden. He required that the students write detailed case histories, even of autopsies, and he taught them pathology, including that of puerperal fever. "For fifteen to twenty generations of students, he was a respected teacher and sometimes their sponsor."[67] Camus argued for an amphitheater for lecture-demonstrations; this was eventually built, in 1808–1809, in the Oratory's former chapel.[68] The midwives practiced bloodletting and vaccination under the supervision of the resident intern.[69]

The decree of 30 June 1802 formalized the students' daily obligations to the patients, hitherto regulated by tradition.[70] Each mother and child was served by one student (art. 19) relayed at night after four hours' duty (art. 22). Tenon had recommended this short timespan so as to assure alertness. The students kept notes for the obstetrician and general practitioner who made daily rounds in the morning (art. 23).

The historian A. Delacoux tells us that Madame Lachapelle preferred to assist in childbirth passively rather than intervene. "She taught first of all the art of observation, in order to help students rec-

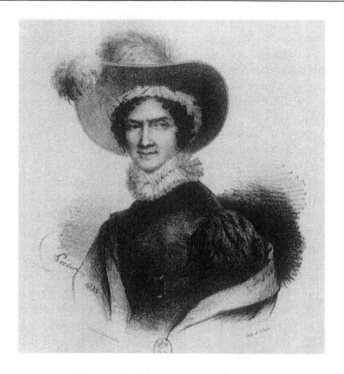

FIGURE 4.7. Marie Louise Lachapelle (née Dugès) (1769–1821). Académie nationale de médecine, Paris.

ognize the configuration, direction, and aim of nature's purpose; the cases where one must be content to wait, or assist natural developments; the cases where one must intervene and change conditions into more favorable ones: these triple indications that the practitioner of obstetrics must always have in mind."[71] After a difficult delivery, and once mother and child were comfortable and safe, she would assemble the students in the amphitheater and discuss the case.[72] Delacoux comments that she was aware of the psychological implications of childbirth. "Before carrying out a procedure, she was always careful to inform the woman of the need and advantage of the intervention, so as to lessen her fears and agitation."[73] She did not like to use instruments or to hurry a woman's labor.[74]

She was evidently not only a gifted teacher but a good administrator. It must have been a high point in her life, at the first commencement exercises, on 13 December 1803, to assemble all the men who had made the lying-in hospital and national midwifery school possible. Chaptal, Dean Thouret, and three other members of the Hospital Council (J. A. Mourgue, Benjamin Delessert, and Louis François Alhoy) attended the festivities, as did the three physicians of the Maternité and Antoine Dubois as commissioner from the medical faculty.[75] Forty-six midwives graduated that day.

The regulations Madame Lachapelle instituted were so farsighted that as late as 1886, the director, Bouilly, noted in his commencement speech that few changes had been introduced in eighty years.[76] And even Florence Nightingale expressed admiration, praising the well-planned details.[77] The midwifery school had become a model throughout Europe. It experienced considerable growth during the Empire (see Appendix C, Table C.1), and by 1814, 1,205 midwives had graduated.[78] But dormitories, infirmaries, and classrooms remained exiguous,[79] admissions subsequently declined, and only seven new students applied in 1845.

Why? The hope that the midwifery school would be self-supporting turned out to be an illusion. Few students could afford tuition and board of 240 francs for six months: in ten years, only fifty-eight paid their own way.[80] It was widely believed that provincial women shied away from the expense, loneliness, and presumed depravity of the capital; they lacked basic education; they knew that provincial customers mistrusted midwives trained in Paris. But the most serious problem was of the government's own making: the Law of 10 March 1803 mandated free midwifery courses "in the busiest hospice of each department," thus echoing the Poverty Committee's recommendations of 1791.[81] The graduates were to receive a "certificate of competency" to practice midwifery in their department. The procedure resembled the registry of health officers, with the same purpose: to make sure these well-trained personnel returned to the provinces, there to help lower the incidence of morbidity and mortality. Yet in direct conflict with the 1803 decree, successive ministers of internal affairs urged the prefects to promote the Paris school over provincial ones,[82] scorning "those small and inadequate institutions" of provincial towns.[83] This contradictory propaganda left provincial women confused, and upheaval at the Paris school added to their misgivings.

Was it urban renewal or the politics of religion that led the Hospital Council, in 1814, to relocate the entire maternity service in Port-Royal and the Foundlings' Hospice in the Oratory? The year 1812 had seen the opening of the avenue de l'Observatoire, a broad, tree-lined street connecting the observatory, via elegant gardens, to the Luxembourg palace. A wide new north-south thoroughfare now separated Port-Royal from the lying-in service at the Oratory. "It is a long way, outside the walls of the establishment, to get from one section to the other," wrote J. P. G. Camet de la Bonnardière (1769–1842), the member of the Hospital Council then responsible for Port-Royal, to the police prefect on 10 October 1812.[84] An unsafe distance for a woman in labor.

Yet it was the sisters' return on 1 October 1814, at the time of the first Restoration, that brought this situation to a head. When resuming control, they insisted on a total separation of the Maternity Hospice and the Foundlings' Hospice, so that innocent babies would again be segregated from their sinful mothers. The sisters' theology shattered the administrator Bernard Hombron's humane vision of women in the ninth month of pregnancy caring for newborns who might motivate them to keep and breast-feed their own offspring.

A total reorganization of the establishment now took place. The Hospital Council decided that Port-Royal had plentiful space for lying-in wards, infirmaries, and the midwifery school, while the Oratory would be appropriate as a foundlings' hospice. Its new auditorium could be used for pediatric teaching and the buildings could accommodate a well-baby clinic and a pediatric infirmary. The vast grounds afforded room for a stable to keep goats. (Eventually asses' milk became popular, and the "Pavillon des ânesses" has only recently been demolished.) A remote structure would house the peasant wet nurses coming to collect their foster children. Significantly, the Foundlings' Home was now christened "Hospice St. Vincent de Paul," with the later addition of "Hôpital-hospice des enfants assistés," its present name.

The separation into two establishments entailed painful dismissals. Hucherard stayed on as director of the Foundlings' Hospice only, to organize the orderly traffic of drivers, wet nurses, and infants. He was told that "the Hospital Council decided on 9 September [1814] that in establishments staffed by sisters there was no need for an administrator: the superiors will fulfill these functions."[85] The spoils system claimed its toll. Thirty-three Sisters of Charity took over nursing care at the lying-in hospital, and twenty seized the reins of internal administration, as well as care of the foundlings. Only the national midwifery school at Port-Royal retained its autonomy, since it reported directly to the minister of internal affairs. The pay scale of the Maternity Hospice staff appears to have remained stable (see Table 4.1). But in infant care, as in nursing, the embattled Catholic religion made a comeback: this meant that citizen-patients again found nurses at their bedsides in the habits familiar since childhood. While this may have been reassuring, another development proved unsettling for the patients: they were unprepared for the large number of medical students who soon crowded around them in the wards.

TABLE 4.1. Pay-Scale, Maternity Hospice Staff, 1806–1815
(in francs)

Obstetrician (Baudelocque)	3,000
Physician (Chaussier)	2,000
Surgeon (Auvity)	1,500
Chief midwife (Madame Lachapelle)	1,500[a]
Pharmacist (in 1806, Nicole)	700[b]
Intern (in 1806, Dufort)	500[b]
Extern	500

SOURCES: Archives de la Seine, Enfants assistés, dossier 5, untitled six-page folio table (internal evidence suggests the year 1806), and ibid., dossier 3, "Project de fixation des traitements . . . pour l'année 1815."
NOTE: In 1815 the doctor was still more highly valued than the surgeon, and the pharmacist than the intern. Madame Lachapelle's salary reflects her importance and the high esteem she enjoyed. All the other supervisory nurses, including the experienced and learned Madame Boivin, received a meagre 350 francs; the domestics lived out and were paid 100 francs.
[a] Plus room and board.
[b] Plus room, but not meals.

Students in the Sick Ward, Medics to the Front

It was in the teaching ward that patients experienced significant tests as citizens. They were now called upon to participate in teaching students how to become physicians. They were asked to exert their minds and express their personalities in helping to create case histories, and they were made to lend their bodies to students and doctors for frequent and detailed examination and probing. How willingly they performed this role, we do not know. Whether they were handled with gentleness or brutality depended on the individual doctors, who ranged from the humane Pinel to the pontificating Alibert and the inconsiderate Dupuytren. All contemporary doctors assumed that, in exchange for the best care, charity patients should serve clinical teaching. As citizens this was their duty. And unless their families objected, their cadavers would undergo dissection. The unprecedented influx of students, for whom the new clinical teaching services held a strong fascination, meant that many hundreds of citizen-patients now underwent examination, and anatomo-pathologic procedures at eventual autopsy.

Medical students flocked to Paris after the Law of 4 December 1794 created the new Health School. The law rescinded all tuition payments, mandated instruction in French, and even provided scholarships for the training of 550 "national scholars" each year.[86] The medical leaders immediately set up juries to select candidates so that the first semester could begin by the end of March 1794.[87] The criteria for selection included a loyalty oath, and the committee was to give preference "to the candidate capable of clear thought, quick and accurate judgment, keen analytic observation, who is able to understand, at a glance, the relationship of complex facts and to draw valid conclusions, who is filled with dedication to science and eager to devote himself unreservedly to his medical studies."[88] The tone and the avowed goals of these governmental instructions are disturbing if one reads them with the patient in mind. Patriotism seems an odd qualifications for a physician, and while intellectual excellence is an essential criterion for becoming a doctor, compassion or eagerness to serve the patient would seem equally important. The official literature did not mention such traits, despite their importance to the hospitalized citizen.

Medical students reached Paris in numbers far exceeding anyone's expectations. From 900 in 1798, their numbers rose to 1,200 two years later and peaked at 3,371 in 1812. An acute shortage of student housing soon developed, as did problems with the students' subsistence and the organization of clinical teaching.[89] Dean Thouret feared that life in Paris under such conditions might bewilder young provincials, and he therefore requested that Parisians offer them housing and help. The students would be financially responsible, argued the dean, since the nation was awarding them a subsidy. However, that sum was so meager and food so scarce that some students subsequently went home.[90] But many retained their wish to be doctors and, since the law proclaimed freedom to practice, they swarmed over the countryside and learned their trade while treating the peasantry. Thus patients in the provinces were at the mercy of quacks and charlatans until the law of 1803 regulated the practice of medicine.[91]

Even though attrition among students in Paris was severe, and the graduating classes numbered less than one fourth the original registered, the Health School, the hospitals, and the patients were overwhelmed by the numbers. No existing amphitheater could hold throngs such as the 876 young men registered for Chaussier's anatomy and physiology course in the summer of 1799, or the 763 wishing to study chemistry with Fourcroy.[92] In the clinical wards, the crowding was even worse. The reformers knew that Desault had accommodated several hundred students at the Hôtel-Dieu in the 1780s. The thousands who arrived required immediate makeshift arrangements, and these, as so often happens, soon solidified into permanent patterns. They put hurdles between student and patient.

For the hospitalized patient, the increasingly structured experience in the official teaching wards was a blessing because it limited questioning and physical scrutiny to the chosen few. New amphitheaters transformed would-be participants into spectators of examinations, of surgical procedures, and of postmortem dissections conducted by professors. Hierarchies of first-, second-, and third-year students, externs, interns, and clinical chiefs rotated through the wards in orderly fashion. But money soon intervened again to pay for clinical instruction: while the law designated only the Hôtel-Dieu and the Charité as teaching hospitals, clinicians offered instruction at the Salpêtrière, St. Louis, the Maternité, the Childrens' Hospital, Necker, and others. These were called "private" clinics and required a modest payment.[93]

Patients were nevertheless often exposed to considerable commotion, particularly at the Hôtel-Dieu, the largest teaching hospital. The nurses had seen this coming, as we know from the prioress' protest in 1788 when she warned that

> the constant presence of the young surgeons . . . is infinitely dangerous, especially in women's wards. . . . Since these young men have been admitted, the Hôtel-Dieu is unrecognizable: our refuges of rest, silence, and calm now echo with loud voices, threats, and sometimes ribald remarks. . . . In former times . . . a young surgeon would never have dared pass by a sister without a deferential greeting: nowadays he keeps his hat on, hums a tune, and feels pleased if he hasn't mocked or insulted her. When a head nurse used to speak in the ward, all listened in silence. . . . the very veil of the approaching sister would calm a dispute. . . . But now that the new rules have promised control to the young surgeons, the accustomed veneration is gone.[94]

Would the jaunty young doctor who slighted the nurse treat the charity patient with respect? The crowded conditions alone made this unlikely. But the relationship of doctors to a significant part of the population changed with the outbreak of war in 1792, warfare that never stopped until 1815.

In 1792, fourteen hundred physicians and surgeons joined the army, and by the end of 1793 six hundred of them were dead. With "the fatherland in danger" because of foreign invasion, the doctor draft law of 7 August 1793 made all young medical men—even barely trained ones—liable to military service. The surgeon-in-chief of the Rhine army, Pierre François Percy (1754–1825), "found the surgeons untrained, weak, easily homesick, and susceptible to typhus and dysentery," so he sent them "to complete their apprenticeships on the battlefield."[95] And that experience, as we shall see in the last chapter of this book, changed their outlook, their attitude, and their medical approach to the citizen-patient, now a sick or dying soldier.

◆◆◆

We have now surveyed the women and men who cared for indigent patients, the nurses, pharmacists, midwives, and students, and seen how their professions evolved from old regime to Revolutionary conditions. The political and moral purpose of the Constituent Assembly to transform objects of charity into citizen-patients was slow to take hold.

The Catholic nursing orders rejected the political message of the Revolution, convinced that their thousand-year-old tradition stood for higher values than the young republic. Progress was made in pharmacy because it could build on an established popular practice of self-medication, and thus a pharmacopoeia in clear and simple French could help patients improve home remedies, hygiene, and health maintenance. Midwifery yielded results for the parturient women patients, whose chances for a normal delivery were enhanced by clean and friendly surroundings and good postpartum care. But what did they learn from the experience? The proportion of women who took their baby home rose but slightly at Port-Royal and we do not know whether the same persons returned later, abandoning more babies to public care.

For medical students the most significant experience with citizen-patients still lay in the future, for it consisted in contacts with thousands of sick soldiers, in Europe, the Near East, and Central America during the Revolutionary and Napoleonic wars. The sick soldiers benefited most from the military doctors' training in surgical techniques and from their familiarity with postoperative wound management and hygiene, since that knowledge could readily be shared with a citizen-patient striving for his own recovery.

Having surveyed the caring professions, we now turn to the world of hospital administration and politics to find out how it viewed and channeled the chances of the poor to turn into citizen-patients.

III

INSTITUTIONS:

The Citizen-Patient and

the Hospital

The Outpatient:
The Strategy of Medical Administrators

Among persons of goodwill . . . there exists a sort of league to prevent the poor from entering [the Hôtel-Dieu]. Any refuge that can replace it is considered a blessing.
    Jacques Tenon, *Mémoires sur les hôpitaux de Paris,* 1788

As we have seen, the transition from the neglect of patients toward attention to their daily medical needs and creature comforts was essentially in the hands of the nurses, midwives, pharmacists, and students. But change would not have come about without the guidance of the Paris hospital administrators and councillors. The administrators, the unsung heroes of this story, were women and men who dedicated their careers to a group of unfortunates, often living among them from the old regime to the Napoleonic era or beyond. They attempted to salvage lives, promote education and training, propel the ailing or recuperating citizen toward independence from public welfare. The hospital councillors joined in the effort. These advocates of the citizen–patient often clashed with medical investigators who made demands on the patients that appeared unwarranted to the reformers.

We shall see that the distressing and confused situation of the hospitals during the Revolutionary decade yielded permanent compromise through administrative solutions. The Hospital Council of the Seine developed a coherent policy and amalgamated traditional practices with creative innovation to keep the citizen–patient *out of* the hospital.

The Crucial Role of Hospital Administrators

The administrators of Paris health care institutions were a group of little-known midwives, religious women and men, physicians, and laypersons.[1] It is difficult to ferret out information about the women

133

in this group. The exceptions are the midwife Marie Dugès and her daughter Marie Louise Lachapelle, and the daughter's rival, Marie Anne Victoire Boivin. Madame Lachapelle stands out as a leader able to harness the energies of the Paris hospital commission during the Directory and to supervise the transfer of the midwifery service from the dangerous Hôtel-Dieu to a healthy setting. The mores of the times did not allow for her membership in committees, but Tenon and Chaptal heeded her opinions, and Dubois, Andry, Auvity, and Chaussier taught at her school. Another woman whose name assured attention was Madame Necker, foundress of the model hospital in pre-Revolutionary Paris.

In contrast to these women, the nuns in executive positions sought and achieved anonymity. The documents rarely mention the fact that the Augustinians of the Hôtel-Dieu not only staffed but administered a hospital for two to three thousand patients, nor do they mention the names of the Sisters of Charity who headed Paris hospitals: Sisters Cassegrain, Braujon, and Clavelot ran Necker Hospital after the foundress's departure; Sister Michelle Michelon headed the Hôtel-Dieu at St. Denis; and Sister Rose Maupetit managed the Beaujon orphanage, which the Revolution transformed into a hospital. Moreover, the *soeurs officières* at Bicêtre and the Salpêtrière were responsible for huge establishments with several thousand inmates each.

The men in this group of administrators include some physicians, such as Dr. Paul Seignette (17 ?–1835), whose energetic initiatives saved the blind children at the Quinze-Vingts Hospice from total demoralization. Among laymen, Bernard Hombron (ca. 1740–1808) stands out for his lifelong dedication to bettering the lot of the babies abandoned in Paris. He began his career as assistant clerk at the Foundlings' Hospice in 1755 and retired as chief administrator of the Maternité Hospice in 1803. For years he advocated the creation of an establishment where single women in the ninth month of pregnancy would care for newborns, thus arousing their eagerness to nurse and keep their own offspring. That vision bore fruit at the Maternity Hospice of Port-Royal, at least for a decade.

Several other men spent their lives administering custodial establishments. The most unusual was Jean Baptiste Pussin (1745–1811), who headed the section for insane men at Bicêtre Hospice in the 1780s and 1790s. His strict, knowledgeable, and humane methods impressed the Poverty Committee site visitors. No less able was his wife, Marguerite Jubline, a coin cutter at the Paris mint and Pussin's assistant.[2] One should also mention M. de Sevelinges, the obscure, but energetic and well-connected, head of the apprenticeship program for orphans, who was able to place hundreds of youngsters in workshops and trades.

Among the five commissioners who served the Hospital Council, two seem remarkable: Louis François Alhoy (1755–1826) acted for several years as assistant headmaster of the National Institution for the Deaf-Mute. Together with the headmaster of the blind, Valentin Haüy, Alhoy submitted to the Council of 500 an ingenious plan for a national tax to finance aid to the handicapped. He later became a trustee of the National Welfare Establishments and wrote a charming book of wretched verse, *Promenades poétiques dans les hospices et hôpitaux de Paris,* dedicated to Chaptal.[3] The other outstanding member of the commission was Dr. Claude François Duchanoy (1742–1827) co-author of a widely known essay on clinical teaching in 1778, author of a project on hospital internships and co-originator of the central pharmacy. He died as dean of the Paris Health School.[4] Thus the Paris health care network was in the hands of women and men administrators who supervised the lives and comforts of the institutionalized sick, ailing, and impaired Parisians. The pattern of that network was elaborated gradually after the Revolution, as a result of a protracted struggle for power in health politics that resulted in a national policy.

Toward a National Hospital Policy

From 1791 to 1796, the cumulative effect of piecemeal legislation created a permanent pattern for hospital administration, first in Paris, then in the provinces. In the end, there developed a compromise that permitted the hospitals to tap local volunteer activity as well as local and national sources of revenue. This compromise inadvertently established two legislative principles, argues the legal expert Jean Imbert.[5] On the one hand, the decree of 25 May 1791 placed the nation's hospitals among the responsibilities of the minister of internal affairs: he stepped into the role of "protector" that had traditionally been filled by the grand almoner. On the other hand, the decree of 25 July 1791 granted the hospitals government subsidies that the communities eventually had to reimburse. Thus the municipalities retained the ultimate financial responsibility for their own hospitals, but the national government ensured their survival. The Law of 7 October 1796, which was fundamental to hospital legislation in France, eventually embedded these principles:

Law on Hospital Administration, 7 October 1796 (16 Vendémiaire, Year V)

Article 1: Municipal administrations shall have the immediate supervision of the civilian hospitals in their *arrondissement*. They shall appoint a commission of five citizens resident in the canton, who shall elect a president from among their number and choose a secretary.

Article 2: In communes where there is more than one municipal administration, this [hospital] commission shall be appointed by the departmental commission.

Article 3: Each commission shall appoint an independent treasurer, who shall report to it each quarter. The commission shall transmit this account to the municipal administration who shall send it, within the *décade* and with its comments, to the central administration of the department for approval, if warranted.

No one foresaw such a compromise in 1789. Imbert asserts that by merely doling out aid, the Legislative Assembly helped the citizen-patient more effectively than the Poverty Committee, whose grand projects were not implemented at the time.[6] In contrast, the Jacobins authorized the sale of hospital property on 11 July 1794 (23 Messidor, Year II) to finance aid to the poor. Substantial real estate holdings were auctioned off until the Convention revoked the measure on 24 October 1795 (2 Brumaire, Year IV), two days before it disbanded.[7] These sales caused hospitals and patients acute distress, yet "no one in the assembly protested against this total spoliation of the charitable patrimony: hastily decreed, under the pressure of war needs, this decision corresponded . . . to the deep convictions of the nation's representatives."[8] The Jacobins were steering France toward a national pattern of hospital administration.

Meanwhile the patients reverted to the status of ailing paupers and the Jacobins adjudged aid on the basis of need, just as the Church had done. Ignoring the Poverty Committee's painstaking analyses, the government again lumped health problems with its enormous load of welfare obligations. Officials doled out an endless stream of funds to beggars, invalids, the deaf-mute and blind, abandoned children, and the victims of fires and natural disasters. The confiscated hospital property financed the Jacobins' largesse. The Convention's approach was thus a step backward, but it led to a pattern that still prevails.

The Convention raised the Relief Committee's funds to twenty million a year, but even the sale of hospital property did not suffice. Eventually the Directory reverted to the ancient principle that the pleasures and gourmandise of the rich should be taxed to relieve the suffering of the poor. On 26 July 1797 (8 Thermidor, Year V), it reinstated a 10 percent amusement tax on theaters, balls, fireworks, concerts, and horse races, using the revenue to finance home care. On 18 October 1798 (27 Vendémiaire, Year VII), the Directory reintroduced the municipal toll (*octroi*), a levy on goods entering Paris and used it once again to finance the hospitals.

In administration as in funding, centralization counterbalanced local power. The reestablishment of the Ministry of Internal Affairs on 2 October 1795 (10 Vendémiaire, Year IV) facilitated the task, particularly owing to initiatives by two early ministers, Pierre Bénézech (1775–1802) and Nicolas Louis François de Neufchâteau (1750–1828). They worked out a compromise according to which the Law of 7 October 1796 (16 Vendémiaire, Year V) gave the municipalities the right to appoint their own hospital trustees; on the other hand, it was not long before the decree of 4 July 1799 (16 Messidor, Year VII) ordered that all nominations to or revocations of membership on hospital councils in towns of over 100,000 inhabitants be sanctioned by the prefect and ultimately the minister. In this permanent arrangement central control counterbalanced municipal contributions of talent, work, and funds.

The quest for power in health politics was protracted. In the troubled summer of 1789, the boards of trustees of the Hôtel-Dieu of Paris and of the General Hospital had tried in vain to resign. The Paris Commune prevailed upon them to continue their services until 15 April 1791, when they gave up their stewardship. By then, the Commune had created eight administrative subdivisions. The sixth of these was the Department of Hospitals and Workshops, under the distinguished physician and botanist Antoine Laurent de Jussieu as deputy mayor. The Commune now claimed the administration of its own hospitals. But a law gave the department of Paris jurisdiction over "public establishments," and these included "education, religion, and welfare."[9] The department therefore appointed a hospital committee of five: the incumbents changed frequently, as Table 5.1 indicates. Its most distinguished and relatively long-lived members were the abbé de Montlinot and Michel Augustin Thouret, colleagues in the Poverty Committee and already expert in hospital affairs; Georges Cabanis; and the mathematician J. A. J. Cousin (1739–1800), a member of the Academy of Sciences.

Thus Paris had two hospital authorities for a while. But the departmental committee controlled the situation, leaving to the municipality nothing but "the servile execution of tedious and irksome detail," Jussieu complained.[10] After the insurrection of 10 August 1792 that spelled the end of the monarchy, Jussieu's subdivision "disbanded spontaneously."[11] From then on, a committee headed by Thouret and

TABLE 5.1. The Evolution of the Paris Hospital Commission, 1791–1801

15 April 1791: Board of trustees of Hôtel-Dieu and General Hospital resigns. Department appoints:				
Cousin	Delachaume	Lecamus	Montlinot	Aubry-Dumesnil
10 August 1792: Monarchy falls. Department loses power.				
13 August 1792: Paris Commune appoints:				
Thouret	Delachaume	Cabanis	Montlinot	Chambon de Montaux and de Jussieu
31 Dec. 1792: "	Levavasseur	"	"	Lecamus
9 Sept. 1793: Cousin	"	"	Daujon	Magendy
9th Thermidor, Year II (27 July 1794): Fall of Robespierre. Paris municipal administration disbanded. Department of Paris appoints hitherto unknown men:				
Lemit		Reverdy		Concedieu
3 October 1794 [12 Vendémiaire, Year III]: "Thermidorian Reaction" takes hold. Minister of internal affairs appoints:				
Thouret		Cousin		Cabanis
7 October 1796, Law of 16 Vendémiaire, Year V: Minister of internal affairs appoints committee of 5 (35 different incumbents from 1796 to 1801).				
January 1801: Minister of Internal Affairs Chaptal and Prefect of the Seine Frochot create General Administrative Hospital Council of the Seine Department and transform the former hospital committee into a salaried commission of 5:				
Alhoy	Duchanoy	Le Maignan	Fesquet	Desportes

SOURCE: Adapted from Archives de l'Assistance publique, Catalogue Fosseyeux, n.s., dossier 17.

Cousin administered hospital affairs in the Seine Department. The membership changed so often that the five seats had thirty-five occupants between 1796 and 1800, and, remarks one observer, "the administrators were there a shorter time than the patients."[12] It was this Parisian model of a five-member administrative committee that the Law of 7 October 1796 applied to the provinces.

As happens so often in France, what looks like drastic reorganization camouflaged unwavering stability. With the reestablishment of the ministries, "welfare and hospitals" became part of the second division in the Ministry of Internal Affairs. One finds the documents signed by familiar staffers: Levéville, the long-time registrar at the Hôtel-Dieu; Guérin, the experienced treasurer of the Hôpital Général; Derniau; Anson; Maison; Levasseur. The same professionals advised them: the notary Girard, the legal counsel Leroux, the appraiser Bertrand.[13] These men had survived the Terror by lying low, and their experience made them indispensable. Their presence presaged a revival of past administrative practices during the Thermidorian Reaction, to be perpetuated under the Consulate and Empire. They helped build the bridge from the old regime to the nineteenth century.[14]

The Paris Hospital Council

The men who now forged the new health care structure were partly reform-minded professionals of the pre-Revolutionary Enlightenment like Parmentier, Deyeux, Hallé, and Cadet de Vaux. But the Revolution also opened fresh careers for talented men like Chaptal, Pinel, and the prefect of the Seine Department, Nicolas Frochot (1761–1828). Some of the leaders had even navigated through the whole Revolutionary decade manning important posts—for example, Thouret and Fourcroy. All now collaborated to organize health care for the poor.

The planning and implementation of this work benefited remarkably from the guidance of Chaptal and the support of Frochot. The latter was the friend and executor of Mirabeau—a connection that endangered his life during the Terror.[15] Installed on 22 March 1800, Frochot assumed responsibility for the administration of health care in the Seine Department.

Frochot says he found a chaotic situation, with demand for hospital admission rising at a time when the persecution of nurses had decimated staffs and the doctor draft had sent physicians into battle. The temporary abolition of the medical faculties from 18 August 1793 to 4 December 1794 had interrupted the supply of educated doctors, swamping France with ill-trained or self-taught empirics. The hospi-

TABLE 5.2. Assignments of Paris Hospital Commission and Council Members,
Early Nineteenth Century

Hospital Council		Hospital Commission
Richard d'Aubigny	ᵇSALPÊTRIÈRE	Desportes
Parmentier	ᵇMENAGES	Lemaignan
	ᵃCHARITÉ (Medicine)	Lemaignan
	ᵃCHARITÉ (Surgery)	Lemaignan
Thouret	ᵃHÔTEL-DIEU	Alhoy
	ᵈVACCINATION OFFICE	[special committee]
Camus	ᵃBEAUJON	Desportes
	ᵇPORT-ROYAL (Maternity)	Alhoy
	ᶜPORT-ROYAL (Foundlings)	Alhoy
d'Aguesseau	ᶜMONTROUGE	Alhoy
Mourgues	ᵃSAINT-LOUIS	Fesquet
	ᶜFAUBOURG ST. MARTIN	Fesquet
	ᵇINCURABLE MEN	Fesquet

SOURCES: N. E. Clavareau, *Mémoires sur les hôpitaux civils de Paris* (Paris: Prault, 1805),
31–32; Seine, CGAHHCP, *Rapports au conseil général des hospices sur les hôpitaux et hospices,
les secours à domicile, et la direction des nourrices* (Paris: Imprimerie des hospices civils, An XI
[1803]), 19–20.

NOTE: Each councilor was responsible for at least one hospital and a hospice or nursing
home. The only specialists were Dean Thouret, the educator, and Delessert, the financier
(although he was responsible for two hospitals). Specialization was more pronounced

tals had been impoverished by the sale of their property, and even
though the law promised compensation, the money could not be put
to use in the purchase of alternative premises, because appropriate real
estate proved hard to find. Frochot thus had reason to worry. But he
disentangled the endowments, revenues, and debts of the hospitals
from those of the city, emerging with the conviction that he could
balance the hospital budget.[16]

He aimed, however, at reorganizing the entire hospital administration. To this end, he sent Chaptal a plan to revive the spirit of the old
regime, amalgamating efficiency with traditional values. "The present
must heed the advice of the past," wrote Frochot. "In administration,
the best argument is experience. The hospitals need a board made up
of paternal citizens untouched by intrigue or greed, whose worth is
guaranteed by their knowledge, virtue, and probity, and whose salary
consists of esteem, glory and the good they accomplish."[17] The wheel
had come full circle: such men, prosperous citizens whose civic pride

TABLE 5.2.
(continued)

Hospital Council		Hospital Commission
Duquesnoy	[a,b] PITIÉ	Alhoy
	[a] COCHIN	Duchanoy
Pastoret	[a] CHILDREN'S	Lemaignan
	[b] INCURABLE WOMEN	Lemaignan
Fieffé	[c] ST. ANTOINE	Fesquet
	[a] ST. ANTOINE	Fesquet
Bigot de Préameneu	[b] BICÊTRE	Duchanoy
Delessert	[a] NECKER	Lemaignan
	[a] VENEREAL DISEASES	Duchanoy
	[d] Treasury	Fesquet
	[d] Real Estate	Fesquet

among the members of the Hospital Commission, who were professional administrators. Desportes was essentially responsible for the senior citizens, and Fesquet for investments and the treasury. The documents speak of nineteen establishments. St. Antoine Hospital, the twentieth, was opened in 1813.

[a] Hospital	[c] Orphanage, nursing home
[b] Hospice	[d] Other

and experience as businessmen or lawyers stood the hospitals in good stead, had served as trustees of the Hôtel-Dieu and Hôpital général. They watched budgets closely, checked supplies personally, set strict rules for staff and patients, stressing orderliness, frugality, sobriety, honesty, and abstinence. They embodied, as the French put it, a "paternal regime." In fact, their tone of voice, as transmitted in the documents, patronizes the poor and was thus no help in creating the citizen-patient.

Frochot also devised an arrangement that endowed the new hospital administration with instant expertise, while at the same time tying faithful servants of the citizen-patient's interests to the new regime. He suggested to Chaptal that the five-member administrative committee that had been struggling to keep the Paris hospitals afloat now be transformed into a salaried commission, to serve under the new trustees.[18] These men included Alhoy and Duchanoy (whom we met at the beginning of this chapter); Dr. Benjamin Desportes (17 ?–

1840), who was in charge of Bicêtre, the Salpêtrière, and the Incurables; Julien Camille Lemaignan (1746–1812), who was responsible for the Charité and Necker; and Jean Jacques Fesquet (1752–1812), who supervised the real estate. We shall study their strategy and stewardship, after we acquaint ourselves with the members of the Hospital Council.

Frochot proposed politically reliable men for the Hospital Council, a move that pleased Chaptal and their master, Bonaparte. Once informed, the government acted fast and issued the decree of 17 January 1801 (27 Nivôse, Year IX) that created the general administrative council of the civilian hospitals and hospices of the department of the Seine and, within two weeks, named its members. They then established the priorities, elaborated the budget, wrote and enforced the regulations, hired the personnel, appointed the medical and administrative leadership, and provided close supervision. As a group, they set the tone that soon pervaded the Parisian establishments. They added up to a successful mix.

Chaptal named Frochot president of the Paris Hospital Council: perhaps a foregone conclusion, but in any case an excellent choice. By the same token, Chaptal denied the presidency to Frochot's rival, the police prefect Louis Nicolas Dubois (1758–1847), also a member of the council, ex officio. So offended was Dubois that he sulked and never attended. Chaptal took clever advantage of this rivalry: in 1802 he assigned Dubois the chairmanship of the Paris Public Health Council (to be discussed in Chapter 10).

Direct links between the Hospital Council and the official world of medicine and pharmacy would be beneficial, Chaptal and Frochot believed. Hence the appointments of Thouret and Parmentier. The presence of F. J. J. Bigot de Préameneu (1747–1825) meant a direct link to the council of state: he presided over the legislative section that was then elaborating the Civil Code. Two other lawyers joined him: H. C. J. B. d'Aguesseau (1752–1826), president of the court of appeals, and C. E. J. P. Pastoret (1755–1840), a former deputy in the Legislative Assembly and Directory, and author of the Hospital Council report of 1816.[19] Experience in finance explains the choice of J. A. Mourgue (1734–1818) and J. P. B. Delessert (1773–1847), both of them well-known philanthropists. Like Chaptal, Delessert was a successful industrialist and, in contrast to his colleagues, a very wealthy man.[20] Several legislators with a scholarly bent completed the council: A. G. Camus, the archivist who wrote the report of 1803;[21] A. C. Duquesnoy (1759–1808), lawyer, deputy, mayor of the 10th arrondissement, and adviser to Lucien Bonaparte;[22] and E. C. Fieffé (1740–1802), mayor of the 8th arrondissement.[23] We know little about

L. T. Richard d'Aubigny (ca. 1750–1824), a council member almost from the beginning (24 February 1801), who was responsible for the Salpêtrière. The councillors took such pride in their work that most vacancies were owing to deaths; Delessert's membership lasted forty-six years![24]

The councillors could thus draw on collective experience in politics, finance, administration, and law. Several had served together in the legislature during the previous decade, some were ennobled under the empire,[25] and personal wealth permitted them all to serve without pay. Their public spirit, and their commitment to welfare work—or was it old-fashioned Christian charity?—appealed to Bonaparte. He counted on them to keep the poor in their place and the expenditures within reasonable bounds.

The councillors met three times a week at their headquarters on the place du Parvis Notre-Dame. They apportioned the nineteen hospitals and hospices[26] among the eleven men, each one being responsible for the smooth functioning of "his" institution(s). The members of the administrative commission specialized in a comparable manner (see Table 5.2). There ensued a friendly emulation that permitted each councillor to spend on his establishment any savings he effected. "It was a memorable day, that 4th of January 1802, when they took this decision," commented Camus, "all the improvements in hospital affairs derive from this working pattern."[27]

"I owe you information, not advice," Frochot told the councillors in his opening speech, on 24 February 1801—an astute initial gambit from an administrator toward trustees.[28] The finances, Frochot explained, were an impenetrable thicket; they required annual budgets and a firm hand. In patient management, clear guidelines were needed to separate the sick from the destitute. A "convenient and appropriate" admitting office should be installed, to end the trek from one hospital to another . . . against which no precaution has so far been taken." Admission must be "strictly regulated . . . and entrusted to diligent and well-trained men, not, as now, to mere students," and discharge must promptly follow recovery, "to overcome at last that misguided complacency that either prolongs the sickness beyond recovery or . . . transforms certain privileged convalescents into nurses." This "misunderstood pity" must cease.

Not only the patients needed firm guidelines, argued Frochot, but the administrators as well: they still assigned adults and children to the same wards, condoned large beds, tolerated uncleanliness. The medical service needed organizing according to general rules. (Frochot was then putting the finishing touches on the internship program, to be launched in February 1802.) The hospices should install workshops to replace those "cafés and numerous cabarets where presumably penniless people . . . buy wine and liquor, and often present the revolting and scandalous spectacle of drunkenness in a house of charity."[29] The councillors must educate those orphaned or abandoned "national children"(*enfants de la patrie*) whose legal fathers they had now become. In conclusion, Frochot outlined "the need for annual tables of admissions, discharges, and deaths indicating the incidence of morbidity and mortality, a comparison of small and large hospitals, of their size, location, and distribution, and highlighting the danger of contact among patients with diverse diseases . . . a code of instruction and a collection of observations. . . . The science of hospital administration remains to be created in France," he concluded, underlining the well-known fact that abroad, in England and Austria especially, great progress had been made.[30]

Had nothing changed, then, since 1790?

◆◆◆

In fact the situation of the hospitalized patient was better than the councillors expected, as they learned from the general report submitted by the administrative commissionners, the men with the practical experience of running the Paris hospitals under desperate conditions.[31] They had hitherto lacked "money, credit, esteem, and authority," but were surprised to find that hospitals and patients had survived the Revolution comparatively well. "Of all public establishments in Paris," they concluded, "the hospitals and hospices have perhaps been least badly treated, either for humanitarian reasons . . . or because the imperious need of the poor became a law in itself and forced successive governments to find precarious and temporary resources." They had been able to pay off all past debts, including those for layettes and trousseaus, the salaries of the wet nurses, and the huge expenses of the central bakery (100,000 francs per year) and pharmacy (200,000 francs per year). They welcomed the new consular regime, but also acknowledged significant change owing to the Revolution, when "long neglected major improvements emerged from the Revolutionary shock. [The hospitals] profited from the timely possibility of total change, without regard for established usage."[32]

The administrators then outlined the hospitals' problems as they saw them: they judged child abandonment and infant mortality to be the pressing priority, attributing the deaths of abandoned newborns to the dearth of wet nurses. They deplored the large numbers of "national children" whom provincial foster parents returned to Paris at age seven, when the payments stopped. These youngsters might have "repaired the loss of manpower caused by long years of war" in the countryside. The commissioners also condemned the custom of allowing impoverished parents to reclaim and take home children whom they had abandoned, letting the city pay for their upkeep. The commissioners protested against the mixture of inmates at the Pitié Hospice, where orphans from respectable families mingled with delinquent boys, "already practiced crooks, thieves or accomplices." An adequate number of qualified teachers should train the boys in useful skills.

They criticized the long waiting lists for the hospices, where from seven to eight hundred indigents claimed admission: "There are now twice as many unfortunates in this populous city." They called for more, and more effective, outpatient clinics; currently these functioned only at the Hôtel-Dieu, St. Louis, and the Venereal Diseases Hospital. They recommended the revival of those "hospitable asylums" where transients had once obtained three days' food and shelter. Like Frochot, they called for a stricter supervision of patients, the segregation of children from adults, convalescents from the sick, and surgical from acute and chronic patients, and for better case histories and statistics.[33]

Faced with so many urgent and all-too-legitimate demands outlined by the commission, the councillors felt a need for initial agreement on their own principles. This stocktaking serves for the historian as a revealing forecast of hospital policy during the Consulate and Empire and beyond. The council grew more conservative with distance from the Revolution, and with the deaths of Camus in 1804 and Thouret in 1810. True, it aimed at the integration of modern medicine and pharmacy into Parisian hospital life, but it also looked to the past, believing that the spirit of Christian charity must be revived, although without permitting the clergy to dictate patient behavior or the nurses to fashion hospital routine. The council did not mean to revert to the old regime, make Catholic orthodoxy a precondition for medical care, or restore altars to every ward, but wished subtly to indicate to the patient population that Christian values had returned. The decree of 4 June 1802 (15 Prairial, Year X) reestablished Catholic worship and provided hospitals with chaplains. The councillors went about this re-Christianization discreetly; for example they named only four chaplains for the 2,000-bed Hôtel-Dieu of Paris.[34]

A symbolic (and inexpensive) gesture signaled the return to tradition: the restoration of the hospitals' pre-Revolutionary names. Thus, the "Hospice of Humanity" resumed its traditional name of Hôtel-Dieu, and the establishment of the Brothers of Charity its logical appellation of "Charity Hospital." The geographically named "North" and "East" Hospitals reclaimed their patron saints St. Louis and

St. Antoine, while the "Hospice du Roule," "South Hospice," and "West Hospice" again displayed the names of their founders, the philanthropist Beaujon, the abbé Cochin, and Madame Necker. Necker Hospital's chapel, Camus reported in 1803, lately used for storage, had been "returned to its intended purpose; after restoring the foundress' name, the council had it inscribed over the entrance door [where it remains], and Madame Necker's portrait has been placed in the reception hall."[35]

But mainly the councillors aimed their conservative message at potential donors: "That source had by then almost dried up," wrote Camus.[36] A decree of 29 September 1802 (7 Vendémiaire, Year XI) reestablished endowments, but with a restricted right to nominate patients for hospital admission. In the provinces, the local hospital councils resisted the move: they wished to retain their freedom of action.[37] By far the most precious traditional Christian contribution to the hospital had been nursing care. Revolutionary history showed that the world was not ready for a lay nursing profession, whereas the Catholic nuns stood ready to resume their demanding profession. Chaptal, as we have seen, recalled them.

The councillors adopted the priorities proposed by Frochot and thus instructed the hospital commission: fiscal responsibility was crucial. They must establish regular budgets, stay within the limits, retrench if necessary, expand where possible. They would investigate every detail of all the operations in the nineteen institutions under their governance; the commissioners were to provide the council with detailed accounts of hospital censuses, personnel, salaries, expenditures for food, supplies, medication, services, and daily patient costs. The council continued to publish these annual surveys.[38]

Frochot began to stem the tide of hospital admissions when, on 19 April 1801 (29 Germinal, Year IX), he widened the Hospital Council's jurisdiction to include scores of centers and schemes for preventive and supportive aid: the wet-nursing office, the city's forty-eight welfare centers, home care, the financial inspection of the city's pawnshop, the Paris vaccination institute, and the treatment of psychiatric patients at Charenton. But the number of persons thus served did not appreciably relieve the demand for hospital services, and Frochot therefore decided to institute a system of medical triage.

Triage: the Identity of the Outpatient

Keep the citizen-patient out of the hospital! Administrators and patients agreed: the hospital was an overcrowded, dangerous, fever-ridden place, and a drain on the municipal budget. The situation urgently required a triage of applicants. Therefore, on 22 March 1802 (1 Germinal, Year X), a modernized central admitting office manned by two physicians, Biron and Chamseru, and two surgeons, Parfait and Prat, opened near the Paris Hôtel-Dieu.[39] It had been "improved to the utmost," wrote the architect, Nicolas Clavareau, in 1803. (He evidently liked his own renovations.) Before the Revolution, this office "must have contributed a great deal to unfavorable prejudice. . . . The quarters were so dark that a light was needed at all times, even on bright days. One can imagine the drawbacks for the health officer and classification of illnesses." Now, wrote Clavareau, "it is bright, clean, with all services properly housed, a large and well-lit registration desk, an examining room, separate dressing rooms for each sex, a washroom for new arrivals . . . a depository for patients' clothes . . . a superb and vast linen department.[40] Open daily from nine to four o'clock, the office processed 34,915 applicants in the first eighteen months. Of these, it hospitalized 22,589 persons, or 65 percent; offered 9,462 persons, or 27 percent, a variety of outpatient services or referrals; and rejected 2,904, or 8 percent. This led to rumors of hardheartedness, which the Hospital Council denied.[41] In the first eighteen months, the four doctors thus saw an average daily total of seventy-six patients if they worked a six-day week, or a daily case load of some nineteen patients for each doctor.[42]

The admitting officers functioned as a "jury and sentinel," wrote Duchanoy. Their scrutiny was needed because a number of malingerers had long been making the rounds of hospitals, "a species of parasite searching for free food and shelter." The doctors kept lists of these persons who appeared to them healthy and feigning illness, their names, ages, and domicile, and even of their chief physical traits, "so as to collect data permitting [us] to recognize them when they would come again."[43]

Even under optimal conditions, the diagnostic criteria at the disposal of the doctor at the admitting office were few, and he was pressed for time. He had to rely mainly on his clinical experience to confirm a patient's symptoms—on signs accessible to his naked eye, such as an edema, fever, or rash, or to his hand when it palpated a liver, stomach, or spleen. The clinical thermometer was not yet available, and it would not have helped anyway, since "fevers" remained ill understood. We cannot tell when the admitting officials introduced percussion, used by Corvisart at the Charité long before 1808, when he publicized it by translating the *Inventum novum* of Leopold Auenbrugger, the discoverer of the diagnostic uses of percussion. Nor do we know how soon the stethoscope surfaced at the admitting office after René Théophile Hyacinthe Laënnec (1781–1826) invented it in 1816.

The four doctors at the admitting office observed prevalent malnutrition and exhaustion, we gather from their reports. They pondered the influence of the "medical constitution," the seasons, the weather, and communicable diseases. In the winter especially, they found that catarrh and fevers spread fast. They still categorized these fevers, according to their rhythms, into quotidian, tertian, and quartan, and, according to obvious symptoms, into putrid, bilious, malignant, and ataxic. They found acute inflammations; sore throats and chest pain; respiratory, circulatory, nervous, and digestive troubles; glandular swellings; cachexias; jaundice; hydropsy; paralyses that followed upon apoplexy; and scurvy that led to "degenerescences."

The admission of surgical patients presented few problems because the excellent French surgeons of the eighteenth century had long ago devised a whole gamut of clinical diagnostic sounds and signs, and thus the doctors at the admitting office could assess fractures, tumors, and ulcers. They sent interesting cases to the Hospice de perfectionnement and to the expanded Charité, while the Hôtel-Dieu admitted patients with "serious wounds, contusions and other accidents, ulcers, all kinds of tumors, lesions of the urinary tract, ophthalmias, some cataracts, and other ophthalmic complaints."[44]

The admitting officials frquently diagnosed scrofula in children; they blamed humid, airless dwellings and malnutrition—in other words, poverty. Initially, they hesitated about whether to assign very young patients to hospitals that specialized in specific illnesses or to send them all to the new Children's Hospital.[45] The physician-in-chief of that hospital, Jumelin, and the administrator, Duchanoy, insisted that all children, even those with surgical problems, belonged in their own special hospital.[46] In vain did the doctors at the Charité object: the Hospital Council countered that patient welfare must take precedence over the requirements of medical instruction.[47] After 1808, even children with contagious diseases were assigned to a special pavilion in the rue de Sèvres.[48]

For the mentally ill, the admitting officials turned into a "sort of legal jury." They knew how to categorize mental illnesses in a general way so as to tell mania and melancholia from mental deficiency and dementia. Before they committed a person who was reputedly insane, they required testimony from a doctor and two "witnesses to acts of madness." In the eighteen months under review, the doctors hospitalized 560 of the 582 persons brought to the office, questioning the petitioners' judgment in only 4 percent of the cases.[49]

Sometimes the requirements of teaching determined the assignment of patients. Thus the doctors stated that "the needs of clinical teaching motivate us to leave few beds empty at the Charité. This hospital has a kind of privilege to select its patients, and to admit only certain kinds of illnesses. Thus 'eruptive' maladies, especially smallpox, are kept away, and almost all interminable chronic complaints, internal as well as external, and, generally speaking, all illnesses not demonstrably curable. . . . women are only admitted to the Charité for clinical teaching, that is, if they present a degree of illness serious enough to warrant observation." In one case, the doctors at Cochin Hospital complained about the monotonous stream of patients with "epidemic catarrh" (influenza?); the central admissions office acknowledged the protest and stated: "As soon as the illnesses of springtime showed more variety, we hastened to respond to the doctors' concerns and offer their skills more diversified cases."[50] Admission to custodial institutions occurred twice a week at Pitié Hospice. There were not enough places and hundreds of eligible aged indigents were waiting their turn.

Within a year, daily census reports from every hospital were reaching the council's headquarters, so that the chart Frochot had called for became functional. In addition, the administrators and chiefs of all hospitals reviewed their patient census every three months to detect persons who had overstayed their welcome.

To their dismay the admitting officials soon discovered that triage accounted for less than 60 percent of all hospitalizations during the first eighteen months. The rest were admitted directly to the several city hospitals on the authority of the respective physicians–in–chief. Surely these 16,143 cases could not all be emergencies, such as traffic accidents, grave injuries, attempted suicides or murders, or imminent childbirth! Rather, their hospitalization remained a local arrangement between patient and doctor for obvious reasons: sick people minded the long walk to the center of town, ambulances were rare,[51] and cabs were expensive. It was simpler to apply directly to the district hospital. A closer look at direct admissions indicates that most of these occurred in a working-class neighborhood at St. Antoine Hospital, where 2,432 persons obtained access, while only 336 bothered to apply to the central office. The only other hospital where "urgent" admissions exceeded those authorized by the bureau occurred at Necker, where 605 persons arrived with an official ticket, as against 966 admitted by the physician in charge: a thirty-year-old tradition of neighborhood service and the fine reputation of the hospital seem the best explanation.[52] The physicians-in-chief, disdaining the opinion of a faraway administrator, preferred to make their own decisions, a lack

TABLE 5.3. Triage of Applicants to Paris Hospitals, Authorized and "Urgent" Admissions, 22 March 1802–24 September 1803 (1 Germinal, Year X–1 Vendémiaire, Year XII)

Hospital	Authorized by Admitting Office		"Urgent" or emergency		Total number admitted
	Number	%	Number	%	
Hôtel-Dieu	9,547	58	6,982	42	16,529
St. Louis	1,913	77	572	23	2,485
Charité	3,310	64	1,884	36	5,194
Venereal Diseases Hospital	2,584	81	608	19	3,192
Beaujon	1,143	59	807	41	1,950
St. Antoine	336	12	2,432	88	2,738
Cochin	858	59	603	41	1,461
Necker	605	38	966	62	1,571
Children's Hospital	1,592	55	1,289	45	2,881
Total	21,888		16,143		38,031

SOURCE: Adapted from Seine, CGAHHCP, *Rapport du bureau d'admission, 1804* (Paris: Imprimerie des hospices civils, 1806), table 4 and text.
NOTE: Discrepancies in numbers of applicants between the CGAHHCP's table 4 and tables 1, 2, and 3 derive from the fact that mental patients sent to Charenton and the Salpêtrière were not included in table 4.

of compliance condemned by Duchanoy.[53] Central triage worked only to the extent that the clinicians collaborated.

Or one might argue that triage—launched as an administrative project—turned into medical policy because the physicians-in-chief at the various hospitals adopted it as well. Thus, as of 1 July 1808, the Venereal Diseases Hospital regulated all its own admissions, followed by Pitié Hospital, opened in 1809.[54] The physician-in-chief selected patients to enhance the quality of teaching at his hospital and to further research.

Triage sharpened attention to diagnosis and led to numerous retransfers.[55] The Hospital Council complicated the allocation of patients by directing that they be hospitalized near their homes, if possible, so that "family, friends, and neighbors, any person who cares, can more easily visit." [56] Eventually, the patient census at the Salpêtrière was almost halved from the 8,000 in Tenon's day, and reduced at the Hôtel-Dieu from over 3,000 to about 2,000. The council accomplished this by the transfer of prisoners to jails and of prostitutes to special wards, first at the Venereal Diseases Hospital, then at the Lourcine Hospital. It removed children with skin problems to St. Louis and healthy children to orphanages. And it transferred all syphilitic patients to the Venereal Diseases Hospital and the mentally ill to Charenton. Mainly, its tough policy of excluding the needy who had no recognizable sickness transformed Paris hospitals into institutions that housed only the medically ill.

The fate of the applicants who were refused hospital beds because they were not sick enough, but whom the admitting officials found ailing and entitled to health care, is intriguing. For these persons, the doctors and the Hospital Council devised alternatives to hospitalization in an attempt to create outpatients, a group of citizens targeted to become partners in caring for their own health. In the first eighteen months, these numbered 9,462, or 27 percent of all who sought admission.

The establishment of a comprehensive network of health care and of supporting agencies for the Seine Department enabled the admitting office to refer 5 percent of the applicants to the district welfare offices in the first eighteen months. There applicants received food, fuel, and clothing, and authorization to obtain medications from the local pharmacist, whom the city would reimburse if he asked. This pattern followed practices that had been well established under the old regime, with a novel emphasis on medications. The admitting office also referred mothers with sick nurslings to the Society for Maternal Charity, and the doctors found that their advice for treatment at home was often crowned with success.[57] New strategies included tickets to the Tivoli Baths in the Seine—baths were believed to be therapeutic—and consultations for orphans serving apprenticeships in the expanded program headed by M. de Sevelinges.[58]

The four doctors at the admitting office found that the most efficient approach was to treat the patients right then and there. Their early experience taught them not to count on regular return visits: the patients' behavior rendered long-term treatment "illusory." The doctors had to devise alternatives, so they turned their office into a multipurpose outpatient clinic.

They dispensed 1,993 "bandages" whose use is fairly clear. Most of these were girdles or braces designed to control the effects of hernias and injuries to the spine. The bandages are described as being simple or double, left- or right-sided, exomphalic (that is, for umbilical hernias), suspensory, adjustable, or belly belts ("*suspensoirs, crémaillère, ventrières*"). In addition, 192 indigent women obtained pessaries to relieve the discomfort of a prolapsed uterus. The doctors added that the availability of the devices at one central dispensary enabled them to send recipients home speedily: in former times these patients

TABLE 5.4. Triage at Outpatient Counseling, 22 March 1802–24
September 1803 (1 Germinal, Year X-1 Vendémiaire, Year XII)

	Number	Percentage
Treated at the admitting office	760	2
Given braces or pessaries	2,185	6
Counseled at the admitting office	4,722	14
Referred to welfare offices	1,795	5
SUBTOTAL:	9,462	27
Dismissed[a]	2,904	8
Hospitalized	22,549	65
TOTAL APPLICANTS:	34,915	100

SOURCE: Seine, CGAHHJCP, *Rapport du bureau d'admission, 1804,* table 4 and
its accompanying text.
NOTE: Discrepancies in numbers of applicants between the CGAHHCP's
table 4 and tables 1, 2, and 3 derive from the fact that mental patients sent to
Charenton and the Salpêtrière were not included in table 4.
[a] An unspecified number of those dismissed were perceived as "malingerers."

would have been admitted to the hospital, where old women who
needed a pessary tended to stay on "as long as possible." Prompt help
"at the source of the complaint" saved hospital days.[59]
 Knowing that the Venereal Diseases Hospital had a waiting list
of from thirty to forty men, the admitting office extended free consultations to patients with syphilitic illnesses. The doctors considered
this measure to be "of great psychologic usefulness," adding that they
had been able to "aid women, hapless victims of their husband's lib-
ertinism, who recoiled from being commingled with public women
[at the Venereal Diseases Hospital]; to help many workers, honest artisans and family men led astray by a moment's weakness, but who
felt the obligation to continue working while pursuing their cure."
The doctors even reported that they "were able to assist families distressed by the horrible effects of prostitution in children of both
sexes."[60]
 In his 1816 report, Count Pastoret tried to picture the fear of venereal disease as unfounded when he explained that consultations were
given every year to "3,000–4,000 persons whose illness exists only in
their imagination or apprehension, who come mainly to dispel preoccupations regarding their health, to know whether they may get married, travel, whether their doctors have really cured them, . . . persons
who have other illnesses than those that motivated their request for

a consultation. This accounts for the presence of 60, 80, sometimes 100 patients, especially men, who are much more numerous."[61]

Expanding its activities further after 1806, the admitting office turned into an emergency hospital, open from 4 P.M. to the next morning. Possibly the administrators knew that Tenon had advocated such an establishment in the center of town with a permanent staff and well-stocked facilities for emergency aid and outpatient treatment.[62]

The concept of outpatient care thus gradually became acceptable to artisans and family men. Yet it remained novel and strange to the experienced administrator Camus, who explained in his 1803 report that an outpatient clinic meant that "patients come to a certain room at specified times, receive advice, medication, [and] linen, in a word, all they need to care for themselves at home." To clarify the advantages further, Camus elaborated: "This diminishes the number of inpatients and permits more individuals to share in the national welfare funds. It permits artisans to continue working in their shops to earn a living and support their families." This revealing passage refers to men who had families to support, who preferred independence to hospitalization and were ready to accept medical counseling and directions for self-medication—citizen-patients. Camus also indicated that suffering from scabies should not be thought shameful, and that the number of persons infected is "much larger than one would think."[63] The message was clear: it urged citizen initiative in health maintenance.

To promote this, the Hospital Council created a fourth outpatient clinic at the Children's Hospital in order to spread the well-established practice of treating ringworm and scabies with sulphurous remedies. We know that syphilitic patients were treated at the admitting office with mercury-based medications, but the reports do not tell us what kinds of medications were available for the other patients treated there.

What of the 14 percent of applicants who received only "oral" advice but no free medications or trusses? They may have been given short shrift. The doctors felt worst about the 5 to 10 percent who were drifters needing a home, food, and a job before health care could be effectively proffered. These homeless patients had fared better under the indifferentiated Catholic charity of the old regime. In contrast, the emergent citizen-patient now found a variety of alternatives to hospitalization, ranging from revived traditional practices to ambitious, innovative projects in medicine, hygiene, and custodial support.

The Revival of Traditional Practices

The agencies supported by the Paris Hospital Council and used for the referral of patients fell into two broad categories. On the one hand, the welfare centers, home care and infant protection agencies, and soup kitchens resumed their traditional activities. On the other hand, innovative ventures such as medical dispensaries, nursing homes, clinics, and infirmaries targeted medical ailments that might become severe if neglected and cause unemployment and thus indigence. By treating serious illness on an ambulatory basis or in the homes of the poor, long hospitalization might be prevented and the citizen-patient returned to gainful employment more quickly. The council also supported small private homes and clinics to relieve the overcrowded public establishments, and it quickly endorsed that famous English import, vaccination.

The welfare centers in the city's districts were the reincarnation of the old regime's charity offices, usually in the same locale. Traditionally funded by municipal, religious, and local donations and served by the Sisters of Charity in or out of uniform, the office contracted for the services of a local doctor and an apothecary. Referrals were useless in the poorest arrondissements. "And yet we were careful," commented Camus, "to refer only residents whose indisposition required merely some food, clothing, and medical attention."[64] In the wealthier arrondissements, for example, near Beaujon Hospital, the welfare center had sufficient funds to cope.[65]

Home care found an eloquent champion in the councillor in charge of the program, the scholarly lawyer and mayor of the 10th arrondissement, Duquesnoy. In his first report, he pleaded that the aged, infirm, and ailing be entrusted to the care of their families, arguing that children, parents, mothers, and spouses made the best nurses. Disparaging all public establishments, he asserted that in the home "everything is done better and to better purpose than in those institutions where the sick, the aged, and [the] infirm are heaped up, left to unknown and often greedy hands. The aid distributed to families strengthens domestic affections. Hospitals destroy them."[66]

When Dean Thouret presented the Hospital Council with a report on the wet nurses' referral service (*bureau des recommandaresses*) on 8 June 1801, he explained that this establishment provided inexpensive services for the legitimate offspring of poor married couples.[67] When these parents' poverty worsened into indigence, they often abandoned their infant. By supporting this referral service, argued Thouret, the councillors would prevent adding to the 5,000 abandoned babies whose legal guardians they had recently become.[68]

The service was situated on rue Sainte Avoye, in the heart of the populous Marais. Headed by Lallemand and staffed with seventeen employees, it processed about 4,500 babies a year in 1801–1813. A physician inspected the wet nurses and the babies who were returned

TABLE 5.5. Infant Mortality in the First Year of Life among Legitimate
Babies in Care of the Paris Wet-Nursing Office, 1799–1813

Year	Infants registered	Deaths	
		Number	Percentage
VII	4,769	1,182	24
VIII	3,863	1,152	33.5
IX	4,213	1,075	39.8
1802	4,583	1,478	32.2
1803	4,916	1,544	31.4
1804	4,854	1,408	29
1805	4,878	1,215	24.9
1806	4,519	1,327	29.4
1807	4,404	1,316	29
1808	4,716	1,280	26.6
1809	4,801	1,194	24.9
1810	5,048	1,480	29.3
1811	5,090	1,407	27.4
1812	4,522	1,104	24.6
1813	4,387	1,107	25.2
Total	57,878	16,222	(average) 28.03

SOURCES: M. A. Thouret and Lallemand, "Rapport sur l'administration
des secours à domicile à l'époque du ler Germinal An XI (21 mars 1803),"
in Seine, CGAHHCP, *Rapports au conseil général* (1803), 11, and Seine,
CGAHHCP, *Rapport fait au conseil général des hospices par un de ses membres sur
l'état des hôpitaux, des hospices, et des secours à domicile, à Paris, depuis le ler janvier
1804 jusqu'au ler janvier 1814* (Paris: Imprimerie de Mme Huzard, 1816), 378.

in ill health—about 150 out of 4,531, or 3.3 percent, in the Year X,[69]
and a total of 1,433, or 2.5 percent, in 1801–1813. The latter figure
included 494 babies whom the parents refused to take back; the wet-
nursing office sent most of them, 456, to a hospice, and 38 to the
Venereal Diseases Hospital.[70]

Perhaps the most sobering remarks in these reports concern the
mortality of infants during the first year of life spent in the country
with a wet nurse—that is, under what contemporaries considered optimal conditions: the results were "satisfactory" for the years VII–IX,
the dean of the medical school believed, for deaths amounted "only"
to an average 32.4 percent.[71] For the years 1801–1813, Pastoret reports
an average mortality of 28 percent, commenting that "this corresponds to the proportions of usual infant mortality."[72]

The wet-nursing office also acted as a clearinghouse for news: it
sent out 4,000 letters in the Year X, not counting correspondence with

the drivers.[73] The office exacted the first month's payment from parents and initiated the baby's return after three months' arrears. After a baby's return or death, the office took legal steps to recover payments. In 1803, the budget consisted of 28,700 francs in wages, 12,000 francs in maintenance, and overdue payments to nurses amounting to 25,000 francs, that is, 38 percent of the total budget!

Reimbursement of overdue nursing fees had been a popular traditional charity. It rescued impoverished debtors, whom the government routinely jailed. These sentences were abolished on 25 August 1792. After help from private donors stopped, the wet-nursing office subsisted on government grants, small at first, but rising to three successive subsidies of 300,000 francs under the Empire. This enabled the office to exonerate more than 6,000 debtors by paying off most of the nurses.[74] But the councillors tried in vain to create an adequate system of medical inspection either at the Paris office or through the mayor or local health officers.

Not all impoverished young couples wanted to send their infant to the country. To help mothers of large families, groups of concerned middle-class women had founded the Society for Maternal Charity in the 1780s.[75] It provided money, regular visits, and a layette to poor families for their fourth and further babies and for orphaned, congenitally ill newborns. The aim was to prevent the abandonment of infants to the Foundlings' Hospice. Under the old regime, help was predicated on a legal marriage and a priest's certificate endorsed by neighbors. The society believed that it had saved many a marriage among the poor and many a father from debtor's prison.

Stressing sensible health practices, the society encouraged its clients to breast-feed. In two and a half years before the Revolution, almost one thousand babies were aided, for two years each, with 192 livres annually. The society's report proudly stated that only two of the mothers died in childbirth.[76] They could not know, of course, that the most important service they rendered was to promote giving birth at home, thus eluding puerperal fever. The National Assembly voted an emergency grant of 1,000 livres per month in July 1790, and of 2,000 livres per month in January 1791.[77] Disbanded in 1793, the society resumed work under the Consulate. In order to find their way into the homes of the poor, its members established close contacts with the city's forty-eight welfare offices. Information surely flowed in both directions—from the homes of the poor via the women in charity work to their husbands on the Hospital Council, and from the council to the welfare offices and to the poor. Certain councillors—Pastoret, for example—were pleased to see their wives bring old-fashioned Catholic charity to the poor. We cannot tell to what extent religious moralizing tinged tangible help.

The council aided another project with a long history that became enormously successful: the soup kitchens that opened, beginning in the harsh winter of 1800–1801, either at the welfare centers, or at independent locations. These kitchens represent an interesting public-private partnership of science with philanthropy. Their reappearance in Paris in February 1800 was spurred by a book. François de Neufchâteau, while still minister of internal affairs, had sent Benjamin Delessert a copy of a collection of essays on philanthropic medical establishments, *Mémoires sur les établissements d'humanité,* which had been edited, at François de Neufchâteau's instigation, by Duquesnoy.[78] In that series, there appeared selections from the *Bibliothèque britannique,* the Genevan journal that kept French intellectuals abreast of new developments in Great Britain, and in other parts of the world, inaccessible because of war. The *Bibliothèque* was publicizing an "economic stove," or stove "à la Rumford," similar to the "Franklin stove," recently developed by the widely traveled Count Rumford. It had multiple advantages and economized two-thirds of the wood.[79]

Delessert had such a stove built, for 600 francs, and sponsored a soup kitchen at the welfare office, 16, rue du Mail. In a pamphlet, he gave the recipe for the soup: barley, potatoes, peas, beans, lentils, onions, celery, leeks, carrots, turnips, sorrel, salt, and pepper. And the recipe for its distribution: this initiative must be privately financed; the poor should pay a small sum for the soup, lest their feelings be hurt, or else coupons should be used.[80]

The Hospital Council welcomed and supported the project. We can conveniently cull information about Paris soup kitchens during the Consulate and Empire from the annual reports of the Philanthropic Society. Several of that society's leaders, Delessert, Parmentier, and Pastoret were also Hospital Council members and met three times weekly in the council office, promoting the project as needed.[81]

The soup kitchens' most ardent advocates, apart from Delessert and Parmentier, were the botanist A. P. de Candolle (1778–1841) and the chemist A. A. Cadet de Vaux. They studied the construction of the Rumford stove and published papers on its design, on the most advantageous fuel, and on the additional uses that the warm stovepipes might serve. These Parisian scientists carefully analyzed the ingredients of the soup, so as to provide the poor with a well-balanced, nutritious, and savory meal. As late as 1814, they were still experimenting with recipes, specifically with the use of bonemeal, advocated by Cadet de Vaux in opposition to the gelatine favored by his colleague

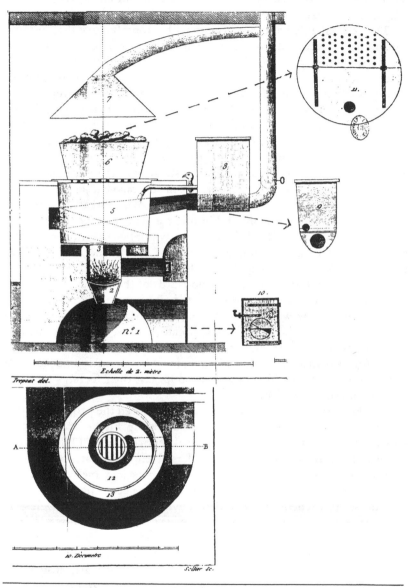

FIGURE 5.1. Design of a Rumford stove. From B. Delessert, *Notice sur les soupes à la Rumfort établies à Paris, rue du Mail, No. 16* (Paris: n.p., Year VIII [1799–1800]). 1–8: general plan. 9: container for additional water (cross-sections). 10: door to remove ashes. 11: wooden cover for casserole. 12–13: heat circulation.

J. P. J. d'Arcet (1777–1844). "We invited several of our members," the Philanthropic Society's report states, "among them the most skillful chemists, to examine this gelatine extracted from bones for its healthful and nutritive qualities." In the interest of taste, gelatine won out over bonemeal soup.[82] But on one important point customers and donors agreed: a minimal payment by the recipients enhanced the worth of a meal. Soup kitchens were enormously successful: at the height of their activity, in 1811, forty-two kitchens operated in Paris. By 1815, they had distributed 12.5 million portions.[83]

Thus, in order to protect and maintain the health of the poor, the Paris Hospital Council helped revive and support a number of traditional practices. However, in the post-Revolutionary context, health care reformers no longer judged it either sufficient or appropriate merely to dispense aid. Hence the appearance of a number of professional projects, all aimed at keeping the prospective citizen–patient out of the hospital: we have already encountered the outpatients clinics; now we shall examine the medical dispensary, nursing home, small private hospital, and infirmary.

Creative Innovation: Prevention and Protection

The Parisian medical dispensaries were the creation of the Philanthropic Society of Paris. Founded in 1780 by seven men, the society grew to 436 members by 1786. Two years later, Louis XVI became a patron, attracting wealthy sponsors from the upper classes, many of them freemasons. One of the society's earliest projects was to support twelve blind children of workingmen with monthly stipends of six livres. It was this stipend, doubled, that gave Valentin Haüy's school for the blind its start. When funds accumulated, the Philanthropic Society decided to aid the work of maternal charity: it adopted as clients women carrying a sixth child, or assisted a baby's widowed parent. By 1786, the Philanthropic Society was supporting 300 eighty-year-olds, 46 blind children, 150 women with a fourth baby, and 36 widows. The society's aid was based on need only and, in contrast to Catholic practice, it occasionally required documentation of physical handicaps: for example, a physician–oculist's certificate to establish that a child was congenitally blind. Disbanded in 1794, the Philanthropic Society resumed work in 1800 with the co-sponsorship of soup kitchens all over Paris. But its most innovative project consisted of medical dispensaries.[84]

In contrast to the haphazard health support and home care tendered at the welfare centers, the program of the Philanthropic Society of Paris proffered first-rate medical treatment by a large staff of young

TABLE 5.6. Philanthropic Society of Paris Dispensaries, Consulting
Physicians and Surgeons, 1803–1815

Physicians	Surgeons
Jean Louis Alibert, St. Louis Hospital	Alexis Boyer, Charité Hospital
Charles François Andry, Port-Royal Maternity Hospice	Joseph F. L. Deschamps, Charité Hospital
Joachim Bourdois de la Motte, Hôtel-Dieu	Antoine Dubois, Maternity Hospice
Jean Nicolas Corvisart, Charité Hospital	Guillaume Dupuytren, Hôtel-Dieu
Jean Noël Hallé, Medical Faculty	Pierre Lassus, Medical Faculty
R. T. H. Laënnec, Necker Hospital	Philippe Jean Pelletan, Hôtel-Dieu
Augustin Jacob Landré-Beauvais, Salpêtrière Hospice	Pierre François Percy, Medical Faculty
C. B. Leclerc, St. Antoine Hospital	
Théodore Nilammon Lerminier, Charité Hospital	
Jean Jacques Leroux des Tillets, Medical Faculty	
Philippe Pinel, Salpêtrière Hospice	
Joseph C. A. Récamier, Hôtel-Dieu	
Michel Augustin Thouret, Medical Faculty	

SOURCE: D. B. Weiner, "The Role of the Doctor in Welfare Work: The Example of the Philanthropic Society of Paris, 1780–1815," *Historical Reflections / Réflexions historiques,* 1982, *9* (1 & 2): 279–304, at 287–288.

physicians and surgeons. It thus carried out the Poverty Committee's intent of targeting illness as a cause of poverty. By 1804, the society had opened five medical dispensaries. Located in the poorer sections of town, they employed an advanced student as permanent resident. A complicated system of membership cards financed these establishments, but the Hospital Council was frequently called upon to supplement their budget. A large (and constantly changing) number of pharmacies collaborated with the dispensaries. What made these establishments especially attractive to young doctors was the distinguished roster of senior consultants, all of them professors at the Paris Health School, who sometimes admitted dispensary patients to the best hospitals. The surgeon Antoine Dubois was evidently most generous in this respect.

The number of citizen-patients seeking these services rose steadily, from 735 in 1804 to just over 2,000 in 1813. The most attractive aspect of these dispensaries was that one-third of the clientele received housecalls—an exceptional service for poor people. Dr. Esparron, one of the young dispensary doctors, explained that when visiting patients in their normal home environment on the sixth floor,

> we know them better and forget them less easily than if we see them in a row of hospital beds. . . . We no longer examine a person only: we study a home, an entire family. . . . An isolated illness stands out, so to speak. Witnesses to its onset give more precise information. One detects causative influences more easily in the locale where the illness developed, and one can better appreciate the health-damaging influence of certain professions, a poorly situated home, a more or less salubrious section of town."[85]

This astonishing statement runs counter to the prevalent contemporary maxims holding that illnesses are best understood in a hospital ward.

Among the young doctors who thus discovered the importance of a personal doctor-patient relationship and the influence of occupation and of living quarters on health were some of the great figures of early nineteenth-century medicine and public health, among them G. L. Bayle, L. R. Villermé, A. J. B. Parent-Duchâtelet, and M. G. A. Devergie.

One of the Philanthropic Society's trustees, P. S. Dupont de Nemours, figured in 1806 that the dispensaries aided poor patients at lower cost than the public hospitals and saved the city of Paris 52,000 francs in 1807 alone—an economy of almost 300,000 francs since 1803.[86] These dispensaries continued to function throughout the nineteenth century (and several are still in existence today). It is sobering to learn that they did not significantly reduce the population of Paris hospitals. We know that medical need grows as facilities expand, because of a greater awareness of what can be done.

Indigent senior citizens were a group of special concern to the reformers. In order to keep the aged out of the public hospices, the council supported a number of retirement and nursing homes, and institutions for senile, demented, but calm old people. These homes were often versions of the manifold Catholic charitable homes and shelters of the old regime. We shall examine two typical establishments, the "Maison du St. Nom de Jésus," a small nursing home, and Petites Maisons, a large custodial establishment.

Founded in 1653 by St. Vincent de Paul, the Maison du St. Nom de Jésus sheltered about forty men and women. Several Sisters of Charity staffed this establishment in the faubourg St. Laurent. Though defrocked, the sisters shepherded their patients through the

Revolution—with the connivance of neighbors and sympathetic public officials, one assumes. The decree of 6 January 1802 officially reopened this "Maison de santé du faubourg St. Martin," popularly known as "Maison Dubois," because Antoine Dubois officiated as attending surgeon. Following St. Vincent's strategy, the home exacted a minimal fee from applicants who shunned outright charity. It also hospitalized the domestics of wealthy employers.[87] (The idea of "foundations" was thus revived, but without those perpetual rights that critics in the Enlightenment found so objectionable.) Payment of one and a half, two, or three francs daily gave patients a choice of rooms, but "treatment and care were the same for all. . . . The large number of applicants testifies to the fact that the public approves of this establishment and appreciates its advantages," commented Camus.[88] It was an early example of a dignified and affordable home for the ailing aged.

Petites Maisons Hospice had struck the site visitors from the National Assembly as a diversified, well-run nursing home.[89] It made the transition to the new era without a hitch because it already dispensed individual attention and medical care and accepted paying inmates. Founded in 1554 by Henri II, the Petites Maisons sheltered 538 women and men in 1790. The rules required that they be at least seventy years old, but the waiting list was so long that some had been admitted only at the advanced age of eighty. Favoritism, on the other hand, routinely circumvented the rules, so that some younger persons also lived there. The residents received a pension (three livres a week in 1788) from which they defrayed their expenses for food and clothing. In this home, forty Sisters of Charity cared for acutely ill patients in an infirmary—a rarity at the time. It had six wards for women (with 9 to 40 beds each, 155 in all) and two wards for men (with 12 and 20 beds respectively). For a fee, traditionally 600 livres per year, forty to fifty mental patients lived in individual cells in a special ward. They were confined by lettre de cachet.[90] In another ward, fifty-two venereal disease patients received medical help. And finally, twenty to twenty-five children suffering from ringworm lived at the nearby Sainte-Reine Hospital and underwent "treatment."[91] The Petites Maisons was thus a multiple-purpose institution. "No praise is too high," wrote La Rochefoucauld-Liancourt in 1790.[92]

Thirteen years later, the municipal government transformed the re-christened Householders' Hospice (*Hospice des ménages*) into a model geriatric establishment housing married or single seniors with some, but insufficient, means. It offered them single rooms, a pound and a quarter of bread daily, three francs and a pound of raw meat every ten days, and two *cordes* (cubic meters) of firewood annually.

Those who paid 1,600 francs upon entering and brought their bed, linen, two chairs, and a chest of drawers received two loads of coal per year.[93]

Repeated inspection resulted in reiterated praise: from Tenon in 1785, Liancourt in 1790, Camus in 1803, Pastoret in 1816. Why? Because the pattern of aid provided specifically for the needs of these citizens and thus stabilized their health: proximity of colleagues assured company, free daily bread curbed hunger; minimal gifts of fuel provided some protection from the cold. The new name, "Householders' Hospice," implied dignity and tried to remove the connotation of mental institution that clings to the name Petites Maisons to this day. The establishment functioned at low cost; supervision assured cleanliness, order, first aid, and referral to the hospital in case of serious illness or accident.

In fact, the private clinic or nursing home for paying patients now gradually became acceptable, even to the middle class. The Consulate tried some interesting experiments: the Retirement Home at Montrouge was set aside for hospital employees in addition to clerics and military men. The reader may remember that it began as a rest home for the Brothers of Charity, and that the Poverty Committee's site visitors were shocked by its luxury. Another retirement home, Ste. Périnne in Passy, required a considerable deposit but offered an assured haven in old age. A model had, of course, long existed in the sumptuous Hôtel des Invalides, where, as Louis XIV had done before him, Napoleon now lodged his veterans in truly royal surroundings.[94]

Finally, Paris boasted several small private hospitals or clinics: one was an annex of the Venereal Diseases Hospital. It had sixty-two beds, cost between 2.50 and 5 francs daily, and shared the medical facilities of the main hospital, including the attentions of Dr. Cullerier, the famous venereologist. [95] Another example was the private mental hospital that Dr. J. E. D. Esquirol opened in 1802, across the street from the Salpêtrière at 8, rue Buffon. Here, some twenty paying patients profited from the expert care of a resident physician, the first well-trained French psychiatrist.[96]

Another innovative strategy that indicates a shift in medical thinking was the isolation of acutely ill patients in an infirmary within the hospice itself. While this was obviously not a means of keeping patients out of the hospital, it did protect them from cursory or thoughtless treatment. The infirmary has a long history, harking back to the medieval monastery, where an ailing monk or nun could enjoy quiet, comfort, and good nursing in a small room set aside for this purpose, the *infirmarium*. Adopted in the lay world, the infirmary first served the privileged few. Thus Tenon mentions two infirmaries at the old soldiers' retirement home (*Maison royale de santé*) and ten "old infirmaries" at the Salpêtrière for ecclesiastics, *soeurs officières,* teachers, governesses, domestics, aged couples, and retired workers (*reposantes*), as well as three for prisoners.[97] We have previously mentioned that Louis XVI, prodded by Jean Colombier, had ordered in 1781 that new infirmaries with adequate nursing and medical personnel for all sick inmates be built in the establishments of the Hôpital Général, but the Poverty Committee site visitors reported that the infirmaries served only a privileged few, who received exceptional rations of meat, white bread, and wine. Insofar as a physician did visit the Hôpital Général, these are the patients he saw. Liancourt wrote of the Salpêtrière in 1791: "Several dormitories have small, rather clean, infirmaries, but only for sisters, servants, and a few privileged women. Paupers are taken to the general infirmary; many old women languish in their dormitory and often die without help."[98] At Bicêtre, Hagnon, the administrator, reported the existence of six infirmaries in 1790, three for inmates and three for the staff.[99] Yet Liancourt noticed no such installations, writing that "Bicêtre's turn had not yet come," and at the Pitié, "an infirmary planned for the past six to eight years is not yet built and, in the meantime, masses of these poor children perish at the Hôtel-Dieu."[100]

It took physicians to perceive the opportunity that these special wards afforded. The title of "physician of the infirmaries" seems to appear first in connection with Charles Jacques Saillant (1747–1804), who served in that capacity at the Salpêtrière from 1782 to 1786 and 1790 to 1791. The Ideologue doctors of the Paris hospital commission, Thouret and Cabanis, surely had ambitious plans when they appointed Philippe Pinel to Bicêtre hospice in 1793 with that novel title. When Pinel arrived at the Salpêtrière as physician-in-chief in 1795, he gave new meaning to the "infirmaries": "A hospital destined for sick women and as large as the Salpêtrière," he wrote, "opens a great career for new research on women's diseases that have always and rightly been considered as the most difficult and complicated of all."[101] With this recognition, the infirmary of this hospice changed into a research and teaching ward. Somewhat later (in 1818), Esquirol pointed out that at the Salpêtrière and Bicêtre, "the mental wards are quite independent from the rest of the establishment. The patients have a special routine, with employees and a special doctor. *These are hospitals within the hospice.*"[102] Similar changes occurred at the Charité and other hospitals, and isolation on small wards ceased to be a favor accorded the privileged. Acutely ill hospice inmates increasingly received medical attention, and professors selected patients for intensive study and teaching. The role of the citizen-patient in the hospital was being further defined.

◆◆◆

Thus the Hospital Council encouraged Parisian doctors and patients to develop innovative ways of coping with illness and ailments, ways that suited the individual patient and socioeconomic situation, rather than relying on routine hospitalization for all applicants. In Marcel Candille's apt phrase, the *"pauvres malades"* [the suffering poor] were gradually changing into *"malades pauvres"* [impecunious patients]. Poverty did not necessarily mean indigence, and a small payment was often considered a sign of individual dignity. The council continued to rely on traditional agencies of health support such as the district welfare offices, home care, and soup kitchens, and to expand diverse ways of keeping the citizen-patient out of the large hospital by promoting new dispensaries, infirmaries, small hospitals, and nursing homes. In this spectrum of possibilities, the role of outpatient was of central importance. It required the recognition that free public care was the citizen-patient's right, balanced by the duty to accept and follow medical directions and to behave in a socially responsible manner. It required a partnership between physician and patient, trust in the doctor's knowledge, intelligence, and persistence in applying advice. The initiative and independence of the outpatient could be an attractive alternative to the more passive role of inpatient, with the added benefit that it was often possible to continue working while undergoing medical treatment.

But whatever their efforts, reformers, physicians, and administrators realized that the hospitals could not be phased out. Not only were too many applicants too sick to be turned away, but a new eagerness in the medical profession oriented clinical investigators toward the hospital ward. Citizens now acquired new importance as inpatients.

The Inpatient:
The Claims of Medical Science

Place hospital patients so that the sequence of their beds represents . . .
the thermometer of seriousness of their diseases.

C. F. Duchanoy, M.D., 1801

Tenon had mentioned a "league among persons of goodwill"
who sought alternatives to hospitalization for the poor in the Hôtel-
Dieu. That "league" of reformers, administrators, and physicians
achieved only partial success in channeling citizen-patients toward
outpatient departments, welfare offices, dispensaries, nursing homes,
and private clinics. But the "league" also helped inpatients: it encouraged administrators to create a dignified hospital environment with
creature comforts for all in a clean and orderly setting. It inspired
physicians to treat poor patients like the affluent, in an individual and
careful manner. Intent on furthering the Poverty Committee's goal, it
created opportunities for work in the hospice, to steer inmates toward
self-sufficiency.

Inpatients were similarly called upon to fulfill the citizen's duties.
They now found themselves assigned to hospital wards, where they
were repeatedly interrogated and examined by inquisitive young men
and subjected to novel procedures, medications, and even experiment.
The bodies of those who died were routinely autopsied. We shall now
explore the changes in the inpatients' experience, assessing the ways
in which they performed citizens' duties. Then we focus on the effects
of specialization and follow the patients from triage at admission to
their accommodations and treatment at the Venereal Diseases and
Dermatology Hospitals and at Salpêtrière Hospice. In a separate chapter we shall look at the experience of young patients grouped according to age: newborns at the Maternité and children at their new special
hospital.

Comfort: The Paris Hospital Council
as the Patient's Advocate

The administrators generally welcomed the new emphasis on medicine at the expense of excessive religiosity and fussy housekeeping. But they resented the doctors' assumption that medical criteria could justify changes in so many aspects of patient care. The documentation reveals tensions that led to a permanent tug-of-war between hospital administration and medical staff. This staff represented "the main stumbling block that has caused all past reforms to fail," warned Duchanoy (himself a physician) in 1801. The hospital commission, he added, had only one wish: "May the day come when the council, cognizant of its great power, uses its moral and permanent authority to bring about reform."[1] It thus appears that the struggle between the Poverty and Health Committees resurfaced in a new guise under the Consulate.

As the administrators saw it, the doctors disrupted hospital routine when they crowded the wards with hundreds of students intent on examining large numbers of patients. Much like the nurses of yore, the administrators complained that doctors interfered in kitchens when they mandated patient diets, and in pharmacies when they scrutinized the compounding of remedies. Medical investigators multiplied their demands for space and renovations as the techniques and instruments for physical diagnosis improved. Anatomists clamored for more autopsy pavilions. While recognizing the validity of these claims, the Hospital Council advocated and protected the patients' well-being, striving to make their hospital stay a more decent experience. The councillors therefore undertook extensive architectural repairs and renovation, purchased new furnishings, provided better food, and paid more attention to hygiene and orderliness.

"The transformation of a convent into a hospital," Tenon had written in 1788, "permits only limited new arrangements."[2] Hospital architecture during our period illustrates how the old order changed slowly into the new. The inpatient continued to experience the ubiquitous presence of Christian symbols—edifying stained-glass windows, high, churchlike ceilings, and Gothic arches. Even if altars and crucifixes had been removed, their outlines remained visible. Although nurses wore ordinary dress, their preoccupation with ritual continued to pervade their medical ministrations. Kitchens occupied more space than pharmacies. Patients might see gardens through a window—a geometric pattern of plots to grow vegetables and medicinal herbs—but only grudgingly were they granted access to them for convalescent recreation. Slowly balconies, cleared of drying sheets, turned into fresh-air promenoirs. And hospital buildings now occasionally housed doctors instead of communities of sisters and the almoner. Gradually, Hygeia displaced Pietas as the officiating goddess.

At the turn of the nineteenth century, only a minority of Parisians were hospitalized in buildings erected recently for that purpose, such as Cochin and St. Antoine Hospitals. These were relatively small, dwarfed by the Hôtel-Dieu and the Salpêtrière. Some originated as nursing homes (Ménages, Maison de la Rochefoucauld), others were adapted from former uses as an orphanage (Beaujon) or the home of a religious order (Necker, St. Magloire, Maison Ste. Périnne). These structures required only normal upkeep and repairs. But all the large hospitals and hospices needed major renovations and these were well under way when the Revolution broke out. The Hospital Council thus built on initiatives of the old regime.

The search for patient comfort befitting the dignity of a citizen can be documented from the work of the three hospital architects of this period: Nicolas Etienne Clavareau (1757–1815), Charles François Viel (1745–1819), and Jacques Gondoin (1737–1818).[3] In *Mémoires sur les hôpitaux civils de Paris* (1805), Clavareau places himself center-stage, and offers the reader an overview of his accomplishments, beginning with the reduction of "all beds at the Hôtel-Dieu and St. Louis to a width of three feet,"[4] followed by the transfer of various services away from the Hôtel-Dieu, thus removing the most serious congestion and fire hazards. This meant structural adjustments at Scipion to accommodate more butchering of cattle, melting of tallow, and manufacture of candles, and extensive remodeling of the former Foundlings' Hospice (whose occupants had moved to Port-Royal) to house the Central Pharmacy.

Clavareau also created amenities at the Hôtel-Dieu: the new women's ward on the left bank, "a superb infirmary with a capacity of 120 beds"; a promenade for convalescents in the place du Parvis Notre-Dame; stoves in all wards; and baths where the transfer of the mental patients to Charenton left unused space and tubs. Clavareau modernized the admitting office, transformed the St. Antoine orphanage, and built the St. Antoine Hospital. Here work had stopped in 1800, Camus tells us:

> It is sad to see solid walls, designed for a useful building, fall into ruin even before they have been completed. . . . [By 1803, and owing to the Hospital Council's initiative,] the former abbey housed the linen department, the pharmacy, lodgings for the hospital director, the doctor, and other impor-

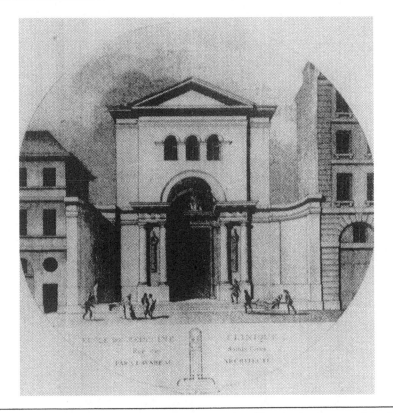

FIGURE 6.1. Charité Hospital. Entrance to the clinical school opened in the former chapel in 1801. From N. Clavereau, *Mémoires sur les hôpitaux civils* (Paris: Prault, 1805).

tant employees. When the buildings are completed and with a few alterations on the main floor, the number of beds can be raised to 300.[5]

Architecture served not only patient comfort, but medical science as well. Clavareau's triumph was the transformation of the Brothers of Charity's Paris headquarters. He built a "clinical school" according to Jean Nicolas Corvisart's instructions, and they fitted the school into the hull of the Brothers' chapel. Even though Clavareau speaks of a "new Epidauros," it was the requirements of bedside teaching, not temple healing, that determined the design. Corvisart omitted laboratories but required autopsy room. A pillared hallway led to an amphitheater that seated 200. (It can still be visited, and it is, by modern standards, exiguous and uncomfortable; in 1800, it was unique.) Camus commented in 1803 on the new setting where the teaching of surgery now took place:

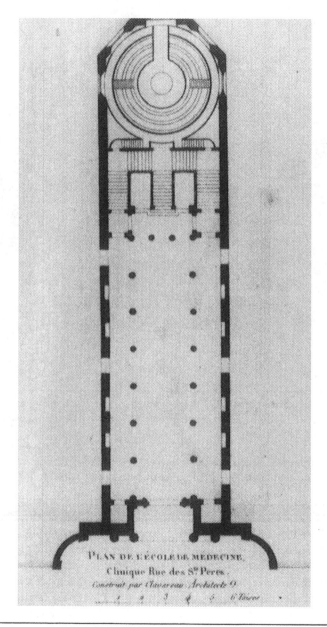

FIGURE 6.2. Charité Hospital. Ground plan of the clinical school opened in the former chapel in 1801. From N. Clavereau, *Mémoires sur les hôpitaux civils* (Paris: Prault, 1805).

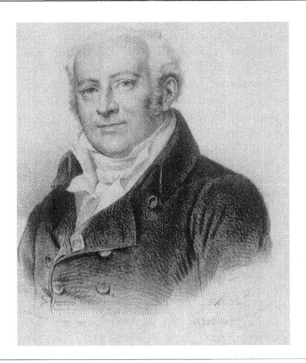

FIGURE 6.3. Jean Nicolas Corvisart (1769–1821). Painting by Gérard, Musée de Versailles. Bibliothèque interuniversitaire de médecine, Paris.

[In the past] two serious problems complicated procedures undertaken on the sickbed. The sight of painful operations and the patients' cries frightened, tormented, and distressed the others in the same ward. The students, eager to watch the operation, besieged the bed, smothered the patient, and hindered the surgeon's movements, risking involuntary accidents. In the operating room built on the council's orders, the patient is appropriately positioned, the surgeon operates unimpeded; the students, seated on benches, are the quiet observers of the surgical intervention.[6]

Forty patients, bedded down in four well-lit wards, now lent themselves to intensive questioning and examination. Soon a clinical society took shape to organize these rounds and protect the patients from the students' excessive eagerness. Therapy included showers, baths, steambaths, and electric stimulation. Clavareau also modernized the Brothers of Charity's hospital next door, transforming the monks' cells into a 60-bed women's ward; by 1803, the Charité Hospital had 230 beds: 126 for medical patients, 104 for surgery.[7]

Clavareau's slightly senior colleague, Charles François Viel, began his career by building Cochin, completed in 1782; then he renovated the Pitié orphanage by erecting one building for 700 boys and an infirmary for 150, with a gallery for convalescents. In 1808 the orphans were moved to St. Antoine and the whole Pitié was turned into a hospital. At Bicêtre, Viel filled up those eight notorious underground cells, eight feet square and eleven feet below ground, and replaced them with eight high-security cells that were both aboveground and salubrious. Equally famous is Viel's great sewer at Bicêtre, a remarkable engineering feat.

By 1789 Viel completed a section for 600 mentally ill women at the Salpêtrière, part of a planned 1,000-patient facility for the insane, epileptics, and cripples.[8] He replaced a cow barn and a pigsty with a new shed and renovated the laundry that served 10,000 persons. He also built a large amphitheater at the Hôtel-Dieu for Pierre Joseph Desault on the left bank; made the Port-Royal Maternity and Foundlings' Hospice inhabitable; helped transform the Capuchin novitiate into the Venereal Diseases Hospital and the Hôtel des Miramiones into the Central Hospital Pharmacy; and renovated the city pawnshop.

The architect Jacques Gondoin modernized the old Cordeliers quarter.[9] He adapted the magnificent Academy of Surgery Building to its new role as the Paris Health School, helped change the former Cordelier convent into an expanded Practical Dissection School, built laboratories, a library, lecture halls. Clinical medicine was establishing itself in the hallowed old Latin Quarter.

The Hospital Council thus discussed, directed, and financed adaptations, repairs, plant maintenance, renovations, and amenities aimed at comfort, cleanliness, and order. We read, for example, in the 1816 report on Cochin Hospital that

> between 1803 and 1805, the council had fifty new bedsteads built, the old doors and windows replaced by new ones, and everything covered with three coats of oil paint. . . . A pharmacy and laboratory were rebuilt, or rather built, and two bathrooms for both sexes, with eight copper tubs. . . . The dining rooms and kitchens were enlarged and furnishing bought or repaired. New pipes were laid and stoves placed so as to improve and facilitate service. The roof, pavement, and walls were entirely rebuilt and all wards scraped and whitewashed.
>
> [No important changes occurred in 1806–1809.] In 1810, the Sisters of St. Martha were called in as nurses. The need for appropriate lodgings and comfort required some new arrangements of space and accessibility, a refectory and parlor, a larger linen-room. Linen, bedding, clothing, and some other things were bought for the Sisters and the entire establishment whitewashed—an expense [that had been] deferred for several years.[10]

At Necker Hospital, Camus reported, "the vegetable garden, tended under Sister Clavelot's care, yielded both greens and economies." At

Cochin, "the garden has been planted to benefit the patients. Last year [1802], fruit abounded and convalescents profited from this handsomely, eating dishes more appetizing than dried beans and prunes."[11]

The reports of Camus and Pastoret focus on achievements, but many projects could not be implemented for lack of money: Bicêtre should not combine the functions of hospital, prison, and hospice: the indigents might be transferred to St. Denis or the prisoners to Vincennes. At the Salpêtrière, the women now busy in workshops had to eat there: a dining hall was needed. This was also lacking at the Incurable Women's Hospice, where the inmates still ate in their wards.[12]

To save money, François de Neufchâteau decided in December 1798 to employ contractors to provision the Paris hospitals. This system seemed preferable to "paternal" supervision by the hospital commissioners or to a half-way measure that allowed suppliers a share in any savings they effected beyond an agreed-upon ceiling price (régie interessée).[13] But were the contractors honest? No historian has as yet examined what deals were cut. Could the council effect savings? The councillors had serious misgivings about buying furnishings and supplies from contractors. For eighteen months, beginning on 10 March 1802."[16] The announcement of a deadline stemmed from Frochot's authority and set a new tone. The manual's minute specifications left service manual (cahier des charges) stipulated the suppliers' obligations precisely.[14] It "gives a faithful picture of all the hospitals' needs regarding service, food, clothing, linen, heating, and all other objects of daily maintenance" and invites comparison with the conditions the Poverty Committee encountered in 1790 and with the suggestions Tenon made in 1786 to improve the inpatients' experience.[15]

A foremost objective was to establish a definitive number of single beds for each hospital: "the double beds still in existence at the Hôtel-Dieu, Bicêtre and other hospices shall be eliminated . . . by 20 June 1802."[16] The announcement of a deadline stemmed from Frochot's authority and set a new tone. The manual's minute specifications left manufacturers and agents little leeway for shoddy work. The following guidelines for single beds provide a telling example: the new beds were to have wooden frames (not metal, as Tenon had advocated) measuring 195 x 81 cm and contain two mattresses, one filled with 19 kg of straw, the other with a mixture of two-thirds wool and one-third horsehair, weighing 11 kg; a bolster filled with goose feathers and covered with ticking, 81 cm in length and 97 cm in girth, weighing 5 lbs.; two white woolen blankets, 290 x 170 cm, weighing 7½ lbs.; three pairs of sheets of Alençon linen, 295 x 168 cm; a feather pillow covered with ticking, weighing 3 lbs., with three pillow covers and two drawsheets. Also, each patient was to be provided with a plate, a bowl, two drinking cups, a basin, a urinal, a chamber pot, a mess kit, a tin spoon, and a metal spittoon.[17]

The laundry and cleaning schedule was equally specific, although skimpy from our point of view: "The covers and beds of the able-bodied inmates shall be washed annually in Floréal," the manual prescribed, "those of the patients and women in childbed in Germinal and Fructidor; the mattresses of the able-bodied beaten once a year, those of the patients twice." Concerning disinfection, the manual specified that "the suppliers must heat the patients' clothing in a special oven to destroy vermin, boil their linen in hot water, and return these clean and white at the time of the patient's discharge."

Food was prescribed with loving care. As in the past, the ingredients of the meat and vegetable broth warranted elaborate attention. The meat received ceremonious treatment: under the eyes of the supplier, double the weight of the cooked meat was to be deposited in the huge pot, with two litres of water per 500 grams of meat, "sufficient salt, and carrots, parsnips, onions, leeks, and celery weighing one-tenth of the raw meat." The pot was then padlocked [eloquent commentary on the prevalence of pilfering], and would simmer for nine to ten hours, so as to reduce the water to a quarter of the original volume. The vegetarian soup, made with barley, potatoes, or lima beans and the same vegetables as the meat soup, contained the luxury of four pounds of butter per one hundred diners. The wine would, of course, be carefully tasted.

Some recurrent complaints finally found a hearing, for the rules specify that the sheets be hung up to dry, "far away from the wards, so that the smell of wet linen is not perceptible there and does not hinder air circulation," and that clean sheets "shall be dry when they are put on the beds." Clearly, nuisances persisted.[18]

The specifications regarding supplies, food, and cleanliness do not differ much from the old regime's attempt to feed its indigent patients frugal rations in decent surroundings and nurse them in a dignified manner. But some differences are striking: first, the single beds and dry sheets. Mainly the invidious distinctions in quality and size of portions are gone, except when ordered by the doctor for medical reasons. Employees ate the same food as the patients. For St. Antoine Hospital, the 1803 report states, for example: "Nurses and maids eat together in the dining hall. . . . Staff members who receive free board eat in the common refectory."[19] Another noteworthy new requirement concerned the role of the doctor. He "alone determines when convalescence has begun," and medical factors regulated all aspects of patient comfort. The doctor decided whether the stove should burn later than usual, when the beds needed a special cleaning or the pots and pans re-tinning. The Sisters are not mentioned in these rules. Frugality persisted, for the budget was tight. The rules specified, for example, that bedclothes and personal linen would be renewed by one-eighth annually. At the same time, however, some traditional measures of economy were forbidden: under no circumstances could convalescents be employed; there would be one nurse per twelve patients, or even ten, if judged necessary. The council expected the suppliers to submit a detailed budget report every month.[20]

The comparative experience of provisioning by the council's own directives rather than by contractors during the initial eighteen months clearly indicated savings of about 20 percent.[21] Accordingly, the council took complete control at the end of September 1803, thereby reducing expenses from 7.7 million francs in 1800 to under 6 million. An agent now traveled to inspect the hospitals' farms and woods, verifying that tenant farmers replanted and repaired their holdings as stipulated in their contracts. In Paris, the hospitals still owned 731 buildings that were impossible to supervise and costly in repairs and taxes, according to Camus, who advised that they be sold.[22] The hospitals' share in the reinstituted municipal toll yielded 5 million francs a year; the amusement tax, 500,000; and investment in the city pawnshop about 200,000. "Under the old regime," concluded Frochot, "the hospitals had perhaps more independence; under the new regime, they have just as much security."[23] But patients themselves might contribute to their own comfort, to the quality of their surroundings, the hospital budget, and to their own progress toward the status of citizen-patients. The councillors expressed three wishes: they wanted to provide cleanliness, order, and work.

Cleanliness is difficult to document, standards being relative and culturally determined. To take one example: the new rules demanded that the floors be swept three times daily. This tells us that, in 1803, they were not found clean enough; but were they properly swept thereafter? Offensive smells, which bothered our forefathers less than they do us, are also problematic. However, when "mephitic" or "putrid" air sent site visitors reeling, we can tell that more sweeping was indicated. To counteract noxious "exhalations" and "miasmata," the administrators practiced fumigation or whitewashed walls, which, Pastoret reports, had not been done in thirty years at the Charité. Neither had the bedsteads been repainted. "Smoke had blackened the walls, windows, ceilings, staircases, reception rooms, doctor's offices, and wards. This gave the hospital an air of sadness that distressed the patients."[24] From time to time, the modern reader is shocked by the primitive condition of old buildings, where "sinks and drainage pipes are urgently needed for each ward [of the new Pitié Hospital], since the soiled water now flows down the stairs and rots them, or through the latrines and fills these up."[25] The need for water is constantly reiterated, but in the context of washing floors and bedclothes, rather than patients. Bathtubs were used for therapeutic, not hygienic, purposes. At the dermatologic center of St. Louis, for example, 120 baths were given daily—200 by 1816—to control eczemas and rashes. Fourteen new copper tubs were in constant use, filled with medicated water. How regularly this water was changed cannot be ascertained from the documents. Personal linen was changed once a week, and sheets once a month, a questionable level of cleanliness by our standards.

In contrast to cleanliness, order is easy to pinpoint. It stemmed from those single, more widely spaced beds of identical dimensions to facilitate nursing, medical rounds, and supervision; identical inpatient clothing so as to intercept unwanted visitors and unauthorized outings; daily charts of admissions and discharges; careful case history and autopsy reports, leading to statistical analyses of morbid phenomena; weekly accounts from each hospital administrator regarding disbursements. "The prefect and the council" concludes Frochot's biographer, "realized with astonished pride that they had created order."[26]

Remunerated labor occupied only 6 percent of the women and 10 percent of the men when the council began its reforms. By 1803, Camus reports, the needs of citizen-patients were better met because workshops for weavers, tailors, and shoe-, button-, and toymakers had been established or reestablished at Bicêtre, apprenticeships for boys at the Pitié were more closely supervised, and a large sewing room had been set up at the Salpêtrière.[27] The savings remained low, as expected, but the councillors argued that work raised morale and improved the patients' "state of mind and behavior."[28] Camus even claimed that "cleanliness, work, and activity introduced into the hospices have lessened the incidence of illness." At St. Louis, where dermatologic afflictions left patients of all ages ambulatory, work was "a great advantage . . . patients who work recover more quickly." Sometimes the inmates volunteered, as when men from Bicêtre whitewashed the walls of the Necker and Venereal Diseases Hospitals at half the price estimated by the painters.[29]

Work was thus more readily available after 1801, but physicians and nurses needed to be reminded periodically that patient welfare must be their first concern. In fact, we find these admonitions reiterated in the "Regulations for the Health Service in Paris Hospitals" of 10 February 1802. These were rules that the nursing orders had long followed, and they echoed the government's draft regulations for infirmaries of 1781, and Drs. Colombier and Doublet's recommendations of 1785. They underlined that patient comfort must override the claims of religion or research.

Object Lesson: The Inpatient in the Teaching Ward

In the first eighteen months of the Hospital Council's existence, the admitting office at the Hôtel-Dieu hospitalized 21,888 women, men, and children, while an additional 16,143 persons gained direct entrance to Paris hospitals, pleading urgency. During the Consulate and Empire, the average total number of annual hospitalizations in Paris reached 32,500, of whom the admitting office processed two-thirds (see Appendix C, Table C.3, for the figures given in Pastoret's report). The new inpatients and the administrators soon learned that physicians and surgeons now applied medical criteria, not only at the entrance door, but at every phase of the patients' hospital experience.

Under the new regulations of 10 February 1802 (4 Ventôse, Year X), the inpatient saw the doctor twice a day: in the morning, the chief made rounds, beginning at seven or earlier; in the afternoon, he usually sent an assistant.[30] The regulations specified that he must serve on the same ward for one year; and for six months on chronic wards (art. 6, par. 114). For the patients, this carried the reassurance that their doctor would stay with them for a long time. With the chief came intern and pharmacist, carrying charts where patients figured with numbers indicating diet and medication. The patient received a regular or fat-free diet, with portions varying from full to three-quarters, half, or one-quarter, including bread and wine. An important new provision concerned the omnipresence, around the clock, of interns on duty. Like the nurse in earlier days, they could "not leave their post under any pretext for twenty-four hours, . . . had to cope with emergencies, care for the wounded . . . and make rounds at specified times" (art. 5, pars. 74–75).

Convalescents could stay a maximum of ten days and go out during their last three days to arrange for living quarters and look for a job (art. 7, par. 121), a thoughtful arrangement pioneered by the Brothers of Charity. The regulations also instituted a quarterly review to be sure that no unauthorized persons lived at the hospital (art. 5, pars. 76–79).

The Regulations mention an "*infirmier*" and "*infirmière*" in passing, without explanation. The Hospital Council, Frochot, and Chaptal counted on the availability of nursing personnel, particularly the Catholic orders. Inpatients experienced a difference in daily nursing care, for the person in charge was no longer a solicitous, often older, woman for whom the patient's meals and comfort were overarching preoccupations. The sight of nuns in religious garb now gave way to that of young civilians in street clothing (white coats were unknown), who proffered medical ministrations. Instead of constant "mothering," the patient experienced the more or less cavalier intervention of young doctors.

Regular meetings of the Hospital Council with the medical staff and the head midwife began on 2 and 5 June 1803.[31] The councillors never conferred with the nurses. The doctors complimented the councillors about the improved quality of the food and then listed their criticisms: the rules were not being observed; patients were not bathed when admitted; there were not enough nurses; the students were inattentive and ignorant; convalescents needed separate wards; amputees should receive special postoperative care; autopsies should be routine; tables of morbidity and mortality should be more regularly kept.[32] If the councillors hoped for new suggestions, they were surely disappointed. Did the physicians in turn ask for the councillors's observations? The answers would have shocked them, for we have every reason to regard Duchanoy's misgivings about the medical service being a "stumbling block" as typical of his colleagues' opinions.

Under the new regulations, inpatients entering the hospital faced probing examination by the head physician or surgeon-in-chief, who "alone confirmed their admission and assigned them to a ward." If denied hospitalization, patients were sent away before morning rounds—that is, before 7 A.M.[33] In practice, mercy often tempered these Draconian regulations. "In case of doubt," states the report of the Year XII, "charity dictates that the patient be admitted."[34] Or, with regard to inmates of the Incurable Women's Hospital: "The council felt it would be inhumane to reverse previous decisions or to demand the expulsion of persons admitted on flimsy evidence."[35]

The admitting interview was particularly thorough for assignment to teaching wards because the young doctor knew that he might have to present the new patient to his chief and colleagues: he needed plentiful information. The only official teaching services were located at the Hôtel-Dieu and the Charité; a third at the Hospice de perfectionnement never opened for want of an appropriate locale. Therefore "France never had a university clinic."[36] But unofficial or "free" clinical teaching proliferated, at the Salpêtrière, St. Louis, Maternité, and Children's hospitals.[37]

Bedside teaching made the inpatient the center of attention. Herman Boerhaave, the admired originator of modern clinical teaching, assigned twelve patients to such a service, Corvisart forty, and Pinel thirty. Students came daily to observe, to learn exactly what changes to look for, to watch and to listen as the professor used the patient to demonstrate the signs and symptoms and explain the natural history of each disease. Pinel suggested that some wards group only patients with the same illness so students could observe the gradations and complications of a single disease.[38] How demoralizing it must have been for patients to learn from their neighbors how their illness might worsen and even prove fatal! But such considerations do not seem to have occurred to the Revolutionary doctors.

Leading clinicians all over Europe made special arrangements for the care of patients in teaching wards, assigning one or two advanced students to look after each patient and report to the professor on rounds.[39] For clinical learning, there was no organization more important than the innovative and exclusive Society for Medical Instruction founded at the Charité on 29 May 1801 by Corvisart. Meant for fourth-year students and their elders, and directed by J. J. Leroux des Tillets (1749–1832) and Gaspard Laurent Bayle (1774–1816),[40] the society provided rigorously structured clinical experience, heralding later nineteenth-century developments. Here the inpatient underwent the strictest admitting interview and continuing close scrutiny. For each patient, the young doctor in charge had to present the supervising professor with a brief, standardized admission record; initial observations (which the mentor would review and, if necessary, revise); daily records on a chart; and, lastly, a summary of the illness and autopsy. By 1818, over five thousand cases had been recorded. Nothing comparable had ever been attempted before. The admission of patients and their assignment to specific wards, long under the authority of a young assistant, developed into the position of chief of service.[41] When autopsies became routine, the full-time positions of prosector and prosector's aide were added to the ranks.[42] Among the earliest members of the Society for Medical Instruction were two outstanding clinical investigators of the early nineteenth century, François Magendie (1783–1855) and René Théophile Hyacinthe Laënnec.[43]

It is thus clear that inpatients paid a price for the good medical care they now received and their new creature comforts. The intern in charge might come several times a day and explain to a group of students the signs and symptoms of a disease they were seeing for the first time: malaria, jaundice, scurvy; ulcers; a fracture or a malformation that required surgery; the manifestations of syphilis or sclerema neonatorum; of depression, delusions, or hysteria. Then the physician-in-chief would come on "grand" rounds and demonstrate the "case," expose the patient's body to general view, palpate, percuss, and auscultate; point, demonstrate, and discuss. He might be gentle and sympathetic, or he might ignore the frightened, shivering person.

These doctors used patients not only to teach their students, but for research as well. Even though the numerical method had been practiced for some years abroad (in Edinburgh and London, for instance), medical statistics could not have emerged without the hundreds of citizen-patients aligned on Parisian teaching wards. Sheer numbers amounted to a qualitative difference.

Did these doctors experiment on their patients? Undoubtedly, as they always do, with regard to medication and diet, trying new drugs and dosages, varied foods or therapeutic strategies. The postgraduate hospital had the traditional mission of checking on new procedures and medications. Did doctors conduct dangerous experiments? That question is not easy to answer. An example concerning smallpox inoculation may be considered typical and illustrate the attitude of both doctors and patients.

A smallpox epidemic in the Year VI prompted the Paris Health School to conduct a public "inoculation clinic"—that is, teach a public course, demonstrate the technique, and make inoculation available to the working class. Medical students supervised the inoculated children and kept careful journals. The report calls this undertaking the "first inoculation clinic ever to exist," a claim that needs substantiation.[44]

This project raises several points germane to the general question explored in this book: the two doctors, Leroux and Pinel, used public wards from the St. Antoine orphanage and the Salpêtrière—young citizen-patients—for their experiment. And they reported their every move to the assembly of the medical school professors and proceeded only with the minister's permission.[45] "We considered the children as appropriate subjects to add to the available proofs that there is no recurrence in smallpox, or only in extraordinarily rare cases," the doctors reported. "We inoculated each of them with fresh pus inserted by six pinpricks; they remained for nineteen days in the infected ward, . . . in physical touch with the smallpox patients, their beds and clothing, and sharing their play and meals. . . . They did not contract smallpox."[46]

At the end of their report, the authors mention further experiments they wished to try, among them "the inoculation of vaccine."[47] This was September 1799: the news of Edward Jenner's discovery had just reached Paris. The medical school launched experiments as soon as vaccine arrived from London.

The smallpox clinic of the Year VI was not the only such experiment conducted under the Health School's aegis that put the citizen-patient at risk. A "ringworm clinic" with six beds was set up at the postgraduate hospital that same year, and another at St. Louis in 1809–1813. There, 795 children were treated with Mahon's depilatory cream, which cured 527, while 196 had relapses.[48] In the Year VII an experiment involving forty patients was tried at Cullerier's Venereal Diseases Hospital: ten patients were inoculated with syphilis, ten with "sporic disease," and twenty used as controls. And experimental therapy for mental patients was carried on at Charenton Hospice (see Chapter 9).

In all these cases, the decision to subject these citizen-patients to new or risky procedures for the advancement of knowledge and for the benefit of society was taken on their behalf by medical men convinced that the action was justified. They took it for granted that inpatients should serve to train young doctors. Trials of new medications and therapies occurred frequently and they involved risks. We have no evidence that physicians, around 1800, felt it necessary to ask for a citizen-patient's informed consent.

The citizen hospitalized at public expense thus performed a hitherto rare public service. We have no documentation about the patients' feelings with regard to their new role: it would be as risky to conjecture resentment as it is to posit pride in a new usefulness. It was undoubtedly frightening to see doctors and students crowd around the bed and proceed to repeated and detailed examinations, and to be carried into an amphitheater for surgery, knowing that, whether one died on the operating table or in bed, one's body would be subject to autopsy. Without doubt the new "hospital medicine" permanently altered the citizen-patient's role, and what had been exceptional gradually became the rule.

From the doctor's point of view, the patient also took on a different "look," as Michel Foucault has so brilliantly argued in *The Birth of the Clinic*. With his "gardener's look," the physician viewed individual patients as specimens that represented stages or aspects of one disease; then, with his "chemist's look," he analyzed and experimented *on* a "case," rather than *with* a sick person. After the patient died, there remained an instructive body.

◆◆◆

"Paris had been the capital of the cadaver ever since the mid eighteenth century," writes Pierre Huard.[49] Cadavers were needed at the Practical Dissection School, across the street from the new Health School: this establishment's enrollment rose from twenty-four students when it was founded in 1750, to 120 students in 1799, working in six new dissection pavilions.[50] At the Hôtel-Dieu, the students' attention had, since Pierre Joseph Desault's day, been directed to postmortem examination, and at the Charité clinical school, after 1800, Corvisart autopsied every dead patient. Xavier Bichat performed this procedure on six hundred patients in twenty-one months: the results of his investigations form the basis of his five books; G. L. Bayle's research on pulmonary phthisis was based on nine hundred cases; and Laënnec undertook twenty-two autopsies in September–October 1822 alone.[51] By assembling a great many pathologic data, doctors gradually came to understand how a disease attacked the bodies of women, men, children, and babies and gained new ways of interpreting the signs and symptoms of living patients in the clinical setting.

The practice of this "pathological anatomy" required appropriate facilities, but exiguous hospital quarters and academic favoritism literally forced ambitious young physicians to find their own locales and means. In the late eighteenth century, Paris had fifteen private dissection "amphitheaters." The best were run by well-known surgeons, such as Desault, who pioneered a dissection course in 1766, first on rue Domat, then on rue des Lavandières, near the place Maubert. He had room for from fifty to sixty cadavers and attracted nearly two hundred students.[52] After him, Philippe Jean Pelletan, Pierre Lassus, Raphaël Bienvenu Sabatier, Alexis Boyer, and Bichat all ran paying dissection schools. These did not require licensing by the police, and neither were they subject to inspection. Those are the main reasons why they were widely criticized for years and finally abolished in 1813. The faculty, from then on, controlled all dissections.

Traditionally, it was "in their rooms or in attic corners that dedicated students . . . were forced to study cadavers they had furtively procured."[53] A teacher rented the upper floor (the least expensive) of some run-down private house, drew the shades in order not to scandalize the neighbors, and set to work. October to March was the appropriate time for these courses, but would-be teachers encountered one crucial difficulty: they had no legal access to cadavers.

The eager researchers' need for bodies was limitless. No expedient could fill it, certainly not the time-honored practice of robbing graves. We read, for example, that Bichat supervised 130 students at dissection, four to one cadaver: surely more than thirty corpses could not regularly be robbed from cemeteries. Such an undertaking was laborious, risky, and expensive. Laborious because digging up a grave in the dark of night is hard, unpleasant work; risky because of a possible confrontation with the police, as happened to Bichat and Dubois; expensive because that is the nature of illegal expedients.

The quest for legal "subjects" has a long history. In 1760, the government empowered the Practical Dissection School to buy two bodies every ten days, for twenty-seven livres the pair. In 1768, the king ordered the Salpêtrière, which was under his jurisdiction, to provide a few cadavers to the Dissection School.[54] But the Hôtel-Dieu, the main potential source of "subjects," steadfastly refused—a stance to be expected from nuns. To a believer, dissection and dispersal of a person's limbs created confusion on Resurrection Day. The nuns deemed dissection an outrage.

Under the Republic, the government did prevail and regulate the supply of cadavers. "The Great Hospice of Humanity [Hôtel-Dieu] and the Hospice of Unity [Charité] are specially designated to supply [the medical school] and the other public establishments," proclaimed a decree of 19 November 1798 (29 Brumaire, Year VII) drawn up by Dean Thouret. "The school shall have first choice in all the other hospices, to obtain all the varieties of age, sex, constitution needed for the progress of its research" (art. 7). Dean Leroux reported in 1813 that "1,320 cadavers were brought to the anatomy pavilions in the seven months when dissections were scheduled. They served the faculty's needs, in lectures, examinations, study sessions, and preparations. They were used in teaching 654 students how to dissect, and 96 students how to operate. If there had not been a shortage of subjects, a much larger number of students could have practiced anatomy and surgery."[55]

If the medical school was short of cadavers, how could the private courses and laboratories manage? The answer clearly emerges from a look at a street map of the Place Maubert area. The addresses of all the amphitheaters: rue des Lavandières (Desault's school), rue des Carmes (Bichat's laboratory), rue des Anglais, des trois Portes, de la Huchette, du Fouarre, du Coeur Volant: these are all located a few steps from the rue de la Bûcherie. A large, heavy door on that street led to the hall where the Hôtel-Dieu collected its dead and sewed them into sacks. Each cadaver fetched twenty francs.

If we examine the registers of the Hôtel-Dieu in the years 1801–1815, we find over five thousand deaths a year. The regulations required that the bodies claimed by relatives be handed to them for burial. Prudence demanded quick disposal of the victims of contagious diseases. But there can be no doubt that thousands of cadavers dissected in the amphitheaters came from the Hôtel-Dieu. These were the bodies of citizen-patients who had served as object lessons when alive. They now served as objects when dead.

The inpatients' new role thus affected their hospital stay at every turn long before they paid the final price. They also helped impart new directions to medicine because their triage into groups created new perceptions for the attending physicians.

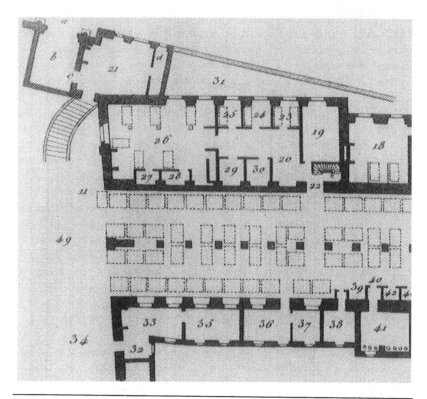

FIGURE 6.4. The morgue at the Hôtel-Dieu, southeast corner, ground floor. From Jacques Tenon, *Mémoires sur les hôpitaux de Paris* (Paris: Pierres, 1788), pl. 9. a: large entranceway, rue de la Bûcherie. b: entrance. c: door. d: storage. 11: door to 25-step staircase from ground floor to cadaver depository. 19: featherbed storage. 21: depository for cadavers. 23: room for two attendants of men's clothing. 24, 25: rooms for saddlers. 26: shrouding room. 27, 28: shrouders' utility closets. 29, 30: room and closet for ward service.

Segregation: The Growth of Medical Specialties

The first specialized hospital to open its doors during the Revolution treated patients suffering from venereal diseases. Over the course of ten years, all of these patients in Paris—men from Bicêtre; women from the Salpêtrière, including pregnant ones; babies and wet nurses with syphilis transferred from Vaugirard Hospital; infected prostitutes and prisoners sent by the police—were sent to the 550-bed Venereal Diseases Hospital in the faubourg St. Jacques. By 1802 the transfers were complete.[56] The new hospital was a model institution, according to Camus, with large gardens and an adequate staff of fifty-nine, under Michel Jean Cullerier (1758–1827) as surgeon-in-chief and René J. H. Bertin (1757–1828) as physician-in-chief.[57]

Given the frequency of simultaneous infection with syphilis and gonorrhoea, it is small wonder that eighteenth-century doctors were unable to make differential diagnoses and called both "syphilis." At the turn of the nineteenth century, admissions to the Venereal Diseases Hospital remained fairly stable, with empty beds a rarity. But numbers are deceptive: patients frequently ran away—no fewer than eighty-nine in eighteen months during 1793–1794. These escapes may well be related to peaks in admissions: fifty-five in the week of 24–31 August 1793, for example. But then, the call for national conscription (*levée en masse*) was issued on 23 August, so treatment for venereal disease may not have been the real objective of all those who sought hospitalization.

While fear of the draft may have motivated admissions, fear of the treatment made patients run away; they knew that physicians used mercury, the specific remedy against syphilis, in large doses and that the side effects were often frightening. These may range from swollen or ulcerated gums and loss of teeth to vomiting, abdominal pain, and colitis or nephritis, to nervous manifestations ranging from tremors to seizures or dementia. C. Berthollier, a recent historian of the Paris Venereal Diseases Hospital, calculates that the average patient received rubs with 120–150 grams of mercurial ointment over forty days, and from two to four "Sedillot's pills" a day (these contained mercury and either sarsaparilla, honey, liquorice, or marshmallow). The exact dosage of mercury is not known but the quantities were high, and even Cullerier recommended hot baths to stimulate sweating and promote the elimination of excess medication.[58]

Once patients began treatment, they had to stay until it was completed. Camus comments: "Supervision is necessarily a bit strict in an establishment such as this. The patients' health demands it, and so do decency and morality. . . . The men are employed in their habitual trades, the women kept busy with spinning, knitting, and shredding linen. *A lock-up room is used to incarcerate persons who create disturbances*" (emphasis added).[59] On admission, a woman would be judged according to her dress and demeanor and assigned to one of three wards: one for prostitutes, one for mothers with infants, and one for other respectable women. Physicians treated them in different ways: as subjects for investigation or with kindness, as citizen-patients.

We owe most of what we know about prostitution in Revolutionary and Napoleonic Paris to A. J. B. Parent-Duchâtelet (1790–1836), who published the epoch-making history of the subject, *De la prostitution dans la ville de Paris,* in 1836. It is a sympathetic account. Parent-Duchâtelet knew the history of prostitution in Paris well. As early as 1780, Police Commissioner Lenoir had founded four "houses" where prostitutes were subjected to medical checkups. Parent estimated that 15,000 to 30,000 prostitutes plied their trade in Paris under the Revolution and Empire, even though only 13,000 of them were registered. He could not say how many of them were infected with venereal disease.[60] The city of Paris and the Revolutionary assemblies repeatedly issued legislation aimed at controlling this contagious infection, but with poor results.[61] The Law of 23 May 1802 (3 Prairial, Year X) established police dispensaries in Paris, and the police rounded up what women they could and forced them to register and undergo periodic examination.[62]

To examine the women, Parent-Duchâtelet tells us, doctors had to be careful to treat them like ladies. They could not use a table for the examination because the ladies would not take off their hats. So they devised an elevated armchair that tilted backward. Visits took about two minutes. That was enough to see whether mouth and throat, vagina, cervix, and anus were free of telltale sores. If diseased, the women would be hospitalized and treated.[63] Thus Paris now had a routine for the identification of infected women. They were incarcerated until freed by the venereologist's verdict, after an average period of 65–70 days, "as if," comments Parent-Duchâtelet, "one had the right thus to dispose of individual freedom and to force people to undergo treatments they find repugnant."[64]

Both Cullerier and Bertin wrote about venereal disease in infants, and Bertin's explicit title indicates the focus of his research on the possible transmission of the disease between infant and nurse.[65] Bertin describes four wards with five to ten beds for mothers (or wet nurses) and double that number of cribs for infants. These numbers indicate that the method tried at Vaugirard in the 1780s was continued here: young mothers with diseased babies stayed on as wet nurses, provided they agreed to service a second infant. Bertin describes the women as "tender, gentle, and sensitive, they devoted all their time to the care of their own infants and those we entrusted to them. . . . They overcame the disgust and repugnance that the infected nurslings aroused in some, and identified with them. . . . If the baby died, they mourned their loss for a long time." Bertin gives mortality figures, for the years around 1800, indicating that only one half of an average of 164 babies survived. But for how long? Nobody knew. "We lose sight of them," wrote Bertin.[66]

◆◆◆

In addition to their special interest in women and babies, the reformers fostered outpatient treatment, and they opened a small private hospital for paying patients. As early as 1790, the duc de la Rochefoucauld-Liancourt had suggested an outpatient clinic where peasants from the suburbs could receive free care, while wealthy patrons' fees subsidized the poor. By 1803 the Hospital Council estimated that at least 10–12,000 Parisians suffered from venereal diseases, and noted that the clinic aided "a large number of patients at low cost, help is never delayed, and the disease is attacked at its origins." [67] But the council noticed that mainly men availed themselves of these facilities, whereas women seemed reticent.

That is one reason why the council decided to open a private hospital for syphilitics. What was working well at the Dubois Clinic, Ste. Périnne, the Maison la Rochefoucauld, and Esquirol's small private hospital now gave rise to an institution for paying customers afflicted with syphilis—an unprecedented development. In 1809 the Hospital Council bought a house adjoining the Venereal Diseases Hospital and secured Cullerier's services as medical director. There were sixty-two beds in twenty-five rooms, fourteen of them single. Patients had to pay the rent, which ranged from 2½ to 3 and 5 francs, two weeks in advance. They had to take all their meals at the hospital and were not allowed to tip employees. Each patient received two clean sheets and pillow cases every two weeks. In the years 1809 to 1813, the census of women grew from 4 to 33, that of men from 43 to 269. This venture was a success, even with women. [68]

Despite the doctors' interest, clinical teaching lagged. Cullerier, a dull lecturer, lacked a professorial appointment and thus could not aspire to a clinical teaching service; his writings concerning surgical cases and the relationship of syphilis to gonorrhoea evidently left students uninterested; but the main reason was that access to his hospital was strictly limited. [69] Porters "prevented patients from leaving and . . . strangers from entering." [70] Few students persisted. And yet the homogeneous inpatient population of syphilitic babies, women, and men would have facilitated research.

Interesting developments also took place at St. Louis, which was transformed during our era into a leading center for dermatology. According to a now familiar pattern, the Paris Hospital Council, wishing to "create order" (and not disinclined to follow past trends), decided on 27 November 1801 that one establishment should henceforth group "chronic diseases, either contagious like scabies and ringworm, or stubborn and cachectic like herpes, scurvy, ulcers, or scrofula." St.

Louis Hospital would best fill this role, it was decided, since its architecture permitted the total segregation of inmates. Patients would be sent there by the admitting office or transferred from other hospitals, in particular the Children's Hospital and the Pitié orphanage. The Hospital Council decided that St. Louis required repairs to improve the water supply; laundry lines far from the inner courtyards; and larger windows that could actually be opened and that were set low enough to permit air circulation between the beds.[71]

In 1803, St. Louis had a patient census of 600–700, and 158 service personnel, two physicians, two surgeons, one pharmacist, and thirteen interns, all living in the hospital "because of the location, and the nature of the illnesses treated there." As for physicians, here was an opportunity to specialize: Jean Louis Alibert (1768–1838) decided on a career in dermatology.[72] He took over the outpatient clinic and founded the first teaching service in dermatology. Alibert's "wish to create at St. Louis a special service and a great school of dermatology were realized in the nineteenth century, more fully than [he] could ever have supposed," concludes a historian.[73]

St. Louis was much larger than Cullerier's hospital, with three times the service personnel, twice as many doctors and thirteen interns. Beyond creating busy outpatient departments for children as well as adults, however, St. Louis did not contribute to liberating patients from routine and demeaning treatment.

◆◆◆

A different picture derives from the study of the Salpêtrière, where we can detect the early practice of geriatic medicine.[74] Upon his arrival as physician-in-chief in 1795, Pinel asked for a census of inmates. They numbered 7,523: Salpêtrière Hospice still housed some 3,500 aged, needy able-bodied women; about 1,100 who were mentally ill or epileptic; well over 1,000 blind, paralytic, or otherwise disabled patients; and an equal number with cancers, ulcers, and open sores; it also provided special accommodation for servants and retired employees. The hospice produced an endless stream of acutely ill patients, who filled the infirmaries, where they were "piled up without order, a prey to the rapacity and ineptitude of subordinate personnel."[75] One of Pinel's first actions was to establish or reestablish infirmary divisions, subsections, and wards so as properly to isolate the acutely and seriously ill from the convalescents. By 1804, the Paris Hospital Council had provided for workrooms for sewing, knitting, and lace-making; arrangements for a little gardening; renovation of the laundry (for fifty thousand sheets!); improved preparation of the food; and a separate dining room for the employees.

A remarkable aspect of Pinel's medical attitude toward the thousands of aged women in his care over a period of thirty years was that he considered aging a natural phenomenon and the frailties of old age as normal occurrences, and he recognized that certain illnesses and impairments become more serious, bothersome, and even chronic with old age. He listed paralyses and hernias, which impede movement; uterine complaints and diarrhoea, which further weaken an aged person; blindness, which entails utter dependency; and consumption and carcinomas, which may hasten death.[76] He also adhered to basic principles that made him an early practitioner of geriatrics.[77] First, he identified certain diseases as specific to old age: pulmonary catarrh headed his list, and for six out of eight patients over 60 suffering from this disease, it proved fatal. Combined with gastric or "adynamic" fever, it killed three out of six patients over 60 and left one in a "long and difficult convalescence."[78] Pinel also knew that some diseases present different signs and symptoms in the elderly; also, they may be multiple and influence each other, so that some symptoms may be masked. He singled out peripneumonia, where often, in the elderly, only slight inflammatory signs are present.

Pinel did not, however, develop a special geriatric therapy. He set down his guiding principles in his essay on "The Clinical Training of Doctors" (1793). Essentially he believed that the physician should not interfere with nature, but should aid her healing powers; supervise the hospital kitchen as much as the pharmacy; prefer natural and mild remedies; administer purgatives, emetics, sudorifics, stimulants, enemas, tonics, and soporifics with low dosages of active ingredients, and resort but rarely to bleeding. He adhered to this plan for patients of all ages. The main exception was that frequently, almost routinely, he ordered one grain of tartar emetic, and very occasionally some opium, quinine, vesicatories, or leeches. Mainly we read about the expectant method and anodyne palliatives to soothe fevers and inflammations: a little diluted wine or absinthe; infusions of lime-blossom tea, chicory, camomile, gentian, or linseed; barley water with honey; plasters with mustard, marshmallow, or theriaca,—and, for one fever patient, lemonade, and snow on the head.[79]

Pinel thus raised the aging and ailing inmates of the Salpêtrière to the dignified status of medical patients. He gave them a physician's serious attention, even though he knew that he could not cure them. They were destined to die in his hospital. He accepted that fact, and acted on his belief in the physician's obligation to attend to the process of dying as a normal manifestation of human existence.

◆◆◆

The hospitalization of venereal, dermatologic, and geriatric patients and their care were a significant development in the social and medical history of Paris at the turn of the nineteenth century. The Hospital Council's policy of purposeful triage furthered medical science, while the council constantly watched over and sought to improve the living conditions, comfort, and morale of the inpatient. But patients could be sorted in other ways than by medical triage, possibly in ways more helpful to the maintainance or recovery of their health and the eventual assumption of their responsibilities as citizens. We now turn to a group at risk of falling ill, namely, newborns and young children, whom the medical administrators and the doctors grouped by age rather than specific illness.

Clinical Specialization: Children at Risk

The direction in which our [modern] agencies have evolved in the past hundred and fifty years was laid down in the program of the Poverty Committee and La Rochefoucauld-Liancourt.

Jacques Dehaussy, *L'assistance publique à l'enfance:*
Les enfants abandonnés, 1951

The babies abandoned to public care constituted the heaviest burden for the Paris health authorities. The newborns at the Port-Royal Maternity Hospital were brought into the world by the same midwife as at the Hôtel-Dieu (Madame Lachapelle), but under healthier conditions and fuller medical attention. Nevertheless, their lives were at risk from the start, because 90 percent of the fatherless newborns were abandoned by their mothers. The wet-nursing office siphoned off the best nurses for paying customers and, as we shall see, artificial feeding made little progress. The councillors concentrated on measures that might save lives, such as prenatal care, the lying-in process, the prompt dispatch of healthy newborns to the country, and neonatal and pediatric services. The immediate task was to save lives, then to provide education and job training, and eventually to salvage citizen-patients. That hope gave meaning to the enormous effort.

Children who survived with foster parents in the countryside were usually returned to the Paris orphanage at age seven. We have no record of adoptions, the Poverty Committee's wishful thought. After at least five years, the children faced apprenticeship leading to independence—if they were healthy. We shall see that responsible doctors watched over them in the orphanage and that Paris opened a special hospital for them in 1802, the first Children's Hospital in the world.

191

Confined and Abandoned

Upon a prospective mother's admission to Port-Royal, she found herself assigned to one of four categories: women whose name must be kept secret, indigent married women, unmarried women domiciled in Paris, and unmarried women without a home address.[1] This traditional reception, similar to that provided for by the regulations at the Venereal Diseases Hospital, left leeway for the subjective judgment of the midwife and the administrators. For the first group, the Code spécial de la Maternité, adopted on 3–5 February 1801 (14–16 Pluviôse, Year IX), specified that secrets about the child would continue to be kept in a locked register in order, writes Camus, to "prevent crime, stop infanticides, suicides, and tawdry scandals."[2] Maternity hospice policy translated the third category into "unwed mothers whose demeanor conveyed seduction rather than profligacy," and the fourth category into "prostitutes."[3] The women remained segregated, and the code specified that women from the first category could not be used for teaching.[4]

All were poor and most unmarried. Births out of wedlock occurred with staggering frequency in Napoleonic France: in Paris alone they amounted to 30 percent in 1806 (6,282 out of 18,667) and rose to 42 percent in 1812 (8,530 out of 20,294).[5] Over one-third of these births took place at the Oratory. Provincial women made up 10 to 20 percent of all patients at the Paris maternity hospice: they traveled to Paris by the hundreds each year in search of anonymity, at a loss where else to give birth.[6] They sometimes arrived so exhausted and bedraggled that they had to be bathed immediately and clad in hospital garb. They "often suffered during pregnancy for want of wholesome and sufficient food," wrote Camus, "needing to regain strength as their term approached."[7] Their babies risked being premature and sickly.

The head midwife sometimes admitted the poorest before the ninth month and employed them in the kitchens and dining or sewing rooms.[8] The women lived in the newborn ward of the hospice—that is, at Port-Royal—under the stern rules spelled out in the code. They slept in one of 130 single beds, in dormitories that accommodated from eight to thirty. They rose at 7 A.M. and went to bed at 8 P.M., did chores, and ate well but were kept strictly in line: they could see visitors in the parlor twice a week, but from behind a partition. The code states flatly: "The pregnant women may not go out."[9] Punishments included deprivation of visiting privileges, since it was "essential that decency be observed."[10]

The pregnant women worked for minimal pay, caring for newborns or sewing; they had to furnish the needles and thread. For pay, they cut and stitched all the clothing for the children under the Found-lings' Hospice's jurisdiction and some for adults, as the following list indicates:[11]

men's shirt	20 sous
women's shirt	15 sous
delivery robe	10 sous
dress shirt	35 sous
day shirt	10 sous
dress	10 sous
pleated apron	10 sous
greatcoat	50 sous
sheet	20 sous
neckerchief	15 sous
petticoat	15 sous

Work helped "order and morality," Pastoret opined in 1816. The strict rules must have created a sober atmosphere, heightened by the antici-pation and anxiety that accompany the approach of childbirth.

When the moment of birth was at hand, the women were escorted from Port Royal to the Oratory. One can measure the distance (ap-proximately three long city blocks), since the buildings are standing today, and one can imagine the excruciating experience of a long walk for a woman in labor. Some, we are told, did not reach the delivery room in time and gave birth in the street. Arrived at the lying-in hos-pital, the woman found herself in "a building in every way perfect," wrote Camus, "with fresh air, quiet, space and a large garden," an impression the modern visitor can confirm.[12] The hospital had well-appointed labor and delivery rooms, and dormitories with 117 beds and 60 cribs, indicating that women stayed longer than babies, or more babies than women died. Madame Lachapelle was obligated by law to call the obstetrician, Baudelocque, later Dubois, if compli-cations arose and surgery was needed;[13] childbirth remained risky, and one out of twenty women at the maternity service died. François Chaussier supervised the women's overall health. The establishment had three adult infirmaries: for ill pregnant women, for midwives, and for wet nurses and domestics. Male servants who fell ill were taken to nearby Cochin Hospital.

A pregnant woman in this situation had probably decided before-hand what to do with her child. Auvity felt that "it was against their wish, yielding to bad examples and perfidious suggestions, that the women abandoned human beings who demanded from their mothers a sustenance prepared for them by nature herself."[14] The low average of 13.8 percent of babies taken home from the maternity hospice rep-

TABLE 7.1. Newborns Taken Home by Mothers, Paris
Maternity Hospice, 1804–1814

	Births	Number	Percentage
1804	1,624	206	12.9
1805	1,701	259	15.2
1806	1,642	218	13.3
1807	1,695	200	11.8
1808	1,690	224	13.2
1809	1,795	265	14.7
1810	1,814	287	15.8
1811	2,395	340	14.2
1812	2,450	323	13.2
1813	2,228	312	13.5

SOURCE: Seine, CGAHHCP, *Rapport fait au conseil général*
(1816), 101.

resents a negligible rise over the pre-Revolutionary era, when the average was 12 percent. Or, to put it differently, about two thousand young women a year—five or six a day—left the maternity hospice as they had come: alone. Pastoret writes that "more than two-thirds" returned to their homes in the provinces.[15] But he did not know either where they went or whether they had a home to return to, any more than we do.

Regarding childbed mortality at the Hôtel-Dieu, the figures are unfortunately inconclusive. Tenon gives the total for 1776–1786 as 1,142 out of 17,876, or 6.4 percent. But this applies only to women who died during the birth process. Once delivered, they were returned to the general St. Joseph ward, and the hospital lost sight of the individual patient. Tenon estimates the total mortality as 10 percent.[16] If we accept his figures, we must explain why mortality should have dropped to 4.4 percent after the transfer to Port-Royal. Credit should go to the supportive, preventive, hygienic, and managerial provisions rather than to sudden advances in medical, surgical, or therapeutic knowledge. Most important was the end of exposure to communicable diseases that made the Hôtel-Dieu such a dangerous locale. Better food, fresh air, and gardens enhanced the women's strength, while cleanliness curbed infection. One may also speculate that a friendlier environment and the serviceability of the numerous midwifery students lowered anxiety, thus aiding the natural process of childbirth by helping the women be less frightened and tense. Since they stayed an average of three weeks at the Babies' Hospice at the Oratory,[17] there was time for new advice to sink in. These factors may have helped

TABLE 7.2. Mortality of Women in Childbirth, Paris
Maternity Hospice, 1803–1813

	Deliveries	Deaths	
		Number	Percentage
1803	1,518	103	6.7
1804	1,624	55	3.3
1805	1,701	76	4.4
1806	1,642	114	6.9
1807	1,695	72	4.2
1808	1,690	60	3.5
1809	1,795	79	4.4
1810	1,814	75	4.1
1811	2,395	107	4.4
1812	2,450	163	6.6
1813	2,228	66	2.8

SOURCE: Seine, CGAHHCP, *Rapport fait au conseil général*
(1816), 100–103.

bring about the dramatic drop in stillbirths from 8 percent of all births
at the Hôtel-Dieu to 4.5 percent at the new maternity hospice (see
Appendix C, Tables C.4 and C.5). The savings in actual lives was
small, not quite one baby each week, yet a halving of stillbirths, to
a yearly average of forty-three, seems noteworthy. Better hygiene,
medical and nursing attention clearly bore fruit.

The worst killer of women in childbed was puerperal fever. Faced
with that disease, the staff remained helpless. They recognized it and
named it and knew it to be communicable, but did not know how to
stop it. Tenon makes the tantalizing observation that mortality from
puerperal fever at the Hôtel-Dieu was extremely high, but "less for
women who gave birth at home." He thus knew that something, or
someone, propagated the disease in the hospital.[18] Camus discusses the
disease at length, musing that "one of the preservative and curative
means seems to be to space the beds far apart on the ward."[19] But
doctors and midwives wiped, rather than washed their hands between
examinations, thus carrying the disease from one patient to the next.

We are fortunate that in preparation for the exchange of accommodations between the Maternity and Foundlings' Hospices in 1813,
the staff drew up a table and a retrospective balance sheet, which are
preserved in the archives,[20] giving us, first of all, the mortality figures
for women in childbirth for 1803–1813 (see Table 7.2). The decline in
mortality from 6.7 percent is spectacular—even although it rose again
to that level in 1806 and 1812, for which puerperal fever may be the

explanation. The low mortality for 1813 remains unexplained. The table also tells us that 2,213 confinements resulted in fifteen pairs of twins and ninety-four stillborn babies, and that seventy-two women nursed babies who soon died. How often mother and child succumbed together, we cannot tell. The table further indicates that of the sixty-six women who died in childbirth in 1813,

2 died before giving birth
2 died while giving birth
13 died 1–3 days after
30 died 3–10 days after
8 died 10–15 days after
2 died 15–20 days after
3 died 20–30 days after
6 died 30 or more days after.

The first two postpartum weeks were clearly critical. Important differences with the pre-Revolutionary period become obvious: only two of these women died in childbirth, and the eleven who died more than two weeks postpartum were cared for at the institution until the end (the causes of their deaths are unknown).

We may conclude that this comparatively small, well-organized, and expertly staffed hospital, with its large gardens, was one of the Revolution's most successful innovations in caring for the health of the citizen-patient. But only the new mother was so expertly served: her abandoned baby fared less well.

Babies as Patients: Neonatology

The initial routine for new citizens did not change under the Code spécial de la Maternité. The clerk approached the mother the morning after delivery to ask whether she wished to keep her baby and what its name should be. The baby had by then been washed—we presume in water, although the famous eighteenth-century midwife Madame Du Coudray added wine. To preserve confidentiality, and for official identification, the clerk assigned the infant a number, which he entered into a ledger and wrote on a parchment attached to the baby's head. It is at this point in their lives, two days old, washed, weighed, named, baptized, swaddled, and labeled, that the abandoned infants were carried in a basket across the grounds to the foundlings' wards at Port-Royal. There the newborns joined abandoned children brought from elsewhere in Paris or from the provinces, often deposited by total strangers.[21]

Beginning in 1798, the newborn citizen was handed over to experts who had hitherto worked in isolation: the midwife and Augustinian nurses at the Hôtel-Dieu, the accoucheur at the medical faculty, the Sisters of Charity, and the "pediatrician" at the Foundlings' Hospice. At Port-Royal the experts collaborated. The key figure in the emergence of an early form of neonatology in Paris was Jean Abraham Auvity (1754–1821). He had joined the staff of the Foundlings' Hospice in 1782 and supported the efforts of Bernard Hombron to move it to a healthier site. Auvity's progressive notions can be identified in the writings of his three sons, who served as interns at the Maternité, specialized in infant care, and dedicated their medical theses to their father, their "guide and best friend."[22] One of them, Jean Pierre, argued in his thesis that, contrary to widely held opinions, the diagnosis of illness in infants is not an impossible task for a good observer. The first years of life are crucial to health and "the care received in infancy usually determines the good or bad, strong or weak constitution of man."[23] The second son, Antoine, advocated feeding babies on demand and criticized regulating the quantity of milk a newborn is given and the number of times the baby is offered the breast. Infants do not vomit from overfeeding, their facial expressions are not altered, and there is "no basis for considering frequent feeding as a mistake." Once they are weaned, the best drink is "water of good quality, with a small quantity of good wine."[24]

After their arrival at the Foundlings' Hospice, whether near the Hôtel-Dieu or at Port-Royal, the babies' first stop was the crib room (crèche), where a triage took place. Sister Claudine Guillot officiated here for fifty-two years, from 1755 to 1807, culling healthy from weak and dying babies. She knew from experience how viable each newborn was. Birthweight was a telltale indicator, with six pounds, or 3,000 grams, considered minimal for survival.[25] Pastoret estimates that, in the course of her career, she handled some 360,000 infants, at least a dozen a day. But under the new Code spécial de la Maternité, it was Auvity who decided officially, during early morning rounds, what each baby's destination would be.

While healthy babies waited in the crib room for transportation to the country, the sickly ones were assigned to the crib room infirmary (infirmerie de la crèche), to be fed "artificially." This method had been practiced since antiquity—witness a variety of feeding horns (cornets) and bottles (biberons) dating back at least to ancient Greece.[26] The problem with these devices was to find a proper opening to funnel small amounts of liquids, slowly, into the baby's mouth. Sponges and rags used for nipples had so often gagged or choked a baby that Auvity in the end forbade their use altogether, and advocated spoon feeding. (That aspect of the problem would only be solved with the advent

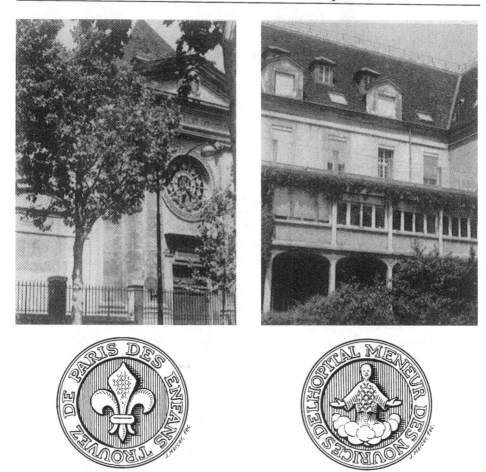

FIGURE 7.1. *Top:* Two views of the Foundlings' Hospice in the former Oratory convent (subsequently known as the Hôpital-hospice St. Vincent de Paul, and now as the Hôpital-hospice des enfants assistés). Photographs by the author. *Bottom:* Two Hospice driver's badges.

of the rubber nipple.) For nourishment, Auvity advocated the milk of cows, asses, or goats. But the infants' weak constitutions tended to reject all substitutes for mother's milk.[27]

The psychologic welfare of the infant was well served by Auvity's orders that babies be picked up and held while being fed. "Among the drawbacks of artificial feeding," he wrote in 1797,

> one must count the lack of gestation (by which I mean carrying in one's arms) so beneficial to newborns. It is certain that the emanations of natural warmth from mother to child during feeding contribute greatly to his

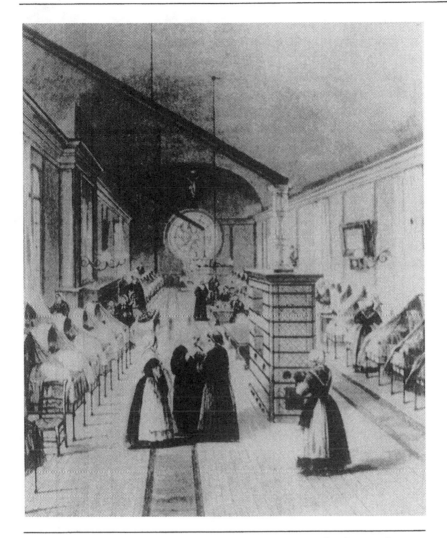

FIGURE 7.2. The nursery at the Foundlings' Hospice in the former Oratory convent. Anonymous illustration inspired by Jean Henri Marlet, *Tableaux de Paris* (1821). Bibliothèque historique de la Ville de Paris.

strength and help prevent the often fatal apathy of artificially fed neonates. This may be the most important cause of the failure of all artificial feeding methods tried with institutionalized infants. This kind of gestation should be considered as a second incubation, of which a baby cannot safely be deprived.[28]

While Auvity judged prompt removal of the baby from town essential, he deemed excessive speed harmful. The following letter from Hucherard, Hombron's son-in-law and successor, to the sister in charge of this service is instructive.

9 March 1813

To Mademoiselle Hubert

. . . starting today, no infant from the cribroom may be handed to country nurses until twenty-four hours after birth, the time needed to expel its meconium;

As clear proof of a measure that you undoubtedly observe, never to hand an infant to a wet nurse until the doctor has examined it, you will in the future, and for each dispatch of drivers, establish a list, to be signed by M. Auvity or his assistant, reading: "Approved. The following infants may be sent to the country." You will carefully keep these lists and send them to me every Tuesday morning.[29]

Auvity and Sister Claudine thus supervised a never-ending flow of about 4,500 infants a year, through the crib room to the countryside, or through the neonate infirmary to recovery, or, for nine-tenths of the sick infants, to the dissection table and the grave.

◆◆◆

Even though expert hands guided delivery, and the maternity hospice was by contemporary standards clean, the infants encountered infection and germs everywhere. The worst killer was thrush, a highly communicable fungus characterized by white pustules. It affected the mucous membranes, particularly in the mouth, with the result that the baby would not suck and died of starvation. Another endemic disease was sclerema neonatorum, a progressive and fatal hardening of the skin. It produced "frozen babies." According to Jean Pierre Auvity, they kept their jaws so tightly closed that it was impossible to feed them. They died of "stupor and torpor."[30]

As far back as 1788, Jean Abraham Auvity had published papers on thrush and sclerema neonatorum in the *Mémoires* of the Royal Society of Medicine; he received a gold medal for the paper on sclerema.[31] The paper on thrush is full of precise observations and empathy, but without a clue as to etiology or therapy. Auvity describes babies with "insomnia, a violent and continuous agitation, tension of the belly, excessive pungent and greenish stools, an angry red anus that sometimes forms gangrenous scabs, these symptoms usually accompany this kind of fever. Its worrisome and rapid progress is evident in the excruciating pain and suffering caused by this most horrible disease."[32]

He detected some infants "infected with the venereal virus."[33] The incidence of venereal disease in these infants was 0.875 percent (see Table 7.4), and it was suspected that some infected their wet nurses.

Many starved because "the venereal chancres on the lips and in the mouth and throat often caused such acute pain that suction and swallowing became impossible."[34] As soon as feasible, these babies were dispatched to the Venereal Diseases Hospital across the street. Triage and segregation helped fight contagion and its fatal consequences.

Auvity focused his attention on the neonate infirmary, to which about one-eighth of the hospice's babies were admitted. It had fifty cribs for acutely ill infants. The supervisor, Marie Anne Victoire Gillain, later Madame Boivin (1773–1841), was a highly skilled midwife who had also acquired considerable medical knowledge. Widowed like Madame Lachapelle at an early age, she turned to midwifery to support herself and her daughter. Madame Lachapelle appointed her supervisor of the babies' division, a job that she held for fifteen years. She must have impressed Chaptal as well, for he sent her on tour through the provinces to test midwives' competence and recruit candidates for the Paris school. She was a learned woman, who published a highly successful book on the art of midwifery, *Mémorial de l'art des accouchements*.[35] She fell victim to the administrative reshuffling occasioned by the separation of the Foundling's Hospice from the Maternité in 1814. Hucherard tried to save her job, but failed.[36]

Madame Boivin's assignment at Port-Royal was both novel and crucial: she headed the special infirmary for newborn babies who were too sick to travel or be breast-fed by sedentary wet nurses. A detailed diagnostic table of their illnesses, covering the years 1808 to 1811, published in Pastoret's report of 1816, is undoubtedly her work. Table 7.4 gives us figures for what we already knew in general terms: the worst killer of infants was poverty. Of all the infants admitted to the infirmary, 631 (34.1 percent) were born too weak to live, undoubtedly the premature offspring of undernourished, tired women. (Most may have breathed long enough to be baptized, a matter of concern to believers, who urged midwives to perform this rite in an emergency.) Of the 1,617 presumably viable infants according to Dr. Auvity and Madame Boivin's diagnosis, 567, or one-third (35 percent), died of thrush; 92, or 5.6 percent, of sclerema; 119, or 7.2 percent, of poorly diagnosed infectious or eruptive fevers, perhaps measles; 34, or 2.1 percent, of convulsions; 154, or 9 percent, of jaundice and diarrhoea, possibly "cholera infantum," the severe diarrhoea prevalent at the Paris Hospice.

Therapy remained entirely empiric, of course, logical by Hippocratic standards, but useless. Against thrush: loving care and good milk; against sclerema: steambaths, sandbaths, "transpiration that softens the flesh." Pastoret reports on an experiment Madame Boivin conducted (with Auvity's approval, we may be sure): she "placed the

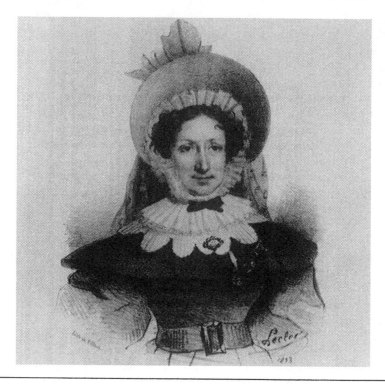

FIGURE 7.3. Marie Anne Victoire Boivin (née Gillain) (1773–1841). Académie nationale de médecine, Paris.

baby near a stove or chimney, gave it dry rubs, let it sleep in the nurse's bed, unswaddled."[37] Contemporary care had no recourse against infection: these babies were doomed.

The medical research service gained growing importance and independence after the Foundlings' Hospice exchanged buildings with the maternity hospice in 1814 and evolved into the modern "Hôpital-Hospice St. Vincent de Paul pour les enfants assistés." In the early nineteenth century, under J. F. Baron (1782–1849) as physician, and Gilbert Breschet (1784–1845) as surgeon, it achieved worldwide renown. It was here that Charles Michel Billard (1800–1832), founder of neonate medicine, was trained. He proclaimed in his treatise on the diseases of newborns that his work was "founded on new clinical and anatomo-pathologic observations made in Dr. Baron's service."[38] That service was crucial to "founding pediatric medicine, particularly for neonates."[39]

For the healthy babies the vital goal was a speedy transfer into the hands of a wet nurse. Hombron and Hucherard regulated a huge na-

TABLE 7.3. Madame Boivin's Table of General Morbidity and Mortality, Neonate Infirmary, Maternity Hospice of Port-Royal, 1808–1811

Year	Admitted to Maternity Hospice	Admitted to Neonate Infirmary	Died in Infirmary		Cured[a]		Sent to Venereal Diseases Hospital
			Number	%	Number	%	
1808	4,296	567	363	65	173	30	31
1809	4,552	563	437	78	89	16	37
1810	4,500	499	385	77	60	12	54
1811	5,150	619	484	78	96	15	39
Total	18,498	2,248	1,669	74	418	18.5	161

SOURCE: Seine, CGAHHCP, *Rapport fait au conseil général* (1816), 123.
[a]"Cured" meant well enough to be discharged. There was no follow-up.

tional network for the selection and transportation of these peasant women so as to cope with the staggering numbers: whereas in the Year VI (1797–1798), 576 babies had left the hospice alive, in 1813 the number was 4,324. Owing to a well-managed exodus, infant mortality at the new babies' hospice declined steadily, from an appalling 83.7 percent in the Year VI to 13.5 percent in 1813. (It even dipped to 9.1 percent in 1811.)[40]

Surrogate Nurture and Foster Care

Wet nurses were the lifeline for several thousand infants abandoned each year in Paris, the "only means of stopping the frightful mortality."[41] Only they could provide the unique natural sustenance the babies needed; all substitutes for mother's milk failed. But the arrival of applicants at the Foundlings' Hospice to collect newborns and take them back to the countryside was irregular, particularly in time of civil or foreign war, during the harvest season, and in winter, when ice and snow blocked travel.

Hombron accordingly established a "sedentary," or residential, wet-nursing service. He experimented with the idea under the old regime, and between 1796 and 1801, he managed to maintain a corps of 250 women. Proudly he showed visitors "the long hallway where good-humored and healthy wet nurses sat in front of their cubicles, each rocking or breast-feeding two babies." It was impossible, he insisted, "to tell the foundling from the woman's child, judging by their health."[42]

Any woman who gave birth at the hospice could join this nursing

TABLE 7.4. Madame Boivin's Table of Specific Infant Morbidity and Mortality, Neonate Infirmary, Maternity Hospice of Port-Royal, 1808–1811

Year	Total admissions	Admitted to the infirmary	Premature, not viable, brought moribund			Sclerema neonatorum			Thrush		
			Cases	Deaths	Cures	Cases	Deaths	Cures	Cases	Deaths	Cures
1808	4,296	567	150	120	30	39	23	16	194	154	40
1809	4,552	563	187	172	15	43	41	2	114	100	14
1810	4,500	499	195	180	15	26	25	1	115	110	5
1811	5,150	619	173	159	14	8	3	5	222	203	19
Total	18,498	2,248	705	631	74	116	92	24	645	567	78
Survival Rates				15%			20%			12%	

Year	Total admissions	Admitted to the infirmary	Jaundice, diarrhoea			Scabies, herpes, ophthalmia, pustules, eruptions			Venereal disease
			Cases	Deaths	Cures	Cases	Deaths	Cures	Cases
1808	4,296	567	48	16	32	70	25	45	31
1809	4,552	563	59	53	6	89	46	43	37
1810	4,500	499	24	22	2	48	22	26	54
1811	5,150	619	74	63	11	65	26	39	39
Total	18,498	2,248	205	154	51	272	119	153	161[a]
Survival Rates				24%			56%		

Year	Total admissions	Admitted to the infirmary	Convulsions			Fracture of limbs			Tumors of diverse kinds		
			Cases	Deaths	Cures	Cases	Deaths	Cures	Cases	Deaths	Cures
1808	4,296	567	11	11	—	6	2	4	10	4	6
1809	4,552	563	12	10	2	1	—	1	6	4	2
1810	4,500	499	12	6	6	1	—	1	20	16	4
1811	5,150	619	12	7	5	3	3	—	10	8	2
Total	18,498	2,248	47	34	13	11	5	6	46	32	14
Survival Rates				28%			55%			30%	

Year	Total admissions	Admitted to the infirmary	Deformities			Hydrocephalus, or hydropsy of the head			Hydrorachitis, or hydropsy of the spine		
			Cases	Deaths	Cures	Cases	Deaths	Cures	Cases	Deaths	Cures
1808	4,296	567	3	3	—	4	4	—	2	2	—
1809	4,552	563	5	2	3[b]	2	1	1[b]	8	8	—
1810	4,500	499	2	2	—	1	1	—	1	1	—
1811	5,150	619	12	11	1[b]	—	—	—	1	1	—
Total	18,498	2,248	22	18	4	7	6	1	12	12	—
Survival Rates				?%			?%			0	

SOURCE: Seine, CGAHHP, *Rapport fait au conseil général* (1816), 123.
[a]Transferred to the Venereal Diseases Hospital.
[b]Sent to the countryside; no follow up.

corps, provided Auvity approved of her milk. She might spend up to fifteen months at Port-Royal, feeding her own infant and a foundling in return for lodging, clothing, food, and 7.50 francs a month, plus a bonus of 3 francs for each child she handed back healthy.[43] She was granted twenty-four hours' rest before receiving a new infant; only on that free day could she go out, for a maximum of six hours, with her own baby,[44] and only twice a month, between 2 and 4 P.M., could she receive visitors in the parlor.[45]

In the Year XI (1802–1803), there were 71 sedentary wet nurses at the Port-Royal maternity hospice. In the years that followed, the numbers first rose steadily and then fell dramatically:[46]

Year XI	71
Year XII	73
Year XIII	97
1806	104
1807	44
1808	23
1809	30
1810	30
1811	30
1812	27
1813	24

Criticism of this service rose in the new century. Drs. Auvity and Andry, and eventually Camus, argued that the women lacked the strength to breast-feed two babies, inevitably favored their own child, and refused to take charge of weak and delicate babies, since these women coveted the premium for handing back a viable infant. Moreover, the change of nurse and of feeding method harmed the child.[47] In the Napoleonic era, Hombron's emergency service became redundant because an annual average of 3,646 peasant women came to pick up newborns and take them home.[48]

The rural wet nurses arrived in the wagon of a Foundlings' Hospice driver (*meneur*), using the rue du faubourg St. Jacques entrance, as specified in the Code spécial de la Maternité, which forbade any communication between these women and the sedentary wet nurses (Title V, ch. 2, sec. 1, par. 8). The code entitled them to eat four meals at the hospice and required them to stay in a day room and sleep in a special dormitory, which contained 120 beds. Auvity gave them a medical checkup, particularly to inspect their milk. He rejected only a few; in 1808 and 1813, in fact, he accepted all of the applicants.[49] A woman who did not qualify had to travel back home at her own expense.

TABLE 7.5. A Wet Nurse's Pay (in francs)

1st month (prepaid)	7
2d month	7
3d month (7f + 8f bonus)	15
4th month	7
5th month	7
6th month (7f + 6f bonus)	13
7th month	7
8th month	7
9th month (7f + 6f bonus)	13
10th month	7
11th month	7
12th month	7
First year total	104
2d year (6 francs/month)	72
3d–7th years (5 francs/month, i.e., 60 francs/year, thus 5 × 60)	300
Total at age 7	476
8th–12th years (40 francs/year, thus 5 × 40)	200
Wet nurse's total income per child	676

SOURCE: Seine, CGAHHP, *Code spécial de la maternité* (Paris: Imprimerie des sourds-muets, An X), Title 5, ch. 1, par. 3, and Seine, CGAHHCP, *Rapports au conseil général* (1803), 170n.
NOTE: Wet nurses' wages were paid each trimester in the presence of the local mayor, who checked on the children. Travel expenses varied in proportion to distance and were 50 percent higher for two months of the winter and three months in the harvest season. The first month's wages were prepaid and included travel expenses and four pounds of bread.

If accepted, a wet nurse registered with the clerk, who recorded her name, age, domicile, and husband's occupation, as well as the number of children she had borne and the number of foundlings she had nursed. With a healthy newborn, she received 7 francs prepaid for the first month. If she kept the child for seven years, her wages totaled 476 francs, and after twelve years, she would have earned 676 francs. At that time she received 50 francs to pay for clothing "for the first communion," arguably a wasteful expense for a desperately poor child.[50]

With a healthy baby, the new foster mother received a layette that included a skimpy twelve diapers, but a lavish seven bonnets or caps. She was handed four pounds of "departure bread" (*pain du départ*) and alotted 20 centimes per day of travel.[51] What innkeeper would feed her for such a pittance? Pastoret comments that "the high price of lodgings, the uncleanliness of the wet nurses, the nuisance caused by all those crying babies relegated this group to disreputable hostelries."[52]

The regulations stipulated that the "drivers . . . shall see to it that the wet nurses . . . give most of their attention to the babies" (Title V, ch. 2, par. 3). One can read this enjoinder as an indication that the babies received short shrift and probably spent most of their waking hours crying.[53]

The nurses traveled in a special wagon redesigned by Mme Fougeret, the founder of the Society for Maternal Charity, which had large suspended baskets that held six babies each. The babies were tightly swaddled and the baskets could be hung from a hook, like so many packages. The council insisted on a new model where each baby had its own basket, so that no more than twenty infants could be transported at the same time.[54] The drivers at first refused, and "it is only by withholding their fees that the council finally forced them to comply."[55] Seven years later, we still find Hucherard struggling to secure the drivers' cooperation. The inference is clear: without government insistence, the newborn babies would be ferried in bare and sometimes roofless wagons, through rain and snow.[56] In the spring of 1814, foreign armies prevented the drivers from approaching Paris.[57] To make sure the drivers did not quit because of bad weather and roads, the Hospital Council established bonuses for men who exceeded their quota. "They could add 500 francs to their annual salary," reported Pastoret; and "they doubled their attention."[58] A driver was allowed to take only nurses, babies, and bundles of clothing. Older children had to be transported separately. This rule indicates that drivers often took on other passengers and packages to supplement their pay.

The driver handled all the administrative and financial aspects of this wet-nursing business. He needed to know how to read, write, and figure, and had to be married and endorsed by the local mayor; moreover, he had to provide a security deposit, which varied from 3,000 to 12,000 francs.[59] But besides material assets, being a driver required a special combination of talents: only a vast network of local intelligence and gossip could facilitate locating hundreds of women who had recently given birth and wished to serve as wet nurses. Yet in a typical year such as 1805, twenty-eight *meneurs* placed 3,127 babies.[60]

For each child the Paris office prepared a document known as a *bulle* with name, date of birth, registration number, and proof of vaccination. The driver used the *bulle* periodically to enter the condition of the child, wages paid, clothing delivered, or, if the child was dead, clothing returned. Hucherard stressed that "the survival certificates are the only documents on which the administration bases the payment of nursing fees." The *bulle* had to be exactly filled out and certified by the mayor.[61]

TABLE 7.6. Distances Traveled and Compensation of Foundlings' Hospice Drivers

	Approximate distance	Approximate travel time[a]	Compensation per nurse and baby (in francs)
Up to 50 km	(−>35 mi)	Up to 7 hrs	3
Up to 80 km	(−>50 mi)	7 to 10 hrs (up to 1 day)	4
Up to 120 km	(−>80 mi)	10 to 16 hrs (1–2 days)	5
Up to 170 km	(−>110 mi)	16 to 22 hrs (2–3 days)	6
Up to 220 km	(−>170 mi)	22 to 32 hrs (3–4 days)	7
Up to 270 km	(−>200 mi)	32 to 40 hrs (4–5 days)	8
Up to 320 km	(−>250 mi)	40 to 50 hrs (5–7 days)	9

SOURCE: Seine, CGAHHCP, *Code spécial de la maternité*, Title 5, ch. 1, par. 3, and Seine, CGAHHCP, *Rapports fait au conseil général* (1816), 110.
[a]Parentheses indicate total travel time, as opposed to time actually spent on the road.

The driver transmitted large sums: a memorandum for 12 August 1815 records 3,363 francs for a driver called Vallée, 10,228 francs for Deteuf, and 10,809 francs for Berthier.[62] The driver's income consisted of 5 percent of all sums remitted to wet nurses, 20 sols for each wet nurse brought to Paris, travel allowances, and a fee for each newborn, weanling, and packet of clothing transported.[63] Distances varied from 35 to 250 miles, which might take a week. Yet despite the hardships, an average of five drivers, with seventy-five rural nurses and their babies, left the Paris Foundlings' Hospice every week according to a schedule closely monitored by the Paris office.

A good working relationship appears to have been established between the Foundlings' Hospice administrators in Paris and at least some of the drivers.[64] Camus's judgment seems harsh when he writes: "It would be wrong to imagine that motives of humanity, welfare, or compassion for those unhappy abandoned children bring drivers and wet nurses to Paris. With very few exceptions . . . they are motivated by sordid self-interest."[65] More equitably stated, the driver was a businessman. The government grew more dissatisfied over time, and in 1819 it created a network of salaried employees for the transport of "national children." Was that system preferable? Would any system work? It might have been more effective to help the pregnant woman so that she could keep her child. That would have meant treating her as a citizen-patient, however, which was not in line with contemporary morality.

The documents dwell on infants, undoubtedly because of the horrendous mortality rate. The surviving older foster children, the ones who might grow into citizen-patients, appear to have been sadly neglected. One inspector commented on the prevalent vagrancy, reporting that the children were routinely sent "to guard cows or gather grass" or "horse dung on the roads, to make manure." [66] Camus spoke admiringly of an offer made by the duc de la Rochefoucauld-Liancourt upon his return from America in 1800 to oversee the foundlings in his department, Oise. He "sent numerous observations." [67] Camus undoubtedly knew that Liancourt followed a practice employed with success by the London Foundlings' Hospital, relying on burghers, parsons, and businessmen as inspectors and mentors. "But can we hope to find throughout France persons willing to shoulder this task?" he queried.

Camus was asking, in fact, whether Anglo-Saxon voluntarism could work in a country accustomed to central management. The answer was no. Parisian expectations seem unrealistic considering the minimal compensation paid to foster parents and the high mortality among the peasants' own children, only one out of four of whom normally survived. But mortality among foundlings was twice as high. As Maurice Garden so dramatically puts it: "The countryside devoured its children." [68]

The vast network emanating from the Paris Foundlings' Hospice would obviously have benefited from close and sustained inspection. This had always been difficult to achieve. Drivers and wet nurses hid sickly children; doctors lacked incentive to intervene. Neither the overworked Sisters of Charity, under the old regime, nor the Paris wet-nursing office proved equal to the task. Eventually the Hospital Council appointed one inspector in 1803, a second in 1804, and a third in 1811. From April to December every year, these men toured France to "ascertain the condition of the children and correct the conduct of drivers and nurses." [69] These inspectors were efficient, but expensive and overworked. They presumably kept an eye on 15,000 nurslings, toddlers, and teenagers. One of them, Boucry de St. Venant, sent a bill for 2,500 francs to the council, which wistfully recalled that in the eighteenth century, the Sisters spent 200 livres and lay inspectors 350 livres a year. Under these circumstances, and by default, inspection fell to the mayors, about whose supervision we have only anecdotal information. [70]

Each year the council had to provide for several hundred youngsters whom foster families returned to Paris. This relatively sturdy lot had survived traumatic transport in infancy and a deprived childhood. They had acquired immunity not only against childhood diseases but against social rules as well. These survivors now joined orphans raised in Paris, and if their health was good, they underwent training for apprenticeship in a manufacture or trade. But some of them fell ill: for them a new hospital now existed in Paris, grouping sick children between the ages of two and puberty. We shall examine this new institution before studying the health of the orphaned child.

Children as Patients: The First Children's Hospital and the Beginnings of Pediatrics

The need for a children's hospital headed the medical reformers' list of priorities once the Hôtel-Dieu's lying-in ward was moved to the outskirts of Paris. Anne Brun, chief surgeon of the Pitié orphanage, had long resisted sending sick boys to the Hôtel-Dieu or Bicêtre because they risked neglect, infection, and apprenticeship in criminality or perversion. He shared the growing general awareness that children should be viewed as a discrete group of patients with needs and illnesses that demanded special attention. They should be hospitalized apart. It would seem that widespread interest in growth and change, in this early Romantic period, favored infancy and childhood as new subjects of study and stirred interest in physical education and the orthopedic correction of deformities. Also, preventive action such as vaccination would be most beneficial if applied at an early age: possibly diseases other than smallpox might be prevented.

The Paris Children's Hospital opened its doors on 29 April 1802 at the former de Maison de l'Enfant Jésus.[71] The government dispossessed the Ladies of St. Thomas de Villeneuve, who eventually moved to Neuilly-sur-Seine, where they are found today.[72] Like the Sisters of Charity at the contiguous Necker Hospital, the Ladies held on to their property throughout the Revolution, when their vast orchards and vegetable plots helped feed their patients.

In 1802, three hundred beds stood ready in accommodations that were separate for children under six and for boys and girls above that age, even in the garden and chapel. The Hospital Council even pushed "precautions" so far as to segregate foundlings from legitimate children, who might thus be safeguarded from "bad habits." Young citizen-patients thus learned at an early age both that the opposite sex offered forbidden distractions and that society discriminated against children born out of wedlock. A former orangery was remodeled in 1808 to allow for the isolation of two hundred contagious patients, initially children with ringworm, scabies, or tuberculosis transferred from St. Louis. All children seeking admission had to bring proof of domicile to facilitate their discharge and prevent their abandonment. The council hired a teacher for instruction in the three Rs and "the principles of religion."[73]

One of the two pediatricians, Jean François Jadelot, who served at the Children's Hospital from 1802 until 1845, described its topography and its medical history in two long articles in 1805.[74] Jadelot's catalogue of achievements rehearses the list of desiderata spelled out by the Poverty Committee in 1791 and by the Hospital Council in 1801. Now the changes had been accomplished: Jadelot describes the vast, airy terrain of five hectares, mostly gardens and orchards, solid, clean buildings, wards of from thirty to forty single beds with appropriate furnishings, adequate spaces between beds, "economic stoves," serviceable toilets. He explains that the Hospital Council had, with guidance from Pastoret, "removed partitions, installed windows, demolished structures that were about to collapse, pulled down high stone walls . . . prepared the material to build two perfectly planned pavilions with four wards. . . . a pharmacy that is very beautiful, and entirely new baths."[75] The children were served soup at 8 A.M., after the doctor's visit, and their daily rations were otherwise as follows:

Bread	360 g
Wine	⅕ liter
Cooked Meat	90 g
Vegetables	60 g
Rice	40 g
Noodles	40 g
Prunes	60 g
Milk	⅓ liter
Eggs	
Biscuits	

For young patients too weak for this diet, bouillon was served every three hours.

The personnel at the Children's Hospital consisted of two physicians, one surgeon, and one pharmacist, assisted by eight interns in medicine, surgery, and pharmacy, six women supervisors of wards, kitchen, and linen, thirty-three nurses, and fourteen male employees. The physicians kept exact charts and histories and "carefully searched the dead bodies for the causes and seats of diseases."[76] The 500 beds accommodated only 1,800 patients a year: hospital stays were long for children who were not only sick, but weakened by poverty, explains Jadelot. Surgery was usually successful. The main problem was the high mortality from communicable diseases: scurvy, poorly defined "fevers," and smallpox (vaccination was far from universal). It may well have been on the pediatrician's initiative that preventive health measures were extended to the Pitié, where in the Year X, out of 1,678 boys, 944 were sick and 14 died. By 1803 all these boys had been vaccinated, the food had improved, and each child had received both summer and winter clothing.[77]

While nosology, etiology, and clinical diagnosis preoccupied the professors and physicians, hundreds of children continued to be treated by traditional methods. In 1803, St. Louis still housed 255 young inpatients, 170 girls and 185 boys. One of their main complaints was scabies, a highly contagious itch caused by *Sarcoptes scabiei*, a mite that burrows and breeds in the skin. Jadelot considered sulphur to be the specific against scabies and used baths with four or five ounces of potassium sulphate in 150 liters of water. Eight to ten baths cured the illness, Jadelot maintained.

The method traditionally used to cure ringworm, or tinea, strikes us as barbarous. While this fungus can occur anywhere on the skin, it often attacks the head. Therefore, at the Ste. Reine Hospice, an annex to the Petites Maisons where this disease had been treated, skullcaps of tar plaster were applied to the children's heads and then used to pull out their hair with the roots. This terrible procedure was repeated six or more times. At St. Louis, doctors preferred a painless remedy proposed by the brothers Mahon. "They used a depilatory cream that works slowly. After a variable time of using their cream on alternate days, the hairs fall out with their roots. If one pulls at them they come out easily." The brothers Mahon received a fee of 1,000 francs a year, plus 6 francs per cured head.[78]

The Paris Children's Hospital grew into an important research and teaching center, first headed by the physicians Mongenot (who served there from 1802 till 1816) and Jadelot and the surgeons Petitbeau (from 1802 to 1810) and René Alexis Baffos (from 1810 to 1840).[79] Although informal clinical teaching began immediately, a chair of pediatrics was not created till 1879, and a separate chair of neonatal hygiene and pathology was only set up at the Foundlings' Hospice in 1914.[80]

Nor is there mention of orthopedics in the Children's Hospital records. The specialty had long existed; in fact, the word was coined by Nicolas Andry (1658–1742), the uncle of the foundlings' pediatrician who wrote a book on the subject.[81] Advocates of corrective gymnastics and swimming tried to straighten crooked limbs, and manufacturers produced corrective apparatus like the famous "Venel's sabot." But this specialty was outside the mainstream of medicine and therefore ignored by its academic practitioners, and such progress as occurred was made elsewhere (for example, in Montpellier). This may well account for Parisians' indifference.[82] In the 1820s and 1830s, however, orthopedics and corrective surgery, particularly tenotomy to correct clubfoot, became all too fashionable in Paris.[83]

Jadelot described the Children's Hospital in the *Journal général de médecine* in 1805 as the optimal place in the world to study "the nature, progress, and treatment of many serious or fatal children's diseases," and he emphasized that "the children are better supervised here than they are in hospitals for adults, and they do not leave this establishment corrupted, as in former times."[84] Pastoret commented in 1816 that "foreigners have, for several years, hastened to visit this hospital. They are impressed with the order and cleanliness that prevail there, with the healthfulness and all the measures taken to help these children grow into useful citizens. They regret not having such an establishment at home."[85]

But the Children's Hospital had its native and foreign critics as well as admirers. The central admitting office was dismayed that in the first eighteen months, half of the children gained direct admission, thus eluding the central triage.[86] To everyone's surprise, the number of child patients dropped considerably in the first few weeks. Camus explained that numerous poor parents, content to see their child hospitalized near their own home, " as though in a kind of pension," did not want to have them transferred to the faraway rue de Sèvres, however health-giving the location, and therefore took them home. On the other hand, Parisian parents knew better than Camus and Pastoret that their children often caught contagious diseases such as measles or scarlet fever while hospitalized. They were frightened by the high mortality at the Children's Hospital, which Pastoret liked to blame on "the excessive affection of mothers [who would not let go until it was too late]."[87] A suspicious medical commission even wondered whether parents did not view the Children's Hospital as "an honest, if not infallible, means of ridding oneself forever of one's children."[88]

On the other hand, many children recovered and went home. Others, with no one to care for them, joined the healthy boys and girls returned by foster parents to the orphanage. They all now prepared for a life of work or military service. We shall briefly review the conditions surrounding their daily lives, focusing on their health and on the children who were sick or ailing—that is, on the citizen-patients among them.

Ailing Orphans: The Raw Material of Adolescent Medicine

Every year 400 to 500 youngsters traveled to the Paris orphanage, the living remnant of about four thousand abandoned newborns who had journeyed to the provinces in the arms of wet nurses a decade earlier.[89] After the Revolution, their legal guardianship had first de-volved upon municipal hospital councils, then upon departments, but in practice on a single council member. In Paris after 1801, first Camus and then Camet de la Bonnardière assumed this responsibility.[90]

The municipal government wanted to group all these children in one institution, but several councillors initially insisted that boys and girls be housed in separate buildings. Other councillors argued, however, that the Pitié and the Enfant Jésus would be better employed as hospitals than as orphanages. Their arguments prevailed. As of 1 January 1809, St. Antoine was therefore enlarged to house all the city's orphans; the Pitié, now emptied of boys, first served as an annex of the Hôtel-Dieu, then as an all-purpose hospital, opened in 1813. Pastoret lamented the move to St. Antoine, commenting that "the Hospital Council greatly regretted that it was compelled to reunite the two sexes in the same establishment, despite its constant effort always to keep them apart."[91] The administration quickly established a "moral" environment, however, by creating separate courtyards and two aisles in the chapel, so that boy and girl worshippers never saw one another. On the other hand, all orphans found themselves on the outskirts of Paris, amidst trees, space, and fresh air.

During the Revolution, orphans had become the objects of patriotic rhetoric demanding the obliteration of social prejudice against them. In a generous effort to make equal rights a reality, the Constitution of 1791 promised that the nation would "bring up the foundlings." The decree of 19 March 1793 proclaimed assistance to be a "sacred debt," declaring: "Abandoned children shall henceforth be known as orphans; no other designation shall be permitted." Various new terms appeared: orphans and foundlings were "national children" (*enfants de la patrie*); the boys at the Pitié were "national scholars" (*élèves de la patrie*). The Revolutionary regime established scholarships for the "children of the country's defenders," boys whose fathers had died in the wars. But the language and inferences used in the archival documentation leave the impression that the change in vocabulary does not seem to have altered widespread condescension toward the "national child."

Child abandonment grew less secretive in the course of the eighteenth century. Dehaussy ascribes this change to the turntables (*tours*) built into the walls of foundlings' hospices, where infants could be safely deposited. The device consisted of an enclosed revolving platform divided vertically by a wooden board. An opening on the street side revealed a mattress and a bell hung nearby. Whoever brought an infant, laid it down and rang. A person in constant attendance (in most places, a Sister of Charity) then turned the table and received the infant.[92] The turntables thus funneled these newborns toward a home; they were no longer "found in the streets, dead or dying from cold or exposure."[93]

Napoleon attempted to settle the legal fate of foundlings, abandoned children, and orphans definitively with the Law of 19 January 1811.[94] Seeking to make abandonment irrevocable, and thus reduce the practice, he designated the turntables as the sole legal means of leaving a baby to public care. (Dehaussy notes that abandonments did indeed eventually decline in the Seine Department, from 5,600 in 1827 to 4,700 in 1837.)[95] The Hospital Council believed abandonment would be sufficiently discouraged if the procedure for reclaiming a child remained complex and expensive. The council therefore issued new rules forbidding that news about abandoned babies be given out to anyone,[96] and on 22 July 1812 it cancelled parents' Sunday morning visits. Pastoret says this restriction "led many parents to withdraw their children: nothing proves better the wisdom of this rule." The Foundlings' Hospice ought not to be considered "an establishment where one could place, visit, and reclaim one's children at will."[97]

◆◆◆

Napoleon had further plans for the orphans of St. Antoine.

The national government had been interested since the eighteenth century in corralling healthy boys for the armed forces. Napoleon created a special corps of *pupilles de la garde* ("boys of the guard") for the consular—then imperial—guard regiment. Furthermore, the Law of 1811 (Title IV, art. 9) required that healthy boys be put at the disposal of the minister of the navy. (One marvels at the grand defiance of reality evident in this, since the French navy had been destroyed by Nelson at Trafalgar in 1805, and the Continental Blockade was crippling the ports.) But the army lured the sturdiest, although we cannot tell how many met the physical requirements.[98] The physician Jadelot commented that "the habit of discipline becomes a need for most of the boys. They find it difficult to cope with the freedom they enjoy upon leaving [the Pitié]. Employers are often ill pleased even with the best apprentices at the hospice, and almost all soon decide to enlist in the army."[99] But we may be certain that the bulk of these youngsters needed a less strenuous way of life, and that a persistent preoccupation of their guardians was that their health and strength be equal to the stress of an apprenticeship.

To teach the children a trade that would make them self-supporting: that was the Hospital Council's fond hope. But conflicting concerns motivated the councillors. They knew that the chances of success were slim because they were dealing with a marginal group of children, often congenitally weak and sickly, children who had never known family life or responsible social behavior, and who lacked motivation to become self-supporting. The councillors persisted in thinking that these youngsters were somehow tainted by their parents' misconduct. This judgmental attitude fostered parsimony. The council spent almost one million francs on these children in a typical year—1809, for example—and it thought this expense excessive. "The dominant concern of the government, until the July Monarchy," comments Dehaussy, "was to reduce [the] cost."[100] From that perspective the council welcomed both the Civil Code's tightened definition of *orphan* as meaning a child both of whose parents were dead and the assertion by the Law of 19 January 1811 that the government was only responsible for orphans "without any means of subsistence" (Title III, art. 6). These definitions permitted the councillors to call on relatives for child support. But insofar as the council shouldered its responsibilities, its best hope was to improve living and working conditions at the Pitié and St. Antoine so that the children could start earning money as soon as possible.

We owe a detailed analysis of the improved accommodations to Jadelot, who served as the children's doctor at the Pitié from 1802 to 1809, succeeding the surgeon Anne Brun.[101] He gives an overall account, with special attention to health conditions. In an essay written in 1807, he described the new three-storey building, which had large, well-aired dormitories with from fifty to eighty beds apiece and schoolrooms on the ground floor. The children now had a dining room rather than eating in the low-lying, humid classrooms. A large space at the southern part of the hospice, now planted with trees and a garden and exposed to the western winds, was turned into a playground for the smallest children. The establishment of the Children's Hospital had made the former infirmary unnecessary, and it was demolished to create more open space.

In his overview of the Pitié in 1807, Jadelot also found the food improved: the orphans ate soup and meat five times a week, vegetables and fruit on the other two days, enough bread, and wine on Sundays. But, adds the doctor, "we are told that they have agreed neither to drink beer nor to eat sauerkraut, as we had hoped, during the recent outbreak of scurvy among them." Clothing had also changed for the better: orphans wore woolen vests, jackets, and pants in winter and twill in summer. They were shod in clogs (the clatter at the orphanage must have been deafening), and in winter in heavy socks that "prevented frostbite, which had tormented them every year." Their linen was changed once a week. All in all, these children were now quite decently housed, fed, and clad.[102] The Poverty Committee's recommendation had borne fruit at last.

In the remodeled Pitié, the northern group of buildings now housed new workshops for shoemakers, tailors, carpenters, locksmiths, and makers of passementerie, such as cords, beads, and gimps, and braids of straw and hair. Skilled artisans supervised the boys under contractual arrangements with masters in town. A placement office for apprentices had been established in January 1802 under M. de Sevelinges (decrees of 16 Nivôse and 4 Ventôse, Year X). Within a year he secured 1,036 apprenticeships,[103] a huge increase over the 120 boys from the Pitié apprenticed in 1790.[104] A typical contract states that "Jacques Bertrand, No. 650, Register 13, born 14 February 1792, was raised by M. Colas, carpenter-driver of Vernon (Eure)." At thirteen years, seven months, Colas placed Bertrand with the shoemaker Depauw in Paris. The contract, signed by de Sevelinges, specifies an apprenticeship of four years, after which the boy would receive 48 francs "to help him find a job." A final word appears in the left upper corner: "*Pupilles, 1811.*" At age nineteen, Jacques Bertrand joined the army.[105] Girls had always been easy to place as servants, seamstresses, and salesgirls. In 1803, two lace-making establishments in the faubourg St. Antoine offered to train a number of them.[106]

The younger, unskilled boys, who lived in a separate building at the Pitié, teased cotton and made the brushes used for carding cloth.[107] They "remained at the disposal of the drivers," to be placed with peasants, but there is no evidence that they were welcome on the farm. When the orphanage was transferred to St. Antoine, a problem arose: there were more boys than the three hundred the buildings could accommodate. That is perhaps why the administration struck sinister bargains with factory owners in the provinces, bargains that totally ruined some orphans' health.

◆◆◆

In keeping with the Industrial Revolution, the Hospital Council embarked on new ventures: in 1802, it contracted with manufacturers of goods such as cotton cloth, blankets, or passementerie to hire a contingent of "younger and weaker" hands, to be replenished as needed.[108] In 1807, for example, 177 boys between the ages of eight and fourteen and a half worked at the cotton mill owned by Lemarrois & Danney at Brionne (Eure). A ledger gives their names, ages, a few words of physical description, and their personality traits. Presumably all could read and over half (98 out of 177) could write. But thirteen-year-old Antoine Caumont, for example, who knew how to read and was "strong, fit, and healthy," was described as "listless, incapable, clumsy, and lazy." No master would hire such an apprentice; this description amounted to a verdict: Bicêtre. And who would want Jean Denis Dubois, aged twelve and a half, who although he, too, knew how to read and was "extremely strong, fit, and in good health," was said to be "very wicked and mischievous [and] . . . pretended to be epileptic?"

In 1810, forty children ran away, and half were recaptured. The mill owner had, by contract, the right to punish them by locking them up on a bread-and-water diet. Yet he hitched them to their work with ball and chain. News of this reached the administrators in Paris. When questioned, the owners justified themselves by saying that they punished first offenders "in other ways," but that chains were the only means that worked with repeaters. The Paris Hospital Council sternly demanded that the "inappropriate punishment" cease forthwith.

Sometimes the boys' state of health was so miserable that even M. Danney called in the local doctor. The surgeon LeBailly examined five boys on 18 February 1806, six boys on 26 September, and ten others on 19 October. His medical diagnoses follow:

Jean Maubert: imbecile

Léger Mongin: has *brought to the factory* a tertian fever and scurvy that have not responded to treatment [emphasis added]

Pierre Lindor came with gangrenous scabs and a cachectic temperament that have kept him in bed continuously. He has therefore done no work. Moreover, he cannot control his bowels

Jacques Dessin vomits every night all that he has eaten

Jean Baptiste cannot control his bowels

In September, LeBailly certified that six boys were unemployable, five because of incontinence and one because of incurable scabies. In October, he found three boys with kidney stones, one with "cold humors," five with myopia, and one with "ophthalmia" who "could not bear the lamplight."

One concludes that these boys were either ill, by modern standards, or in very poor physical condition and distressed or depressed by their state. The third certificate is marked "returned to the hospice." Relations between Danney and the Paris foundlings' administration had never been of the best. They ended abruptly when the supply of cotton to France ceased, cut off by the British blockade. Without warning, Danney returned sixty-two boys, to be followed shortly by the rest.[109]

The orphaned boys' health had been a serious worry for all reformers ever since Tenon first reported on the Pitié in his *Mémoires*. When the duc de la Rochefoucauld-Liancourt visited the orphanage in 1790, he came away exasperated. "Every step taken in these hospices increased one's conviction that they are a hotbed of outdated prejudice," he commented. Excellent reasons are always given to prove that any change would be for the worse."[110] He would have approved of Jadelot's efforts to improve the boys' health. As a physician with a medical degree from Nancy and experience in military medicine, Jadelot was better trained than Brun. He also had an easier task, because various transfers had halved the number of boys at the Pitié to between five and six hundred. They were even taken on outings on Thursdays and Sundays, to some "military exercises," and for frequent swims in the Seine. They were made to go bareheaded all year and to wear their hair short. This custom was presumed to have "saved them from many colds, ophthalmias, earaches, sore throats, and toothaches." Spartan toughness had become fashionable.[111] In his essay of 1807, Jadelot quickly reviewed a variety of childhood diseases, such as measles, scarlet fever, whooping cough, and croup. He recorded less scrofula and fewer gangrenous ulcers of the mouth and aphthae, and only one epidemic of scurvy, in the winter of 1803. But he continued to see boys with fevers, anginas, pleurisies and peripneumonias, ophthalmias, rheumatism, and gout.

More interesting than this conventional report is Jadelot's attempt to relate the children's ailments to the exposure, posture, and effort required in their work. First he noted that these demands were imposed too early in the lives of young children. But mainly he analyzed the medical problems connected with these apprenticeships, particularly as they affected circulation and respiration. Makers of shoes and trimmings sat in a bent-over position all day. This compresses the belly and impedes circulation, reasoned Jadelot, and may cause palpitations, aneurisms, and hepatitis. The bonnet makers used a loom that required moving a heavy lathe: this strenuous and repetitive motion interfered with the lesser circulation and caused palpitations, choking, and nosebleeds. Although many young workers suffered from these problems, few of them died: but autopsy confirmed the diagnosis of aneurism. In this connection, Jadelot admiringly refers to the work of Baron Corvisart, a senior consultant at the Children's Hospital, who was, of course, the ranking expert on diseases of the chest. The hospice substituted English looms, which were easier to move and thus lessened the incidence of heart trouble among apprentice bonnet workers. Tailors and weavers who used the "flying shuttle" were not bothered by problems of posture. Carpentry is the healthiest trade, Jadelot observed, "it develops strength without excessive fatigue and is unquestionably preferable to all others."[112] Respiratory problems prevailed, particularly among bonnet workers and the younger children who plucked cotton. But the worst endemic problem Jadelot observed was anthrax, caused by infected wool or hair that the children processed. It was usually fatal.[113]

The Pitié required a medical examination upon admission and excused weak boys from strenuous apprenticeships. Jadelot himself kept an eye on the relation of the boys' health to their work. He used less activist therapy than Brun, and although he sometimes recommended leeches, vesicatories, quinine, or camphor, he often prescribed antiscorbutic liquids, mouthwash, wine, good food, baths, and rest. Jadelot concluded that

> the children are, from the point of view of their health, as well as their condition allows. The diseases specific to artisans affect all apprentices who work in the same professions. The children suffer from no communicable diseases other than those prevailing in all establishments that house a large number of persons their age. . . .
>
> The children are cheerful and content with their fate; they usually grow up to be quite sturdy workers. And when they leave, having learned a profession and knowing how to read and write, they become useful artisans, and readily turn into excellent soldiers.[114]

It is typical of the trials and errors and mixed motives of the administrators that in 1809 all the new facilities at the Pitié went to waste when the establishment was turned into a hospital. Yet Dupoux concludes that "all in all one must admit that the Hospital Council made real progress in the first ten years of its tenure. Starting from the chaos of the Revolutionary years, the council made quite successful efforts in bringing order into the administration, lowered infant mortality (without, however, overcoming it) through rapid placement with wet nurses, struggled against the carelessness of drivers, organized the inspection of wet nurses, and established regulations for apprenticeships that, although not perfect, brought some initial results."[115]

◆◆◆

The Hospital Council thus organized care for children at risk —in many ways the most promising group of dependent citizens in ill health—whom the French government hoped to turn into productive adults. The Poverty Committee also reached out to citizens whose sensory or mental faculties were impaired at birth or by accident, and this book next explores the uncharted ground trodden by a government that sought to extend an equal right to health care to impaired children and adults. To assess the extent to which Revolutionary achievements in this field fit into the overall story of the citizen-patient during our era, we shall therefore now look at the historic and conceptual background of new theories and the consequent innovative methods of teaching and therapy for the deaf, the blind, and the mentally ill.

IV

OUTREACH:

The Impaired Citizen-Patient

CHAPTER EIGHT

The Schooling and Health of the Deaf and Blind

From now on there will be no more deaf-mute, but only deaf who talk.

Jacob Rodriguez Pereira, ca. 1750

The world of the blind, filled with hands begging for alms, was transformed by Valentin Haüy into a world where those hands read and work.

Lieutenant Guéhenno, blinded in battle, 1918

It was logical for the Revolutionary reformers to include the handicapped in their plans for health care of the indigent: the logic derived from the Poverty Committee's mandate. And the young seemed particularly worthy of support and education, in the hope that many might progress to the status of citizen-patients. Educators, physicians, and administrators collaborated to create appropriate institutions for congenitally deaf and blind children, now considered national wards. This chapter highlights persistent questions. Are handicapped children patients who need medical attention or students with learning disabilities? Should they be raised in segregation? Should deaf children learn to speak and lip-read the national language or have a sign language of their own, which the whole population should learn?

During the Revolution and Empire, three boys dramatized these questions. Jean Massieu (1772–1846), star pupil among the deaf, was the true creator of French sign language; Louis Braille (1809–1852), a student at the National Institution for the Blind in the early nineteenth century, invented the six-dot cell that radically changed communication among and with the blind; and Victor, the "wild boy of Aveyron" (178 ?–1828), helped his doctor devise a new method of educating the mentally retarded. The Revolutionary mandate of their right to

225

equality gave these young men's experience historic dimensions. We shall explore the institutions for the handicapped created in the Enlightenment and later nationalized; the problems these institutions encountered in obtaining funding and providing health care; the role of physicians; and the prospects for helping impaired young citizens lead a productive life.[1]

The Enlightenment and the Handicapped

In Western culture, the deaf and the blind have always been considered dependents, along with minors, cripples, and the mentally retarded; the medieval world pronounced the deaf "dumb" on Aristotle's authority. The blind, on the other hand, sometimes secured awed attention as prophets and poets who could "see" into the future. In medieval France, Saint Louis (King Louis IX) endowed a hospital for "fifteen times twenty" blinded crusaders, and his Quinze-Vingts Hospice[2] was soon imitated in Padua, Venice, and elsewhere.[3] But not until the Renaissance did Western man cease to consider serious handicaps as divine punishment and begin to devise therapeutic strategies to remedy them.

The eighteenth century took a lively interest in this question: the role of the sensory organs in conveying impressions that the mind can transform into thought fascinated philosophers, especially after John Locke had formulated the problem. The Enlightenment wanted to understand how a deaf or blind person's perception is impaired, how a cognitive faculty can malfunction, how to use a contrived environment to educate the handicapped. Although several Renaissance philosophers mention teaching the deaf how to speak,[4] it was Pedro Ponce de Leon (1520–1584), a Spanish Benedictine monk, who first seriously attempted it.[5] "The Arte to Make the Dumbe to Speak, the Deafe to Hear"[6] became fashionable in France after a Portuguese Jew, Jacob Rodriguez Pereira (1715–1780), won the approval of the Academy of Sciences in 1749. His system included a manual alphabet and writing, but mainly instruction in speech. He refused to publish his method without a government patent and consequently the details remain unknown,[7] although the Academy's approval indicates widespread interest (witness also Diderot's *Letters* on the deaf-mute [1751] and the blind [1749]).

Methods for teaching the blind were devised beginning in the Renaissance—for example, by Nicholas Saunderson, professor of mathematics at Cambridge (1682–1739) and by the philosopher-physician Gerolamo Cardano (1501–1576). "Reading" with the fingertips proved promising, and inventors experimented with maps, abacuses, chessboards, and piano keys.[8] Meanwhile growing agitation in favor of the Rights of Man charged these philosophical discussions, humanitarian efforts, and technologic innovations to improve the quality of life for the handicapped with political significance.

The reformers championed the right of the handicapped to their share of equality. The deaf, the blind, and the retarded required assistance, but only until they learned to work for a living. Literacy and job training would make them self-supporting. Toward this end the pedagogues of the Enlightenment elaborated carefully structured programs, expecting the individual children to fit themselves into those schemes. They had a famous model in Rousseau, who never asked Emile what *he* wanted to learn. The authoritarian aspect of producing citizen-patients appears most clearly in these programs.

In contrast to academic education and manual training, the children's physical growth received scant attention, and their emotional development none at all. When the student records discovered some years ago in the cellar of the National Institution for the Deaf are finally analyzed, they will harbor few revelations about the children's physical and psychologic adjustment to their handicap.[9] As for the blind pupils, we barely know their names. Psychology had not reached the point where anyone charted the normal or abnormal progression of the individual child, and "follow-up studies" did not exist. Philippe Ariès's thesis that the "idea of childhood" emerged gradually at that time applies to health care as well.[10]

It is thus remarkable that a few handicapped children and their unusual teachers charted new directions for special education during this era. These educators observed, listened, and permitted the deaf, blind, or retarded child to help shape the instructional paths and materials. The French national establishments for the deaf and blind, created by the Revolution, led a stormy existence owing not only to social upheaval and economic distress but also to their headmasters' political decisions and personalities. In fact, no three men could have been more different than the abbé de l'Epée, the abbé Sicard, and Valentin Haüy.

Methods of Teaching the Deaf and the Blind

The abbé Charles Michel de l'Epée (1712–1789) founded a school for deaf children in 1755.[11] At first he financed it with his own funds, then the king awarded him an annual stipend and the Philanthropic Society regularly contributed small sums. In 1784, he published a book on "The True Manner of Teaching the Deaf-Mute, Confirmed by Long Experience," which won him international fame.[12] Although he knew of previous experiments involving lip-reading and speech, he preferred using "methodical signs," fingerspelling (which he called "dactylology"), and written communication. He based his method on the theory that the deaf have their own well-developed language, made up of gestures, signals, and pantomime. He incorporated this "language of the deaf" into his method, which he demonstrated at frequent public sessions in order to attract funds. He saw the teacher as an interpreter and hoped to develop a "universal tongue." But his major preoccupation was to teach religion: "spiritual instruction . . . is my chief goal," he wrote.[13]

The abbé's method was to be influential but controversial.[14] For example, he confidently entitled chapter 14 of his book "That There Is No Metaphysical Idea That the Deaf-Mute Cannot Perceive Clearly by Means of Analysis and Methodical Signs." There follows his well-known example of explaining "I believe." He relates this term to four others: I say "yes" in my mind; I say "yes" in my heart; I say "yes" with my mouth; but my eyes do not see.[15] Did his students really understand?

The method implies that a congenitally deaf person perceives and thinks like one who hears. Surely the fact that these children could learn proved that they were intelligent. Whether this function was not impaired in some is impossible to tell now. But the abbé knew that the intelligence of most would always be limited and that he could not train writers, but only "copyists."[16] Yet he died, on 23 December 1789, believing that his handicapped wards could face the future with confidence.

To die in 1789 believing one's life's work secure was a blessing, and the abbé de l'Epée furthermore expected that his assistant Salvan would succeed him. But another, similar school had been founded by the archbishop of Bordeaux, Champion de Cicé, in 1783, and he had sent the able young abbé Roch Ambroise Cucurron Sicard (1742–1822) to be trained at the Paris institution.[17] As soon as Michel de l'Epée died, Sicard announced his candidacy and demanded a public contest where each candidate would be judged by the performance of a student whom he selected. Sicard's Jean Massieu easily won against the pupils of the abbés Salvan, Masse, and Perennet. Jean Massieu made Sicard famous.

Massieu had five deaf-mute siblings. Imagining that he might acquire hearing and speech by imitation, the boy knelt for morning and evening prayers and moved his lips in imitation of others. Hired as a shepherd, he counted the animals on his fingers and made a notch on his staff when he reached ten. He yearned to go to school, but his father and the schoolmaster refused. "The signs I used were very different from those of educated deaf-mutes," he later reminisced.

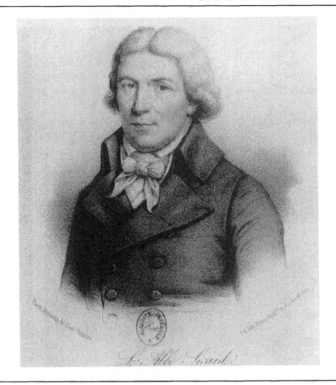

FIGURE 8.1. Abbé Roch Ambroise Cucurron Sicard (1742–1822). Bibliothèque nationale, Paris, Cabinet des estampes.

"Strangers never understood when we expressed our thought through signs; but the neighbors understood."[18]

In his well-known "Course of Instruction of a Deaf-Mute," published in 1800, Sicard acknowledged Massieu's key role. He had found Massieu in the woods near Bordeaux, a creature "with merely animal habits, astonished and frightened by everything. . . . Whatever he saw seemed dangerous, each movement he was *ordered* to do, a trap. His shrouded and expressionless physiognomy, his timid and shifting glances, his *inane and suspicious* looks, his difficulty in acting normally . . . everything seemed to indicate that Massieu could not be educated." In fact, it was Sicard who learned the signs of the deaf from Massieu. The abbé reported quite candidly that "every day [Massieu] learned more than fifty words, and not a day passed when he did not *in turn teach me* the signs for the objects I taught him to write." A unique collaboration thus evolved: "I taught him the written signs of our language, Massieu *taught me the mimed signs of his.* Thus we prepared to converse, eventually, in that pantomime I was perfecting, while my student unveiled its elements through his gestures." Sicard concluded: "Neither I nor my famous teacher [de l'Epée] are the inventors of the language of the deaf (this must be admitted). And just as a foreigner cannot teach a Frenchman his national language, so *it is not the business of a speaking man to invent signs* and give them abstract meaning."[19]

Sicard went far beyond the simple theory and pantomine elaborated by the abbé de l'Epée and constructed a "theory of signs" about which he would discourse for hours.[20] Adroit and adaptable, he managed to avoid any compromising political commitment during the Revolution.[21] He died knowing that he had long ago destroyed a rival whom he had resented ever since a public controversy in the winter of 1784, and whom he had conclusively humiliated in 1814 by refusing to vote for even an honorary reinstatement as headmaster: Valentin Haüy (1745–1822), the teacher of the blind.

◆◆◆

Haüy, the son of a weaver, had been educated by the Premonstrant priests in his native Picardy and at the Collège de Navarre in Paris.[22] He earned a living as translator and was named royal interpreter in 1783. His expertise familiarized him with the problems of conveying the meaning of words to persons who do not understand them. He tells the story of watching some blind street musicians perform, and how they used the senses of touch and hearing to compensate for their disability. The experience stimulated Haüy to devise the method he explains in his "Essay on the Education of the Blind: A Treatise on Various Ways, Tested by Experience, of Enabling the Blind to Read with the Help of Touch, to Print Books in Which They Can Study Languages, History, Geography, Music, etc., and to Perform Varied Tasks on Simple Machines, etc." (1786),[23] a book whose title summarizes the curriculum of the school he founded in 1785. He hoped that some of his students might become teachers of sighted as well as blind pupils, perhaps translators like himself. A choir and a small orchestra attempted to earn money for the school, and so would weaving, rope- and mat-making, bookbinding, and especially printing. Haüy even projected the production of books in foreign languages and of sheet music.

Haüy was sensitive to blind children's psychologic needs, although he neglected their physical development. He mixed blind and sighted students and instructors, let boys and girls learn, work, eat, and play together and approved when fourteen of them intermarried—for which he was widely criticized. Subsequent directors of his school discarded many of his principles, only to reinstate them eventually.[24]

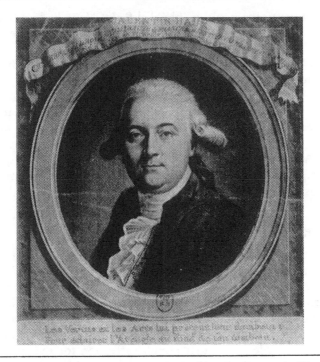

FIGURE 8.2. Valentin Haüy (1745–1822). Etching by Baron de H—, Berlin, 1806. Bibliothèque nationale, Paris, Cabinet des estampes.

The technology to implement his method remained Haüy's life-long preoccupation. Recalling his boyhood experience in the paternal weaver's shop, he tinkered with tools, machines, maps, musical notation, and type for the workshops of his school—a professional attitude reminiscent of the craftsmen who engraved the plates for Diderot's *Encyclopédie*. He devised a multiple spinning wheel with spindles whose speed each blind worker could control, thus eliminating the frustration that a uniform speed might impose on blind children.[25] For printing he used a method where strong, wet paper is pressed down over large metal characters, thus producing text in relief. His response to the objection that books thus printed were too voluminous (which they are) was to set to work experimenting with a "method of abbreviations"—that is, shorthand.[26] When the newly invented semaphore caught his imagination, he wrote a "Short Historical Memoir on Telegraphs" (1810).[27] But communication with the blind progressed, not by such minor improvements, but by methodologic quantum jumps—to Braille, then phonograph records, and now tapes and electronic aids.[28]

In contrast to the wealthy abbé de l'Epée, Haüy had no funds. He joined the Philanthropic Society in 1786, securing twelve livres a month to support the education of twelve blind boys in his school at 18, rue Notre Dame des Victoires.[29] The number of children soon grew to forty-eight.[30] Invited to present his method to the Academy of Sciences on 16 February 1785,[31] Haüy received a favorable verdict from a review committee composed of the geologist Demarest, the oculist Demours, and the two foremost architects of social medicine in France, Félix Vicq d'Azyr and the duc de la Rochefoucauld-Liancourt.[32] A royal audience followed on 26 December 1786, when the king "deigned grant marks of kindness" to Haüy and his students,[33] so that, as one historian put it, "the enterprise was launched."[34]

The Revolution: Recognition and Funding

The outbreak of the French Revolution brought worsening circumstances because wealthy patrons, including members of the Philanthropic Society of Paris, faded away. Eventually the handicapped needed to find a new basis of support within the democratic context.[35] In this endeavor, the deaf led the blind. The abbé Sicard was installed as headmaster of the abbé de l'Epée's school for the deaf in Paris on 6 April 1790.[36] He hoped that popular affection for the late abbé de l'Epée might provide the basis for a public subsidy and was encouraged when a delegation from the Paris Commune proposed to the National Assembly on 18 February 1790 that the "adoptive children of M. l'abbé de l'Epée" become wards of the nation "for reasons of equity and social justice."[37] Seeing that the school's enrollment had already fallen from sixty to forty-five,[38] Sicard decided to orchestrate an appearance of the deaf children before the National Assembly. On 19 August 1790, and again on 21 July 1791, he brought his students Laurent Clerc (1785–1869)[39] and Jean Massieu to a public session and staged a dramatic display of Massieu's talents: "What is an aristocrat?" a deputy asked the twenty-seven-year-old star pupil, who wrote in response: "An aristocrat is a man critical of good laws who wants to be sovereign master, and very rich."

Massieu then asked that the assembly "instruct its Poverty Committee to study the situation [of the deaf], watch over their future, and assure their well-being."[40] He won public recognition in 1795 when a parliamentary decree elevated him to the rank of Sicard's assistant.[41]

Massieu's mention of the Poverty Committee was surely prearranged, for this committee chose Sicard's friend Prieur de la Marne as *rapporteur* of its draft legislation. Two letters in the archives, dated 26 and 29 June 1791, indicate that Sicard coached Prieur, supporting the surmise that an unsigned, undated manuscript "General Plan of a School for the Deaf-Mute" in the archives of the National Institution for the Deaf is in Prieur's hand.[42] Thus well prepared, Prieur presented the Poverty Committee's bill to the National Assembly on 21 July 1791. He analyzed Sicard's school, methods, curriculum, and needs. He praised French sign language and reported that skilled volunteers were already teaching the mechanical arts, drawing, sculpture, engraving, and botany. The deaf students printed the *Journal des savants* and the *Journal d'agriculture,* earning 3,000 livres a year. A projected orchard and hothouses could boost their revenue to more than 6,000 livres. A few years' help from the assembly would make the deaf self-supporting.[43]

Prieur then proposed an annual budget of 12,700 livres for the salaries of ten staff members and an exceptional allocation of 8,400 livres for twenty-four one-year scholarships of 350 livres each. The assembly adopted this bill, proclaiming "that it owed special protection to the establishment for the deaf-mute," which should serve as a "training school for teachers." As for the abbé de l'Epée, he had "earned the special thanks of humanity and of the fatherland."[44]

The possibility of merging the institution for the blind with that for the deaf was first mentioned on 26 August 1790,[45] and the Poverty Committee visited Haüy's establishment on December 6, perhaps to determine the feasibility of this arrangement.[46] In fact, the idea of associating a blind with a deaf person was not novel: Diderot mentions it in his Letter on the Blind.[47] The Constituent Assembly faced adjournment in September 1791, and the hard-pressed deputies, wishing to provide for the blind as they had for the deaf, welcomed a stratagem whereby the two groups could be lodged in the same building. "Yes, gentlemen," the *rapporteur* exclaimed, "the deaf-mute will understand the blind man's conversation and the blind will learn the sign-language of the deaf-mute. . . . Two souls locked into imperfect prisons will overcome the insuperable obstacles that nature has placed between them." This picture was rendered even more appealing by the suggestion that funds for the blind be taken from the Quinze-Vingts Hospice, an institution with an endowment accumulated over half a millennium.[48] (The subsequent nationalization of the Quinze-Vingts undercut this maneuver.)

The decree of 28 September 1791 proclaimed the French nation's obligation to persons born blind and established the National Institution for the Congenitally Blind. It directed Haüy to transfer his students into the Célestins convent, a damp building near the Bastille,[49] into which Sicard had moved the deaf in 1790.[50] Haüy was to appoint his staff "jointly" with Sicard, sharing one administrator and expenses, so that the Célestins would be "a single and integrated establishment."

These administrative arrangements worked poorly, and yet the two national establishments survived and have trained and graduated deaf and blind students from 1791 to this day.[51] The legislature treated the two institutions almost evenhandedly,[52] and this attitude persisted in the Jouënne decree for the deaf (5–8 January 1795),[53] followed by parallel provisions for the blind (on 28 July 1795).[54] But national goals for the handicapped remained ill defined because of uncertainty about their numbers, funding, teacher training, and the confused guidelines laid down by the ministries.

No one knew the numbers of dependent handicapped children in France. Assembly debates kept referring to 4,000 needy deaf-mutes, whereas the abbé de l'Epée had suggested 25,000.[55] The earliest national estimate of blind children, dated 1828, mentions 20,000 blind children under the age of fifteen and 40,000 blind Frenchmen in all.[56]

Raising money for the handicapped from private sources became impossible as the Revolution gained momentum. Therefore the decrees of 1791 included 24 scholarships for the deaf, later increased to 60 for each national school, in Paris and Bordeaux, to which Chaptal added another 20. Yet few believed that 120 scholarships, or even 140, could solve the problem. In fact, the question of creating six, eight, even ten schools for the deaf was raised several times during the lengthy preparatory legislative debates, but to no avail.[57] As for the blind, their scholarships remained at 30: Haüy failed to demonstrate the need for more.

In addition to problems of numbers and funding, it soon became clear that more teachers would be needed. Both Sicard and Haüy saw themselves as models and offered to spread information throughout the country. Some deputies explored the schools' mandate of teacher training. The regulations of both institutions, laid down in 1791, specified that during their vacations teachers should "acquaint various parts of the kingdom with the special programs. . . . They shall try to stimulate the creation of similar establishments in their native provinces." And at the December 1792 meeting of the Legislative Assembly, Maignet, deputy from Puy de Dôme, proposed the creation of a national program with twenty places for instructors, who were to be trained for three years, and an additional six places for foreigners.

The French government from then on usually spoke in the same breath of "the deaf-mute and the blind." The government found it impossible to decide whether these children should be treated as students or as patients, whether it should provide for compensatory education or for health care. Therefore the Daunou Law of 25 October

1795 (3 Brumaire, Year IV) included schools for the handicapped in plans for national education,[58] while the Law of 7 October 1796 considered the establishments for the handicapped as part of French hospital administration.[59] The Consulate found a clever solution by creating a separate group of "welfare institutions." The notion harked back to the old regime, allowing the government to appoint a board of wealthy trustees. For decades the government pretended to have solved the dilemma, at least for the blind, by appointing physicians as headmasters of their institutions. It was only in 1837 that Dr. Guillié dissociated the two jobs, thus freeing the school from the hospice connotation. Some of the headmasters acted merely as administrators, others paid heed to the needs of deaf and blind youngsters for spacious surroundings and for attention to their physical and psychologic health.

The Health of the Handicapped: The Struggle for Air and Space

With the children's subsistence thus minimally assured by the National Assembly, their guardians could turn their attention to housing, daily routine, education, and job training. The goal was to produce self-supporting citizen-patients. But in the Revolutionary and Napoleonic period, we find many of the children and their teachers living under conditions that actually impaired their health, engaged in a protracted struggle for air and space, and subjected to Spartan regulations and to what amounted to a prison term for the blind under Napoleon.

Sicard maneuvered to his establishment's advantage. The Célestins convent, although spacious, was inappropriate. A report in the National Archives, dated 15 October 1790, reveals that the government chose it for the handicapped because this former church property was unsalable but permitted "the merger of the two institutions at little cost."[60] As for directing the two headmasters to share one administrator and agree on personnel, expenditures, and repairs—it requires little imagination to conjure up countless causes of annoyance, friction, altercations, trouble. Somehow they coexisted under these conditions for three years.

In the meantime, the political sky was darkening. After the declaration of war in the spring of 1792 and the fall of the monarchy in August, the situation grew tense. Sicard became increasingly suspect to the radical inhabitants of the "Arsenal section," who believed that his primary motivation was that of a counterrevolutionary Catholic cleric. Haüy turned into an ardent Jacobin, active in revolutionary committees. During the subsequent seven years, as power in the government shifted back and forth between Right and Left, each headmaster was several times arrested, interrogated, and jailed, and Sicard narrowly escaped death in the September massacres. Each was convinced that the other had instigated the incidents.[61]

Tension mounted at the Célestins as the Year II wore on. Then a chance development brought relief: the Arsenal barracks needed more room for military purposes, and the deaf and blind had to move out. Sicard maneuvered adroitly: a decree of 5 March 1794 transferred his school to the former Magloire seminary, high on the montagne Ste. Geneviève, to what is still the National Institution for Deaf Children, 254, rue St. Jacques (familiar to modern moviegoers from François Truffaut's *The Wild Child*). A visit to the present-day institution, with its gardens, nurseries, hothouses, and flowerbeds, essentially unchanged since the Revolution, and a chat with the young gardeners (whose adeptness at lip-reading nowadays enables them to converse with complete ease), quickly convinces one that horticulture has special meaning for these handicapped youngsters. In this instance, the institution successfully applied the traditional notion that working the land has therapeutic value, especially for the handicapped; gardening and agriculture still receive special emphasis in their training, and these citizen-patients are readily placed in good jobs, for which the government gives them preference.[62]

Sicard's skill in defending his palatial new home can be documented from an incident in 1808. Would Sicard consider moving to the Petits Pères and yield St. Magloire to the Sisters of Charity? "No sacrifice would be too great if the government so desires," Sicard wrote. Having visited his intended new abode, he told the minister of religion the same day: "That building is a real cesspool, whose foul air is surely pestilential for those condemned to live there. . . . [It] has no garden, and the deaf-mute seem to need pure and salubrious air more urgently than others, and sufficient open space for physical exercise. . . . I doubt, monseigneur, that there is in this capital any building . . . that suits us as well as the one we inhabit."[63] The minister of internal affairs reported to Napoleon that "the superior general of the Sisters of Charity, the abbé Sicard, and I met at Saint Magloire and agreed." The deaf did not need to move.[64]

Sicard managed to stay in office even under the Jacobins, taking the "minor oath" of allegiance. He eventually won the trust of Chaptal, who, as we shall see, promoted him to a position of authority and influence.[65] Haüy, in contrast to Sicard, put patriotism before common sense. Writing to the Committee on Public Safety on 21 May 1794, he praised his own parsimony and requested transfer of his school to the vacant maison des Filles Sainte Catherine on rue des Lombards in the densely populated heart of Paris, halfway between the Hôtel de Ville and the Halles. He argued that "the Working Blind and their teachers are true sansculottes and enemies of luxury. They like to be housed in classrooms and workshops. And may I add that this building is perhaps the only one in Paris that would require no expense to adapt it to the uses of the National Institution for the Working Blind."[66] The term "working blind" (*"aveugles-travailleurs"*) was Haüy's invention. He dreamt of self-supporting citizen-patients. His proposal to move to the "Catherinettes" proved irresistible to the legislators, hard-pressed at the height of the Terror. Haüy thus condemned his blind children, many of them in poor health, to residence in constricted quarters that lacked air and sunshine. One of them, Galliod, later commented: "For almost a year, we could not resume work, owing to the prevailing scarcity."[67] Haüy lacked Sicard's thespian skills, political adroitness, and administrative ability. He had no expert associates, only subordinates.

The Spartan regulations and demanding curriculum for the handicapped were elaborated in 1791 by the duc de la Rochefoucauld-Liancourt, with help from Prieur de la Marne and an assist from Sicard.[68] These Regulations imposed the regimen of the seminary: the children rose at five o'clock in the morning (six o'clock in winter), and, after washing, chores, prayer and breakfast, went to classes from ten until two. After dinner and a brief recess, they attended more classes, from three until supper at eight . . . another recess, and to bed at ten. The regulations applied to the blind as well as the deaf.

Instruction for the deaf focused on vocabulary, grammar, speech, "signing," and religion, with regular master classes and weekly public demonstrations led by Sicard. La Rochefoucauld-Liancourt's rules alerted the staff constantly to expect student misbehavior. Thus we read: "The porter shall always keep the doors locked and shall only open them for a student on the written order of the headmaster or administrator," and "the masters . . . shall not leave the students, day or night. They shall eat together at common tables and share the same food." And even misconduct after dark could be prevented, because "all dormitories shall be lit at night. The proctors shall have their beds at both ends of the dormitories."

In January 1800, Sicard tightened discipline further, including uniforms, short hair (*"cheveux coupés en rond"*), surveillance, denunciation, and punishment. The regulations threatened that "if a student does any damage, or refuses to fulfill an assigned task, the supervisor reports the incident to the director who decides on the punishment . . . ranging from deprivation of [the] wine alotted on *quintidi*

and *décadi,* to a diet of bread and water, to several days in the disciplinary room, to dismissal." One cause for dismissal was for a student
to be found in the garden alone. These rules remained in force well
into the nineteenth century.[69]

La Rochefoucauld-Liancourt was most concerned that the children
should learn a trade (the Poverty Committee had seen too many
young idlers at Bicêtre and the Salpêtrière). Thus we read in the duke's
regulations that the two institutions should provide "a moral education, and training that will enable [the children] to live from the
products of their own hard work" and that "the two families of the
deaf-mute and the blind" were to manufacture "bed-frames, chairs,
tables, linen, clothes, and all the furniture for the two institutions.
Each worker shall receive one-quarter of the price for his work."
The deaf children soon printed numerous government documents and
worked at gardening, shoemaking, joining and cabinetmaking, printing, lithography, bookbinding, and wood carving, thus implementing
the government's plan to transform its wards into citizen-patients. Activities for the blind were more limited, as we shall see.[70]

Fresh air and physical exercise received some attention, at least for
the deaf boys, who were taken on outings twice a week. The girls
remained cloistered. To take blind children on walks evidently seemed
too complicated. Several legislators proposed healthful measures:
Maignet, the deputy from Puy de Dôme, suggested in 1793 that all
schools for the deaf add two nurses, a pharmacist, and a health officer.
All students should be inoculated, he proposed; and "several times a
week, teachers should lead the deaf to the countryside and show them
how the land is cultivated and emphasize repeatedly the advantages of
this earliest of human professions."[71] The suggestions were ignored.

Distractions were rare, and the deaf and blind children lived a miserable existence, particularly during the Directory. The archives are
filled with appeals, especially from Haüy, for more (or at least more
usable) beds, mattresses, pillows, sheets, blankets, curtains, comfort-
ers, towels, aprons. On 15 June 1796, for example, he warned the
minister that "our housekeeper has neither bed nor sheets for any
additional student you may send." On 31 May 1797, he described
the "shocking conditions prevailing in the establishment"; on 13 July,
he asked that the minister stop all new admissions "until the Treasury
pays the overdue scholarships, since no supplier will extend any more
credit." The minister appointed a team to investigate and the ensuing report called for the immediate emergency disbursement of six
hundred francs to the butcher and baker, to "assure two weeks'
supply. . . . But clearly this is only an expedient."[72]

Sicard did not plead, but struck a political note, writing to Lucien

Bonaparte in August 1800, soon after his reinstatement: "The buildings at the institution for the deaf-mute need inspection: the roof is in very bad condition and dormitories need to be built. Classes are held where dormitories should be, and meals are served in what ought to be classroom. The whole establishment makes a dreadful impression on the many visitors who come there."[73] Under such conditions, even fresh air and space to play and a normal diet and hygiene were luxuries.

The blind children were less trainable than the deaf. A payroll statement for the Institution for the Blind, dated fall 1794, lists four teachers in addition to Haüy, who was employed at that time as interpreter to the Committee of Public Safety. Two foremen supervised the small printing press and two governesses the needlework. Eight blind assistants helped the four music teachers: a violinist, a singing teacher, a cellist, and a clarinetist. It is difficult to ascertain whether they succeeded in teaching the children a trade. The few accounts we have of public performances to raise money leave the reader with a painful impression: one visualizes the short plays, heavy on moral lessons, awkwardly acted; one imagines two string instruments and a clarinet accompanying the thin voices of pale, undernourished blind boys and girls. The spectators' donations were surely motivated by pity.

While Sicard was outlawed in 1797 and in hiding, Alhoy, the acting administrator, proposed a decentralized, collegial administration with much less emphasis on discipline, supervision, and punishment.[74] One speculates sadly that the deaf students' lives might have been happier had their teachers been less regimented. However, Sicard returned. Also, Alhoy joined with Valentin Haüy to propose a remarkable tax scheme to aid the handicapped: grateful godparents of each baby born healthy would donate fifty centimes to help the deaf and blind. This humane project was discussed in the Legislative Body on 5 October 1799, and the Council of Five Hundred took it under advisement. But it foundered in the commotion caused by Bonaparte's coup d'état.[75]

For the deaf and the blind, the coup d'état meant a new administrative status as a part of "welfare institutions,"[76] and in 1805 Napoleon appointed Sicard to the board overseeing this unit. Sicard had longed for the position. This is apparent in the *Almanach national,* where he had annually entered his name ahead of his institution's administrative council. Now he was able to turn the clock back and tighten the rules, emphasize religious training and regimentation, and block experiment and innovation. Characteristically, one of his first moves was to invite Pope Pius VII, who was in Paris for Napoleon's coronation, to visit the Institution for the Deaf. Wishing to be even-handed, the pope also visited the blind: he found them relegated to the Quinze-Vingts Hospice, where he met only Haüy's successor.

For indeed the new welfare structure permitted a cunning political move, which amounted to incarcerating the children and led to Haüy's exile: the purpose of this move was to integrate Valentin Haüy's school into the Quinze-Vingts Hospice, a forbidding, dark former barracks, surrounded by a high wall, located on the eastern fringe of Paris.[77] It is difficult to reconcile Chaptal's concurrence in this obliteration of Haüy's school with his imaginative and generous intervention during these same months in the reestablishment of the nursing orders, the creation of a midwifery school, the reform of hospital administration, and the formation of a public health council in Paris. Archival documentation solves that puzzle, for it reveals that it was not governmental penny-pinching, Sicard's prodding, or Haüy's opinionated pride, but a totally incongruous political circumstance that proved to be the real cause of Haüy's downfall.

Haüy was a founder of the revolutionary religious sect of theophilanthropy,[78] a group under surveillance since 1797,[79] which was suppressed by Joseph Fouché, the minister of police, on 2 October 1801 (12 Vendémiaire, Year X).[80] That Haüy was the real target of this measure appeared obvious to knowledgeable observers. Haüy protested (which annoyed Bonaparte), and thus, on 15 February 1801, some thirty blind children, henceforth the "second-class blind," were carted off to the Quinze-Vingts Hospice.[81]

Haüy went down fighting, in a futile struggle to retain his teaching staff, maintain his children's identity as students, and cling to his role as headmaster.[82] After a series of incidents, in which Haüy's rigidity played to the government's punitiveness, Chaptal abolished the position of headmaster.[83] A comparison of payroll statements for Haüy's school for 1794 and 1808 indicates that the "National Institute for the Working Blind" had made way for a simple category of "young blind" among the inhabitants of the hospice; the staff of twenty persons to educate the children had shrunk to six, the most notable victims of the cutbacks being Haüy's prize pupil, Lesueur, two workshop foremen, and the four music teachers: they remained at the hospice, but lost their jobs; the monthly expenditures had been reduced from 1,550 to 550 francs, and government scholarships were abolished.[84]

"Disgusted by this state of things," according to Galliod, and despite an annual pension of 2,000 francs, Haüy withdrew to a private school for the blind that he had founded on rue Sainte Avoye at the time of the forced transfer to the Quinze-Vingts. His fame among foreigners, at least, persisted—witness the example of Dr. Joseph Frank of Vienna, who wrote in 1804: "Before visiting the Quinze-

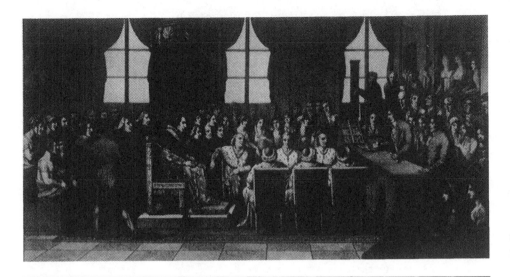

FIGURE 8.3. Pope Pius VII visits the blind students, 28 February 1805. Postcard sold at the time to commemorate the event.

Vingts, I wished to acquaint myself with the method of teaching the blind. Therefore I first went to a different institution, namely, a private one directed by Monsieur Haüy (the brother of the famous mineralogist)."[85] We know of only two prominent blind pupils whom Haüy trained during this time, Alexander Rodenbach, later a well-known writer and public official in Belgium,[86] and Alexandre Fournier who accompanied him to Russia.[87] For in the end Haüy accepted the invitation of Czar Alexander I to establish an institution for the blind in Saint Petersburg. He stopped in Berlin, where he met young Johann August Zeune, who would soon open a school for the blind,[88] and thought it politic to pay his respects to the comte de Provence (the future Louis XVIII). In September 1806, Haüy reached St. Petersburg, where he would struggle for eleven years to run an establishment that never really existed.[89] Letters to his son Just indicate that he endured the poverty and humiliation of a refugee existence in wartime.[90]

After Waterloo, Haüy yearned to return home. He approached the administrative board of the welfare establishments in Paris, asking to be reinstated as instructor of the blind, *honoris causa*. Two trustees, Malus and Germain Garnier, favored this kindness. The board refused, one of the remaining three members being the abbé Sicard.[91] Haüy persevered, but no French régime in the nineteenth century acknowledged his achievement.[92] On 25 August 1817, he returned to Paris, "aged, disillusioned, embittered,"[93] to live with his brother, the famous abbé, at the Jardin des plantes. On 22 August 1821, a ceremony in his honor was held at the Institution for the Blind. One of the young participants was the thirteen-year-old Louis Braille, who was to make Haüy's institution world-famous and who would be buried in the Pantheon on 22 June 1852.[94]

◆◆◆

In reviewing the experience of the deaf and the blind during the Revolution and Empire, we find a paradoxic outcome: while Haüy's difficult personality and inept maneuvering resulted in a political failure, his methodology was innovative and experimental and created an environment in which Braille could pursue his discovery. Sicard, on the other hand, although successful and much decorated, was a grammarian who lost himself in the intricacies of vocabulary and syntax. He refused to listen to opponents of the manual alphabet and his insistence on mimicry of spoken French delayed acceptance of French sign language for over a century.

Like many powerful and aged men, neither Sicard nor Haüy trained a successor. Haüy, as we have seen, lost authority over his school for political reasons. Sicard ruled his establishment in an autocratic manner. A dissenter, the abbé Roch Ambroise Bébian (1789–1838), Sicard's godson, left France because of disagreement over teaching methods. He later complained that "some of [Sicard's] disciples adhered to his method with the fanaticism of a sect." Bébian was an advocate of signing and later headed an institution at Rouen.[95] A student of Bébian's, Ferdinand Berthier (1803–1886), also an advocate of signing, taught at the Paris institution for forty-five years, ending up as dean. Another graduate, the abbé Charles Louis Carton (1802–1863), moved to Bruges to head a school for the deaf in newly created Belgium.[96]

It is suprising that the medical profession was so slow to indicate its concern for the children living in the new institutions. But there were exceptions. Dr. Paul Seignette (17 ?–1835), administrator of the Quinze-Vingts while the blind students resided there from 1802 to 1815, saved their morale and their school.[97] When he arrived, he found that Bertrand, the teacher who had succeeded Haüy (the headmastership had been abolished), had reduced classes to two hours a day. "The rest of the time was spent spinning wool," a monotonous, unhealthy task that did not produce much money.[98]

Seignette realized that the first necessity was to revive a positive outlook on the children's part. Encouraging Galliod, the blind musician, and Lesueur, the printer, Seignette visited classes and workshops and "promoted the study of varied subject matter. His presence encouraged the students. . . . The best among them came to him in the evenings when his office turned into a classroom. He helped eagerly, lending them the classics."[99] Seignette thus emerges as one of those unsung heroes among the administrators who helped the handicapped survive the Revolution and Empire.

In 1815, Louis XVIII made good on a promise to Haüy and assigned the blind children a new home, the former St. Firmin monastery near the Pitié Hospice. Dr. Sébastien Guillié, the new headmaster, soon installed dormitories with large windows, courtyards for exercise, and two large dining halls. He did appreciate the need for living space and fresh air.[100] He took credit for renovating the school, even though he merely resurrected Haüy's methods and dusted off his equipment.[101] He used Haüy's relief maps, looms, and tools, but made no progress in teaching the blind how to write and discontinued musical notation, relying on auditory memory. An admirer of Pestalozzi's method, he favored the so-called Lancaster system of mutual instruction.[102] Guillié also called for a "moral reorganization," dismissed forty-three students, and cleared the library shelves of books "offensive to modesty and religion."[103] He replaced these with works on history, geography, and mathematics. He was advised in this housecleaning by one of the trustees, his "excellent friend, the abbé Sicard."[104] He established seven workshops and classrooms, an infirmary, and servants' quarters. Classes were held from seven in the morning till eight at night, with schedules that favored a mixture of intellectual with manual training. Pierre Henri, the biographer of Louis Braille, characterizes this regime as "desperately hard."[105]

Guillié's successors accused him of having selected the new building for the wrong reasons—namely, the strict separation of facilities for boys and girls. Such segregation seemed vital to Guillié, and he appointed an adamant Breton spinster, Zélie de Cardeilhac, as headmistress for the girls. "Formerly," he wrote in 1817, "marriages between blind persons were favored, but couples are no longer allowed to live at the Institution."[106] The new tone differed from the easygoing family atmosphere that Haüy had created for his "children"; the youngsters now led a Spartan existence, occasionally brightened by supervised outings and summer vacations.[107]

One did not need to be a physician to observe that Saint Firmin was cramped and humid, yet the government only took notice when two medical inspectors visited in 1821 and 1828 and reported that "mortality is high among the students. Their health is endangered by that building."[108]Eventually their report reached the Chamber of Deputies, which finally voted the credits of 1,600,000 francs needed for a new building. It was the poet Lamartine, a deputy, who helped bring about this hoped-for event when he told the chamber that he went to visit "that narrow, dirty, dark building, those hallways cut in two to form veritable cells dubbed 'studios' and 'classrooms,' those many twisted, worm-eaten staircases that seem a challenge to blindness." Lamartine concluded that if the whole Chamber had visited the institution, "the whole Chamber would vote the credits requested by the minister."[109] The legislature appropriated the funds on 18 July 1838, and in 1843, Haüy's students moved into their present palatial home, 56, boulevard des Invalides. A life-sized statue of Valentin Haüy now greets the visitor in the middle of the courtyard.[110]

Guillié made one decision crucial to the lives of the blind everywhere: in the summer of 1819, he admitted Louis Braille. The boy did not especially impress him, and yet, at the age of fifteen, Braille devised his ingenious new method. It was based on a complex arrangement of punched dots devised by a retired artillery captain, Charles Barbier de la Serre.[111] Braille's simplification of this system amounts to an original discovery: his six-dot "cell" permits the formation of all the letters in the alphabet, all the numerals, and even accents, symbols, and musical notation.[112] The students enthusiastically adopted the new method, but the institution opposed it at first. It had invested so much money in material for printing with embossed letters! For fifteen years Braille struggled, first against Dr. Pignier, then against his successor, P. A. Dufau. Finally, the vice-principal, J. Guadet, fully described and praised the new system in his speech at the opening of the new building in 1843. Louis Braille had revolutionized the lives of the handicapped. More than anyone else, he smoothed their way toward being citizen-patients.

◆◆◆

So did "Victor," the twelve-year-old mute "wild boy" caught in the woods of Aveyron in the fall of 1799. Physicians and other Parisian scientists became keenly interested in studying this child, who had survived in the "state of nature." The most actively involved group, the Society of the Observers of Man (1799–1805), consisted of about sixty Ideologues: naturalists, linguists, philosophers, physicians, explorers, archeologists, historians, economists, classicists, and writers, Sicard among them. This short-lived society epitomized contemporary curiosity about the globe and its creatures, human origins and growth, and normal and abnormal development. But these Ideologues wished to do more than study: as pointed out in the first chapter of this book, they yearned for public service, in this case as rescuers of a handicapped child. They studied the "wild boy of Aveyron," wondering whether he might grow into a citizen-patient.

Sicard had a logical claim to a boy who was selectively deaf, and mute, and his flair for publicity heightened his eagerness. The child arrived rue St. Jacques in the summer of 1800, and the Society of the Observers of Man set up a study commission consisting of Pinel, the distinguished naturalist Georges Cuvier, and Baron M. F. de Gérando, philanthropist and expert on deaf-mutism. Pinel, chosen as reporter, read a careful appraisal to the Society on 29 November 1800 and offered his conclusions in May 1801. He tested the boy's five senses, his affects, and his thought processes, finding "dissonance" between the senses of touch and sight, and inappropriate bursts of laughter, all of which reminded him of children on the mental wards of Bicêtre and the Salpêtrière. Describing fifteen such children under his care, he concluded that attempts to "civilize" the boy were futile and asked rhetorically: "Is it not most probable that the boy from Aveyron resembles children or adults fallen into a state of dementia or idiotism?"[113]

Less than six months after Pinel's report, Sicard announced to the Observers of Man that the physician of the deaf, Jean Marc Gaspard Itard (1775–1838), had studied the boy, whom he called Victor, and stood ready to share his observations.[114] Itard eventually published three long essays.[115] As Pinel's student, he shared the conviction that the mentally ill—including retarded and mentally defective children—are patients whom the physician can study and help. Convinced of Victor's intelligence and daily witness of his capacity for affection, Itard devised ingenuous methods to stimulate the boy's senses and to educate him. He seems to have developed a deep personal attachment for Victor. For five years he tried, but success was slight, and eventually Victor's puberty proved so explosive that Itard had to desist.[116]

Victor never led the life of a normal adolescent and never spoke a word. But he patiently helped Itard construct a method and refine the materials needed to teach a retarded child his letters and numbers, basic notions of shape, size, color, and socially acceptable behavior. He also demonstrated his capacity to feel a wide range of emotions. Although lack of human contacts had hindered his social development, life in the woods had sharpened his wits and stimulated his agility. Itard concluded that Victor was a retarded, but not an idiot, child.

Itard was left with a lifelong concern for problems of deafness and mutism related to impaired mental functions, and he permanently established otology as a branch of medicine.[117] He was the creator of special education for handicapped children like Victor, and he inspired Edouard Seguin (1812–1880), who brought this specialty to the

United States, as well as Maria Montessori (1870–1952), who adapted Itard's method for the kindergarten education of the normal child.

Cardinal de Rohan's Debt

When, under the Third Republic, the lay Society to Aid the Blind lobbied for higher government subsidies, they used a novel argument: the state owed the blind a *debt* because, on the eve of the Revolution, the buildings of the Quinze-Vingts had been sold for 6,312,000 livres by their official protector, the Grand Almoner of France, Cardinal de Rohan (of "Affair of the Queen's Necklace" fame).[118] Supporters located a phrase in Finance Minister Necker's famous budget of 1781 stating that the Quinze-Vingts were due 250,000 "to constitute a perpetual annual payment for *part* of the sales price of the land and buildings formerly owned by the hospice."[119] Louis XVIII had reinstated the Grand Almoner as trustee of the Quinze-Vingts,[120] and under the Republic, it was argued, the finance minister was his successor. By 1903, this obligation had become an "I.O.U.," a "public debt—none more sacred."[121]

The Law of 14 July 1905 on "aid to the aged, infirm, and incurable" raised the number of blind eligible for government help from three to six thousand. The 1909 budget carried two special provisions: one to create more workshops and studios, the other for research to *prevent* blindness, a strategy of which Valentin Haüy never dreamt.

◆◆◆

This chapter has analyzed the endeavor of the French government to assist handicapped children and enable them to acquire an education and learn a trade. Such an official undertaking, novel at the time, has become a permanent part of modern governments' definition of their duties toward the impaired citizen. Debate continues about the methods used to teach the deaf and the blind, and the authoritarian organization of institutions in Napoleonic France has its critics. But about the generous motivation there can be no question. We now turn to an even more complex range of needs, those of the mentally ill.

Humane Treatment of the Mental Patient

An understanding of the varieties of madness teaches one to identify the almost certainly curable cases, the doubtful ones, those where relapses are to be feared, and those without any hope of cure.

Philippe Pinel, "Memoir on Madness: A Contribution to the Natural History of Man," 1794

A new and humane approach, formulated, developed, and publicized during the Revolution and Empire, applied the Poverty Committee's mandate to the mentally ill, as it did to the deaf, the blind, unwanted children, and the elderly during this era. The living conditions, diagnosis, and therapy of the institutionalized mentally ill underwent considerable change. Modernized legislation eventually followed. Mainly, the women and men who had been considered incurably mad found themselves transformed into mental patients, whom physicians perceived as curable by nonphysical, psychologic means—dubbed "moral treatment." Madness turned into "mental alienation"—an aberration that skilled therapists might rectify by leading patients back into the "normal" world and motivating them to become citizen-patients.

The condition of the mentally ill in four establishments located in the Paris region can serve to illustrate the changes that occurred during the era surveyed in this book. First, treatment at the Paris Hôtel-Dieu, as condemned in Jacques Tenon's *Mémoires sur les hôpitaux de Paris,* exemplifies how the impecunious "mad" were dealt with in all of western Europe whenever fear of the madman and humoral theorizing led to activist physical therapy. Second, some innovation bore fruit at Bicêtre Hospice, where an uneducated but skillful "governor," Jean Baptiste Pussin, applied the instructions elaborated by the royal inspectors Colombier and Doublet in 1785. It was at Bicêtre, during the Terror, that Philippe Pinel discovered the large group of institutionalized mentally ill men whom he observed along with Pussin's management of that ward. These observations led Pinel to his basic theoretical formulations and to his practical, humane approach. We shall study the patients' condition at Bicêtre through analysis of two recently discovered documents, Pussin's "Observations" of 1794 and 1797 ("Observations du citoyen Pussin sur les fous") and Pinel's "Memoir on Madness" of 1794 ("Mémoire sur la manie pour servir à l'histoire naturelle de l'homme").[1]

Moving to Salpêtrière Hospice, we enter a world of elderly, ailing, or sick women that we have already analyzed, and we know that by 1804, the accommodations, food, and laundry—and thus the morale—of the women were greatly improved. It was in infirmaries for more than 1,000 mentally ill women, in his thirty-bed teaching ward, and through his textbook on "Philosophic Nosography" that Pinel introduced thousands of medical students to a humane medicine that was based on the observation of patients' behavior as well as of their physical signs and symptoms. Young doctors would take this new approach toward the citizen-patient to the battlefields and to the bedside of patients throughout France.

Finally, we obtain perspective on the condition of the French mental patient in the nineteenth century from a look at Charenton asylum. Here the Brothers of Charity provided expert custodial treatment to wealthy men under the old regime; in the nineteenth century, Charenton evolved into the public asylum of the Seine Department under the Law of 1838. That law is still in force, and Jean Dominique Esquirol (1772–1840) was one of its chief architects. The evolution of the management and care of the mentally ill from the late eighteenth to the early nineteenth century can thus be told in the light of these examples.

Traditional Custody of the Mentally Ill

It is true that of all the handicapped, impaired, and impoverished Frenchmen in need of public care, the mentally ill were the least likely to reach the level of citizen-patients. And yet attention focused on their management and cure, thus leading to the emergence of psychiatry in France during the Revolutionary period. This development resulted from the confluence of three trends. First, the indigent mentally ill were now seen as entitled to decent accommodations and support within the public hospital system. Second, many of these patients were now perceived as curable, so that appropriate therapeutic strategies would be well worth pursuing. And third, doctors now granted a major place to the "neuroses" in their general nosologic framework, thus including mental derangement within the spectrum of diseases and eventually including psychiatry within the field of medicine.

In medieval and early modern times the "mad," such as the demented elderly and village idiots, seem to have been tolerated and largely ignored. They were maintained for motives of Christian charity, but expelled if they became a menace. Neglect of the mentally ill sprang from ignorance, and from indifference to deviant behavior. But behind this indifference lurked fear. Fear of malevolent magic spawned accusations of witchcraft against odd old women; religious fanatics interpreted witchcraft as heresy, and the Catholic Inquisition developed a textbook for the interrogation of witches, the *Malleus maleficarum,* while Protestant purists gained comparable expertise at spotting the devil and his cohorts. The history of hysteria finds plentiful material in witch trials. The Enlightenment, spurning superstition and religious bigotry, sought a new explanation for deviant behavior but continued to restrain violent madmen and confine them in the local fortress, the town wall, the prison. The horror stories of madmen loaded down with heavy chains have obscured the fact that these victims were few in numbers (which does not, of course, make their fate any less pitiable).

Although neglect and fear gradually waned, parsimony has always prevailed in the public care of the mentally ill: medieval law courts already emphasized that the care of "lunatics" and "fools" was their families' responsibility. A family with means had two choices: their deranged relative could live either in their own home or in an institution at the family's expense. The study of custody for the insane in the early modern period reveals two important distinctions: one economic, the other religious. Wealthy mental patients enjoyed comforts that public funding could not afford; that difference between rich and poor has never been bridged. Equally stark is the contrast between Catholic and Protestant countries: monastic orders specialized in psychiatric nursing, but in Protestant countries the Reformation had disbanded these. In some cases, national institutions developed, as in the Holy Roman Empire; in others, notably in Great Britain, the mentally ill languished in the poorhouse until the eighteenth century, when voluntary hospitals and private "madhouses" assumed the role of caretakers.

In France, as we have seen, wealthy Frenchmen who were mentally ill were often confined by *lettre de cachet* and cared for by the Brothers of Charity and similar orders. The inmates lived under strict, but thoughtful, supervision, some in closed wards, some in locked cells. If one of them fell ill, he was sent to the infirmary; if unruly, he could be put in solitary confinement, "in a room that was more solidly built

TABLE 9.1. Violent Madmen, Mad Women, Imbeciles, and Epileptics Confined in the Jails and Hospitals of Paris, 1788

	Mad (agitated)		Imbecile (senile)		Epileptic		Total
	Men	Women	Men	Women	Men	Women	
In municipal hospitals							
Salpêtrière ⎫ "General Hospital"		150		150		300	600
Bicêtre ⎭	92		138		15		245
Hôtel-Dieu	42	32					74
Charité of Charenton (Brothers of Charity)	1		77		4		82
Petites Maisons	22	22					44
							(1,045)
In the clinics of the Faubourg St. Jacques							
M. Massé, Montrouge		2	16	2			20
M. Bardot, rue Neuve, Ste. Geneviève			5	4			9
Widow Rolland, route de Villejuif			4	8			12
Mlle Laignel, cul-de-sac des Vignes				36			36
M. des Guerrois, rue Vieille Notre–Dame				17			17
M. Teinon, rue Copeau			5	1			6
							(100)

In the clinics of the Faubourg St. Antoine

Mme. Ste. Colombe, rue de Picpus			28			28	
M. Esquiros, rue du Chemin Vert			12	9	2	23	
Widow Bouqueton, au Petit Charonne		3	10	20		33	
M. Belhomme, rue de Charonne	2		15	16		33	
M. Picquenot, au Petit Bercy	1		5	1	1	7	
Widow Marcel, au Petit Bercy				2		5	
M. Bertaux, au Petit Bercy	3		2	1		6	
Convent for men, Picpus			2	3		3	
M. Cornillieux, Charonne			1	1		2	
						(140)	
In the clinics of Montmartre							
St. Lazare, Faubourg St. Denis		5	17	15		17	
Mlle Douay, rue de Bellefonds						20	
M. Huguet, rue des Martyrs			6	3		9	
						(46)	
Total	163	214	346	286	22	300	1,331

SOURCE: Adapted from Jacques Tenon, *Mémoires sur les hôpitaux de Paris*, 218. See also J. Postel and C. Quétel, eds., *Nouvelle histoire de la psychiatrie* (Toulouse: Privat, 1983), 117.

than others, but not detrimental to health."[2] The supervised freedom that William Tuke presumably inaugurated at his asylum for Quakers, at the York Retreat, in the 1790s thus had a well-tested, if unacknowledged, Catholic antecedent. The brothers' paying patients ate well: we have published menus to prove it. Most important, the inmates could count on the services of physicians who treated them according to the latest medical theories and therapeutic practices—if we are to believe Paul Sérieux and Lucien Libert, two Catholic scholars who sought, in the early twentieth century, to undermine the prevalent conviction that the French Revolution decisively improved the lot of the mentally ill. These authors assembled evidence of the professional excellence with which the Brothers of Charity cared for their inmates for moderate fees. The brothers provided medical care and consolation (which Sérieux and Libert equate with "moral treatment").[3] Tenon, in contrast, mentions annual fees of 6,000 livres.[4] Other documents suggest that the brothers operated under exclusive, lucrative government contracts regulating the lives of the mentally ill confined by *lettre de cachet* at the family's or the government's direction and expense.

In France, lay and private nursing homes for the mentally ill are known to have existed in the eighteenth century—primarily, perhaps exclusively, in the cities. In Paris, there were eighteen of them in 1789.[5] Best known among these is the establishment owned by an ex-cabinetmaker, Jacques Belhomme. We are told that he was uninterested in the recovery of his paying guests and that political suspects found shelter at Belhomme's home during the Terror, under cover of mental illness, provided they paid a huge fee. Documentation on such services is scarce, given the secrecy required under the circumstances.[6]

As Tenon's table indicates, the Parisian establishments were all small: the largest had thirty-six inmates, the smallest, two.[7] Almost two-fifths of the city's senile elderly (267 out of 632) who could afford the fees found shelter in these private nursing homes, whereas agitated and epileptic patients were cared for in municipal hospitals, with the exception of 16 out of 377 agitated, and 22 out of 322 epileptic patients. (Note the discrepancy in numbers between men and women categorized as epileptics: we cannot explain this difference.) In contrast to the notorious British madhouses, where public supervision seems to have been ineffective, so that rapacious and ruthless owners brutalized inmates, the French nursing home had always been strictly controlled by the police, and researchers have registered no complaints about patient management.

While *lettres de cachet* for the confinement of the well-to-do mental patients were usually based on thorough investigations, the indigent did not rate such caution. At the time of Louis XIV's notorious roundup of beggars and vagrants in the 1650s, hundreds of mentally impaired indigents were caught in the net and imprisoned in Bicêtre and the Salpêtrière, and in workhouses (*dépôts de mendicité*). The mentally ill thus constituted a considerable proportion of the inmate population. Their arbitrary imprisonment caused the champions of the Rights of Man to include them in their crusade for the liberation of all persons they believed to have been wrongfully confined by the absolute monarchy.

The Revolutionaries' quest for the freedom of these prisoners was sometimes ill-informed, as the following episode indicates. The National Assembly's committee on *lettres de cachet* readily assumed that innocent persons had been arbitrarily jailed on the pretext of madness, so the Assembly decreed in March 1790 that each confined mental patient be interrogated by a judge and visited by a physician. One can follow the Revolutionaries' trend of thought in the correspondence between the mayor of Paris, Jean Sylvain Bailly, and the future Jacobin Bertrand Barère de Vieuzac, a member of both the Committee on *lettres de cachet* and the Poverty Committee.[8] They were mightily surprised when their site visitors to Charenton reported that the Brothers of Charity ran a model hospital, took excellent care of the inmates, housed them appropriately, and fed them well. Every single inmate was patently mad, and confined according to a legal document. And not one of the eighty-seven patients asked to be released![9]

◆◆◆

Mental illness was poorly understood in the eighteenth century. The ascription of sanguine, choleric, melancholic, or phlegmatic "temperament" remained the rule, and a division of patients into manic and melancholic, demented and idiot categories. Most physicians believed that some physical or physiologic disturbance caused the observable morbid psychologic phenomena. They subscribed to the theory of an excess or deficiency of nervous sensitivity or irritability, or a disturbance in the circulation of fluids or vapors through blood vessels or the nervous system. Such physicalist theorizing had the advantage of dealing with quantifiable entities and held out the hope that active therapeutic intervention would be of help in mental illness.

Not all physicians reasoned in this manner. Many were familiar with the psychologic theories of John Locke, David Hartley, and the abbé de Condillac, men who defined thought as the result of sensation, reflection, and the association of ideas. For them, mental illness could be caused by a malfunction in such associations. But for all physicians equilibrium or balance—whether expressed in physical or psychologic terms—meant normalcy or health, disequilibrium meant illness.

Traditional treatment of mental illness aimed at restoring balance and health by evacuating "peccant" humors and spirits, and relieving the pressure of excessive nervous fluid on the brain. This could be achieved by the administration of purgatives, emetics, sudorifics, and diuretics, or venesection, for which leeches were often substituted. Evacuation could also be achieved by using mechanical devices such as the rotating machine advocated by Erasmus Darwin: their centrifugal action would expel harmful fluids through every opening in the human body.

In Paris under the old regime, the only place for treatment was the Hôtel-Dieu. Chapter 2 alluded to its special wards for mental patients: Ste Geneviève for thirty-two women and St. Louis for forty-two men, the first located in the northwestern corner of the enormous women's fever ward on the third floor, the latter in the upper ward built upon the Pont-au-double. In the women's ward stood several bathtubs used to immerse the insane, a procedure that had always been found soothing for them. Tenon describes patients, three or four to a bed, who "press against each other, gesticulate, and quarrel, and are then garroted and restrained." [10] The depleting treatments often weakened violent patients into compliance, so that they were pronounced cured and dismissed. Or, after two six-week sessions failed to provide a remission of symptoms, the patient was declared incurable and relegated to Bicêtre or the Salpêtrière for life. Pussin expressed anguish about a totally debilitated patient arriving at Bicêtre from the Hôtel-Dieu: "I have noticed that excessive bleeding is dangerous for most madmen, because it causes the illness to degenerate into imbecility. Inmates often arrive from the Hospice of Humanity [the Hôtel-Dieu] whom bleeding has reduced to such a state that they are even unable to eat." [11] With good care, Pussin restored the young man to health. But such conservative treatment was rare, whereas drugs were abundantly used.

These drugs were as varied as the pharmacopoeia, further diversified by superstitious beliefs. Among plant extracts used as calmants, opium ranked first, and "laudanum" was to have a great future. Next to the poppy, the extract of thorn apple (stramonium) was favored for its calming effect, as were henbane and belladonna. Camphor, already known to the Chinese, was used as a sedative, and antispasmodics included castoreum and musk, asafetida, valerian, mistletoe, and peony. As purgatives, doctors counseled rhubarb, senna, and jalap; as emetics, ipecac and tartar. Given the prescientific state of pharmacology, it is not surprising to find favorite remedies such as hellebore, mandrake, and theriaca Andromachi, or Venice treacle, prescribed for multiple and contradictory purposes. The Paracelsian iatro-chemists favored copper ammoniate and zinc oxide as antispasmodics, and tartar emetic. Further to stimulate evacuation and restore mental health, doctors recommended irritant procedures—namely, moxibustion, cauterization, and blistering; the application of setons and cups, preferably as close to the brain as possible to favor exudation, after producing inflammation and "laudable" pus. One concludes that the absence of doctors from eighteenth-century asylums may in fact have promoted the patients' recovery![12] In fact, medical scientists increasingly tried to free patients from activist therapy, just as advocates of the Rights of Man planned to liberate the unjustly confined mentally ill.

Before turning now to Pussin's and Pinel's contributions to transforming the insane into mentally ill patients with a good prognosis for recovery, it may be important to point out that humane—that is, nonviolent and decent—treatment of these men and women was not uncommon on the part of physicians of the Enlightenment. Joseph Daquin of Chambéry (1732–1815), the author of a work on insanity entitled *Philosophie de la folie* (1791), advocated humane methods, few drugs, therapeutic bathing, and electric therapy.[13] Vincenzo Chiarugi (1759–1820), physician-in-chief at the Bonifazio Hospital in Florence, followed strict rules never to let his staff mistreat a patient. He described and pictured restraints that would hold but not hurt in his treatise on madness entitled *Della pazzia in genere ed in specie* (1793).[14] William Battie (1703–1776), the first British doctor to devote a whole book to mental illness, stated as early as 1758 that "management did much more than medicine."[15] In Geneva, Abraham Joly (1748–1812) "abolished the use of chains and other barbarous means of coercion at the city hospital,"[16] as did a Dr. Gastaldy at the Providence Hospital in Avignon,[17] and Johann Theobald Held (1770–1851) in Prague. A search would undoubtedly reveal numerous physicians as well as laypersons who treated the mentally ill in a humane manner.

We saw in Chapter 2 that the Poverty Committee site visitors were surprised, in May 1790, to find that the insane at Bicêtre were well-treated, and that Pussin maintained calm and order.[18] Thouret was one of those site visitors, and it was undoubtedly on his recommendation that, on 6 August 1793, the Hospital Commission appointed Pinel "physician of the infirmaries" at Bicêtre, a novel title that marks a moment in the history of medicine, as noted earlier. (Other friends and colleagues may have promoted Pinel: the philosopher Cabanis, the mathematician Jacques Cousin, or the medical scientist and powerful politician François Fourcroy.) The hitherto "incurable" indigent patients housed in the hospice, particularly those lodged in the infirmaries, including the insane, now came for the first time under a full-time resident physician's care. It turned out that the conditions in that particular mental ward, the personality and methods of the governor, Pussin, and the professional bent of the new appointee led to a new, humane approach on the part of physicians toward the mentally ill indigent patient.

From Madman to Mental Patient at Bicêtre during the Terror

Even before 1793, the two hundred indigent men incarcerated at Bicêtre and judged to be incurably insane experienced significant changes in the way they were treated, housed, clad, and fed. That was because Pussin was determined to improve management. He had come to Bicêtre as a patient and thus understood the inmates' wants,[19] and he made considerable efforts to fulfill the desiderata outlined in the "Instructions for Governing the Insane and Working for Their Cure" promulgated by Colombier and Doublet in 1785.[20] Fresh air was no problem at Bicêtre, clean water came from the famous Great Well, and Viel's new sewer assured good sanitation. Madame Pussin's vegetable garden and cooking skills helped produce the "succulent and tasty soup" Pinel found "as good as any citizen may desire."[21] The inspectors had admonished that "harsh treatment and especially blows should be considered an outrage."[22] Pussin agreed and wrote: "I have never used anything but repressive measures without mistreatment, and yet I have always managed to impress [the patients], and even to gain their confidence . . . they are the first to protect me." For the patients' daily care, he favored using former inmates, a practice frequently followed at that time.

Pussin knew that violence could be counterproductive in the management of the mentally ill. He asserted that "the memory of mistreatment leads them to watch for the moment of vengeance as soon as the opportunity arises and when one expects it the least. What is more, while they are consumed by this thirst for vengeance, anything one undertakes for their cure is, if not harmful, at least absolutely useless."[23] The inspectors asked for "exemplary punishment" of employees who disobeyed the rule against violent treatment of patients.[24] Pussin agreed again, stating that he would never permit the insane to be beaten. When he formally announced this policy the guards protested, but Pussin stood firm.

> The attendants tried to rebel against me, saying that they were not safe and objecting that if I myself was not spared, they were all the more ex-

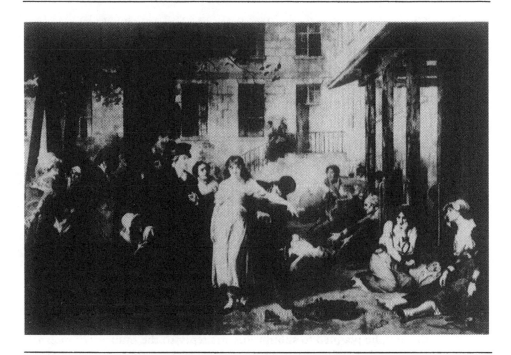

FIGURE 9.1. *Pinel délivrant les aliénés*. Philippe Pinel (1745–1826) delivering the mental patients at the Salpêtrière Hospice from their chains. Painting by Tony Robert-Fleury, Charcot Library, Salpêtrière. Bibliothèque interuniversitaire de médecine, Paris. (The title of the painting gives the masculine "aliénés," even though a young woman is being freed.)

posed, etc. But, despite their clamors, I persisted in my resolve and, to reach my goal, I was forced to dismiss almost all of them in turn when they disobeyed. It is thus not without trouble that I realized my purpose, but I finally managed to see to it that the servants never beat any of the insane, even when victimized by their violence. I know that those who care for the insane run great risks, but I am also certain that the danger is less when gentleness rather than severity prevails.[25]

Pussin makes a statement of great historic interest in this connection: "I have tried so hard to improve the condition of these unfortunates that in the month of Prairial of the Year V [May–June 1797], *I managed to eliminate their chains* (used until then to contain the furious) and to replace them with straitjackets that permit freedom of movement and the enjoyment of all possible liberty without any added danger."[26] Pussin thus first unshackled the mentally ill at Bicêtre, and Pinel followed suit at the Salpêtrière three years later.[27] Yet it is Pinel's "gesture" that is everywhere commemorated—for example, in Tony-Robert Fleury's tableau *Pinel délivrant les aliénés* in the Bibliothèque

Charcot at the Salpêtrière (Fig. 9.1), which shows Pinel ordering the chains struck from a young woman. (The huge painting by Charles Muller that hangs in the hall of the Paris Academy of Medicine, on the other hand, commemorates an event that never happened at Bicêtre.)[28]

Our acquaintance with the details of custody and treatment on the St. Prix ward derives from a two-part document written by Pussin, discovered in the Archives nationales in 1978.[29] Immediately upon Dr. Pinel's arrival at Bicêtre on 11 September 1793, and at his request, Pussin prepared a "Table of the Madmen Admitted to Bicêtre on the 7th Ward, between 1 January 1784 and 31 December 1792" (Table 9.2). It breaks down each year's group by ages and categories, followed by observations remarkable for the physical criteria that guided Pussin's triage of inmates and his decisions regarding their accommodations and management. His rule of thumb shows shrewdness, kindness, and, when he thought it necessary, an unshakable firmness.

The second part of Pussin's report dated 1797, includes an additional table indicating the patient census, mortality, and cures from 1793 to 1797 (Table 9.3).[30] This document was also composed at Pinel's request: he asked nine questions about patient management and therapy; he planned to submit Pussin's reply to the minister of internal affairs and thereby obtain Pussin's transfer from Bicêtre to the Salpêtrière (where Pinel had been appointed physician-in-chief). Eventually, in 1802, the government granted the request.

◆◆◆

Pussin's "Observations" clearly show the influence of Colombier and Doublet's guidelines on policy at Bicêtre Hospice. But mainly they reveal a sharp contrast between Pussin's ideas of 1793 and 1797: Pinel's nineteen months' presence transformed Pussin into a good observer of individual inmates' behavior. At the earlier date, ancient popular notions of temperament and a telltale physique dictated Pussin's prognosis and led him to isolate, and sometimes to restrain, "redheads and black beards," whereas he believed that "blondes are gentle and usually degenerate into imbecility." Safety and order on his ward being his prime concerns, Pussin warned that "madmen whose principle of madness is pride or religion are . . . usually very dangerous." By far the most interesting and possibly original observation—one that even includes a differential diagnosis, a recognition that mental illness can recur at more or less regular intervals, and a plea for therapy—reads as follows: "The most agitated madmen are usually those whose recovery is most likely. They can be divided into two groups: the first and larger group is certain to recover its common sense to-

TABLE 9.2. Madmen Admitted to the Seventh Ward at Bicêtre between 1 January 1784 and 31 December 1792 (old style)

	Ages						
	15	20	30	40	50	60	Total
Madmen entered in 1784	5	33	31	24	11	6	110
Discharged cured	2	13	20	9	4	1	49
Died	3	18	9	15	7	5	57
Remaining at year's end		2	2				4
Madmen entered in 1785	4	39	49	25	14	3	134
Discharged cured	2	15	13	8	1		39
Died	2	19	32	14	13	3	83
Remaining at year's end		5	4	3			12
Madmen entered in 1786	4	31	40	32	15	5	127
Discharged cured	4	17	16	14	4	2	57
Died		10	23	15	10	3	61
Remaining at year's end		4	1	3	1		9
Madmen entered in 1787	12	39	41	26	17	7	142
Discharged cured	5	7	18	9	6		45
Died	6	29	19	16	1	7	88
Remaining at year's end	1	3	4	1			9
Madmen entered in 1788	9	43	53	21	18	7	151
Discharged cured	4	15	10	7	10	1	47
Died	5	26	37	13	8	6	95
Remaining at year's end		2	6	1			9
Madmen entered in 1789	6	38	39	33	14	2	132
Discharged cured	2	18	14	10	4		48
Died		18	24	20	10	1	73
Remaining at year's end	4	2	1	3		1	11
Madmen entered in 1790	6	28	34	19	9	7	103
Discharged cured	5	11	16	4	3	1	40
Died	1	12	12	9	6	5	45
Remaining at year's end		5	6	6		1	18
Madmen entered in 1791	9	26	32	16	7	3	93
Discharged cured	3	15	12	6	2		38
Died	4	18	14	8	5	3	42
Remaining at year's end	2	3	6	2			13
Madmen entered in 1792	6	26	33	18	12	3	98
Discharged cured	3	1	5	4	3		26
Died	1	8	17	9	6	2	43
Remaining at year's end	2	7	11	5	3	1	29

SOURCE: Archives nationales, Paris, 27 AP 8. (Translated by the author.)

TABLE 9.3. Madmen Admitted to the Seventh Ward at Bicêtre between 1 January 1793 (12 Nivôse, Year I) and 21 September 1797 (the end of the Year V)

	Ages						
	15	20	30	40	50	60	Total
Madmen entered in the last nine months of the Year I	1	13	13	7	4	2	40
Discharged cured	1	4	6	2		1	14
Died		3	4	3	3	1	14
Remaining at year's end		6	3	2	1		12
Madmen entered Year II	3	23	15	15	9	6	71
Discharged cured	1	11	5	1	2	3	23
Died	1	9	7	10	6	3	36
Remaining at year's end	1	3	3	4	1		12
Madmen entered Year III	4	20	24	15	5	4	72
Discharged cured	1	5	8				14
Died		8	11	11	3	4	37
Remaining at year's end	3	7	5	4	2		21
Madmen entered Year IV	5	18	18	14	7	3	65
Discharged cured	3	2	5	1	1		12
Died	2	7	3	9	2	2	25
Remaining at year's end		9	10	4	4	1	28
Madmen entered Year V	3	16	26	17	4	1	67
Discharged cured	1	5	2	2			10
Died		1	3	2	1		7
Remaining at year's end	2	10	21	13	3	1	50

SOURCE: Archives nationales, Paris, 27 AP 8. (Translated by the author.)

tally. The second group also recovers, but relapses at intervals, and it is this group for whom renewed treatment would be of greatest urgency."

Pussin's rather crude visual impressions of 1793 contrast with an interest in prognosis and therapy evident in his "Observations" of 1797: "When they are young and under thirty years of age," he comments in the later part of the document, "it is rare that the strength of their temperament does not bring about a favorable change. . . . Above the age of thirty, this kind of cure is rare."[31] This conforms with experience in present-day psychiatric wards: a first schizophrenic illness is likeliest to remit in young patients; life in the asylum tends to hasten the death of the elderly. Pussin blamed the food shortage for the increasing mortality.

Most remarkable is Pussin's advocacy of "psychologic" therapy as the only effective means of treatment: "My experience has shown, and shows daily, that to further the cure of these unfortunates one must treat them with as much kindness as possible, dominate them without mistreatment, gain their confidence, fight the cause of their illness and make them envision a happier future. I have always fought this illness by psychologic means and thus known the happiness of some favorable results." He also advocated work as therapy for convalescents. Pussin reports that he headed a quiet ward as a result of these policies and comments: "The regulations are so well observed that most of the time one does not seem surrounded by madmen. Strangers have often told me of their surprise."[32] Pinel would repeat this observation.

◆◆◆

The insane men at Bicêtre would have continued to live under Pussin's intelligent custody, unknown to Paris and the world, and psychologic treatment would have received no publicity during the French Revolution, had not Philippe Pinel taken up the cause of the mentally ill. Pinel and Pussin learned a great deal from each other. While it is surely commonplace for a supervisor to learn from a physician, it is remarkable that a highly educated forty-eight-year-old doctor should apprentice himself to an unschooled superintendent. But Pinel brought qualifications to his new job that transformed what might have been routine activity into a creative moment in the history of medicine. Because of his excellent classical and modern education, supplemented by twenty years of self-directed study of the medical sciences, Pinel was able to transform his observations at Bicêtre into a theoretical formulation for academic psychiatry, into a practical and humane policy for the asylum, and into a clinical method sensitive to the psychologic aspects of illness. Since he was touched by the miseries and indignities of mental illness and a believer in the rights of man and the duty of society to help the disadvantaged, he appeared at Bicêtre at the right moment to champion the cause of the mentally ill.

Educated by the Doctrinaires in southwestern France,[33] Philippe Pinel earned his M.D. degree in Toulouse in 1773. Discontent with its mediocre medical faculty, he spent four years of self-directed medical study in Montpellier, where an affluent and powerful medical milieu offered rich stimulation.[34] Pinel paid daily visits to the Hôtel-Dieu St. Eloi, taking notes on the physical and mental state of patients over a continuous period of time. (He tells us this in a manuscript of 1793.)[35] After four years at Montpellier, Pinel walked to Paris, in quest of a meaningful career. He encountered the frustrations that the restrictive rules of the old regime imposed on medical men until the Revolution opened the way to an appropriate appointment, fifteen years later.

The inmates confined in the 7th ward at Bicêtre faced an unheard-of experience, beginning in September of 1793, when the new doctor engaged them in serious conversation day after day, in their cells, or perhaps on a bench in one of the courtyards. He wanted to know how each inmate was feeling about himself, and about his life in the hospice. What had brought him there? When? From where? Where had he been born? Did he have a family? a wife? children? Had he ever been sick? With what illness? Had others in his family been sick? How had the Revolution affected his livelihood? his politics? his religion? his safety? What exactly had precipitated his psychologic illness and when exactly had it started? What were his symptoms? his fears? his hopes?[36]

The new doctor would gravely note the answers, and, while listening intently to each man, he would be searching for gestures, postures, and facial expressions revelatory of moods and affects. These personal revelations and observations impressed and shaped the thinking of a physician who stated publicly in December 1794 that "a large gathering of madmen inspires an undefinable thoughtful tenderness when one realizes that their present state derives only from a vivid sensitivity and from psychologic qualities we value highly. . . . Man is most often led from the free use of reason to madness by overstepping the limits of his good qualities and of his generous and magnanimous inclinations."[37]

A set of case histories resulted from Pinel's notes, observations, and convictions that would soon be cited throughout Western psychiatric literature. We meet the clockmaker infatuated with perpetual motion; the patient who imagines himself to have been guillotined but pardoned, only to have the executioner put the wrong severed head on his shoulders; "the madman who believes he is Louis XIV and who often hands me dispatches for the governments of his provinces" and the "white-haired seventy-year-old . . . who believes he is a young woman . . . [who] obstinately refuses other than feminine clothing . . . [and] is flattered by the polite behavior of the staff"; and a man who "believes that an order from heaven commands him to bestow the Baptism of Blood and merciless immolation upon all those whose happiness in the next life he craves."

While listening and observing, Pinel was also considering criteria of classification so that he might "enrich the medical theory of mental illness with all the insights that the empirical approach affords, or rather . . . perfect the theory and provide practice with the general principles that it lacked."[38] In pursuit of this goal, Pinel discriminated between continuous and remitting mental derangement; he was particularly struck by periodicity in the attacks and searched for regular patterns. He also recognized that the beginning and termination of violent bouts of excitement could be seen as moments of special importance in mental illness: these bouts were often a sign of a crisis marking the approach of recovery, and precautions must be taken to prevent harm to the patient and to others. The attendants had to be especially alert to premonitory symptoms. The patient's age and the violence of attacks seemed important criteria of curability. Pinel concluded that total insanity was rare: usually only one mental faculty was involved. He especially noted the dangerousness of what he called "reasoning madness," where logical thinking was intact, even though the patient's premises were delusional. He noted that some patients are very dangerous, observing without protest that three of these inmates had been chained for fifteen, twenty-five, and forty-five years respectively. The community needed to be protected from the violence and cruelty of totally psychotic madmen.

Pinel believed in firm management to deal with obstinate behavior. He cited the history of a man "appalled by the abolition of the Catholic religion in France" who was "ceaselessly terrorized by torments concerning the next life. Thinking about the mortifications of the saints' penitential lives, he obstinately refuses any kind of food and appears close to death." In such cases "one of the major principles of the psychologic management of the insane is to break their will in a skillfully timed manner without causing wounds or imposing hard labor. Rather, a formidable show of terror should convince [them] that they are not free to pursue their impetuous willfulness and that their only choice is to submit." With Pussin as his model, and in order to save a life, Pinel thus stressed the role of the asylum superintendent as a figure of authority—a formulation that has generated much adverse comment in the modern "anti-psychiatric" literature. Pinel's opinion represents the consensus of informed specialists at that time, shared, for example, by William Tuke and Johann Christian Reil. But Pinel's opinion about the authority needed by the head of the asylum is by no means the most important message that his early formulations convey. Apart from his exemplary empathy, Pinel's main message is that each patient, even though poor and forlorn, is worthy of the doctor's prolonged attention because each person is unique and needs to be studied with care in order to be helped. It is thus a democratic message. And Pinel's initial 20 percent rate of cure means that he was able to help at least forty men leave the Bicêtre mental ward and attempt to take charge of their lives as citizen-patients.

The utterances and behavior, signs and symptoms of the Bicêtre inmates were duly recorded by the doctor, who tells us that he took notes daily. Unfortunately these are lost. Thus one remarkable document of those days becomes all the more precious: it is a "General

Table of the Madmen at Bicêtre Numbering about 200," an autograph manuscript sheet in Pinel's hand, measuring about 15 square inches, first published in 1913 and translated here for the first time (Table 9.4). Here Pinel jotted down his initial thoughts about classification that would not only facilitate a conceptual approach to mental illness but also permit the grouping of patients into small, homogeneous units and thus open the way to innovative therapeutic strategies.[39]

One new conceptualization of great importance for a novel therapeutic approach to the mentally ill citizen-patient resulted from Pinel's special interpretation of the periodicity he frequently observed. He did not presume to know its cause—it still baffles investigators. But instead of merely citing conventional coordinate factors such as the seasons, the sun, and the moon, instead of merely observing more or less regular alternations of rationality and insanity, he conceived of the periods of madness as interruptions in a person's rational life. During periods of rationality, the therapist could attempt to engage the patient in dialogue, establish a relationship of trust with the healthy part of the patient's personality, and thus create the therapeutic process. This was a crucial concept, new to psychotherapy. No less a thinker than the philosopher G. W. F. Hegel (1770–1830) appreciated the innovative nature of this approach when he wrote in 1817:

> When the madman learns to respect his therapist, he becomes conscious of his subjective state, in collision with objective reality. To have discovered this remnant of reason in the insane and maniacal, and to have conceived of it as the germ of their cure, and to have conducted treatment according to this principle, this conception should mainly be attributed to Pinel, whose writings on this subject are the best available.[40]

Hegel thus perceived the dialectic process at work in the mentally ill patient.[41]

◆◆◆

Not content with his tentative theoretical formulations, Pinel reworked and honed his data and his literary style and, in the subsequent six years, he eloquently argued the cause of the mentally ill. On 11 December 1794, he read his "Memoir on Madness: A Contribution to the Natural History of Man" to the Society for Natural History, and the society, recognizing the political importance of Pinel's plea for the rights of the mentally ill, voted to send the essay to the Committee of Public Safety.[42] (To date the essay has not been located in the committee's papers.) Twelve days later Pinel was appointed to a professorship at the Paris Health School, thus acquiring a student audience, which soon reached many hundreds of young men. For them he com-

TABLE 9.4. Pinel's General Table of the Madmen at Bicêtre Numbering about 200

Considered

1° according to the nature of precipitating events
2° according to the particular type of their insanity ["*manie*"]
3° according to their personality of their usual behavior

I. Known Precipitating Events

Family Problems
financial upsets, jealousy, forced divorce, loss of a dearly loved child are often causes of insanity, and there are 27 madmen of this kind at Bicêtre

Love
there are 8 gone mad because their sensitivity is too acute and 5 because of passionate excesses; the latter commit indecent acts at the sight of women

Devoutness or Fanaticism
there are 18 some of whom believe they are gods or prophets others commit puerile religious acts and sometimes exhaust themselves through abstinence and fasting

Revolutionary Events
there are 27 whose reason has been deranged by the events of the Revolution, either through the loss of their fortune, or fear of the draft, or other accidents

sunstroke

sequelae of acute illness

TABLE 9.4. (*Continued*)

II. Particular Type of Insanity

Regular Attacks	Irregular Attacks	Continuous Psychosis ["manie"]	Epilepsy with Psychosis ["manie"]
these are the rarest cases	these are the most usual cases; there are 32 of these, and in 29 the attacks have become less severe and less frequent; the other 3 have grown worse. in general irregular madness is most susceptible to cure	this kind of madness is quite usual and suggests a cause more difficult to overcome; there are 31 of these madmen. several are insane from devoutness, love, or excessive ambition. they give the least hope of cure	the hospice for the insane houses 12 epileptics whose attacks are followed by a psychosis that lasts a variable number of days. this psychosis is very dangerous and resembles bouts of rage; experience teaches that it is almost always fatal
1 is mad 3 summer months			
1 mad in the morning and calm at night			
1 mad every other day			
3 mad 6 months and 18 months calm			
1 mad only 3 weeks a year madness recurs in spring and fall and sometimes in winter			
for 8 years, mad 6 months every 2 years, and for the last 10 years always mad			

III. *The Varieties of Insanity*

Lesion of the Understanding with Violence Grandiose Words or Actions	*Violence without Lesion of the Understanding. Madness One Might Call Reasoning*	*Melancholia–Maniacal Misanthropy*	*Idiotism Imbecility*
one notices that periodic insanity with the most violent attacks is the most susceptible to cure and that time alone renders the attacks less frequent and gentler; there are 29 of this kind; in continuous insanity the grandiosity is less violent, as in the 31 above.	there are certain madmen who are very dangerous and yet seem entirely rational when one speaks with them; they would commit the most violent actions if they were free; this kind of insanity is periodic, regular, or continuous. there are 10 of these in the hospice	madmen of this kind generally live retired in their cells and one cannot extract a word from them; some are quiet and content not to reply when spoken to; others respond with a kind of fury, and some do not even want to permit the opening of their cell door. There are 17 well-defined misanthropes in the hospice.	this madness is often no more than a gentle dream-like state. blond men are most subject to it; in the hospice there are 31 tranquil and nonviolent imbeciles and 18 subject to dangerous attacks

SOURCE: "Notes inédites de Pinel, présentées par R. Semelaigne," *Bulletin de la Société clinique de médecine mentale*, 1913, 6: 221–27. Pinel's manuscript notes, included in this article in a photograph, are translated here by the author of this book.

NOTE: The following is written near the top of the original table:

cretins. doctor in Lausanne has done research on localities in the Valais. has collected several skulls which he compared to other Valaisians. cretins and conical—not noticeable in skulls of other Valaisians. "one cretin" strongly attracted to first, all skulls flattened toward the temples and conical—not noticeable in skulls of other Valaisians. "one cretin" strongly attracted to women to the point of attacking them physically. with a normal woman[,] offspring not always cretin. cretins often in sexual orgasm between the ages of 18 to 25 because strongly driven to sexual activity and unable to satisfy the urge posed a textbook that surveyed the whole field of medicine and presented the "neuroses" (the future psychiatry) as a major "class" of diseases. This textbook on "philosophic nosography" went through six editions and served as every French medical student's guide for a generation.[43] In 1796–1798 Pinel read three papers to the outstanding young investigators grouped in the Society for Medical Emulation,[44] and these papers became chapters in his treatise on mental alienation (1800).[45] In the meantime, he had been appointed physician-in-chief at the Salpêtrière, where he wrote his third book, on clinical medicine,[46] which was meant to complement his book on nosography with case histories collected at the sickbed. It was at the Salpêtrière that Pinel trained his main disciple, Esquirol, and where he succeeded in transferring his trusted collaborator, Pussin, in 1802. These three men's achievements, taken together, constitute complementary parts of nascent psychiatry in France. Pussin contributed native wisdom and the model of the authoritarian administrator. Pinel made the study of mental illness respectable in medical and academic circles, acceptable in the Academy of Sciences, and intriguing to a wide reading public. He projected the image of a wise, gentle, sympathetic doctor. Esquirol saw mental illness as a problem that called for a national solution based on clear, legal concepts.

Esquirol was thirty years younger than both Pussin and Pinel, but he was acquiring professional experience that would soon dwarf Pussin's innate gifts, and eventually he would rival his teacher.[47] From the beginning of his career, Esquirol set a pattern that differentiated him from Pinel: he opened a private hospital and his medical thesis dealt with a psychiatric topic. Upon Pussin's death in 1811, Esquirol replaced him. Esquirol personifies the final phase in the evolution of psychiatry in Paris during the Revolution and Empire, and his influence on the treatment of the mentally ill citizen-patient in nineteenth-century France was of the greatest importance.[48]

In March 1802, Esquirol established what can be considered a laboratory for methods to be used for citizen-patients hospitalized in the asylums of nineteenth-century France. His maison de santé was located at 8, rue Buffon, across the street from the Salpêtrière and managed under Pinel's supervision. We know from a recently discovered patient register that an average of twenty-five patients lived with him in the first six years.[49] These paying patients are dubbed "rich" in the contemporary literature, in contrast, no doubt, to the thousands of poor at the nearby Salpêtrière. But nowhere is a fee mentioned, and the register lists quite ordinary individuals, such as a lemonade dealer, several soldiers, and medical students, among Esquirol's patients. We shall therefore include Esquirol's private charges among the "citizen-patients," pointing once again to the importance of these persons' desire to get well and resume their productive lives. In contrast with the *maisons de santé* of the past, a resident, qualified physician was in charge here. We shall look at the first six years.

In this small hospital, Esquirol tried out his method: among a total of 151 patients, he diagnosed 28 cases of mania, 20 cases of melancholia, 19 cases of dementia, 3 each of delirium and hysteria, 1 of lethargy, and 4 he cryptically labeled "alienated." Their length of stay varied from eleven days to life. In agreement with his colleagues elsewhere, Esquirol believed that the first essential step was to remove the patient from home and familiar surroundings, to *isolate* the man or woman in the hospital for treatment. But it was the initial encounter with the director of the clinic, Esquirol believed, that should impress, if not frighten the patient. Again he had models, notably Francis Willis, the man chiefly responsible for the management of King George III's bouts of mental illness. Esquirol lived at his own institution and knew his patients well. He sought to re-socialize them gradually, carefully orchestrating their treatment. The ruling principle in this *maison de santé* was awe of the director. Although he never permitted patients to be beaten or intentionally hurt, he used *"des secousses,"* or shocks, "physical or psychologic, that shake and one might say threaten the machine [i.e., the body], and forcibly redirect it toward health."[50] His means are mild if compared to the chamber of horrors that J. C. Reil imagined—although the famous German physiologist fortunately never had occasion to carry out his ingenious strategies for stimulation, excitement, fear, terror, pain, deprivation, and total subjection to the asylum director. Esquirol speaks a different language than Pinel.

◆◆◆

Pussin's transfer to the Salpêtrière finally occurred on 19 May 1802, after a direct appeal from Pinel to Chaptal. It was Pinel's hope that Pussin would apply "the same principles to the women patients" that had worked so well at Bicêtre. Pinel had initiated efforts to have Pussin transferred to assist him as early as 1797, writing to the minister of internal affairs, François de Neufchâteau, that Pussin, who "combined a rare intelligence and several years' experience with humane feelings and an unshakable firmness, would also know how to handle the servants and to dominate the minds of certain mental patients." Mainly, he would free Pinel from administrative duties that interfered with teaching, research, and writing: "I have now worked at the Salpêtrière for three years," Pinel concluded. "I have been unable to undertake the therapy of madness or even to make any exact observation of this illness because of the disorganization prevalent in that part of the hospice."[51]

Pussin's transfer coincided with the Hospital Council's decision to transfer the treatment of all mentally ill women to the Salpêtrière. Most of the women came from Charenton, the former *charité*, temporarily used as the city's public asylum. And some were the last remaining mental patients from the Hôtel-Dieu. The Hospital Council allocated funds for appropriate renovations, to improve furnishings, clothing, utensils, and diet, according to a now well-established pattern. Pussin therefore had to arrange for triage, assignments, and transfers of patients and personnel. He did not make himself popular. It is surprising to find him listed as "physician of the madwomen" in the hospital budget for the Year XI, where his wife figures as supervisor in the same division.[52]

Given the persistent struggles for power within the Salpêtrière, a hospice the size of a village, the multiple regulations, and the traditional favoritism, a newcomer with special ties to the chief was an easy target of envy and spite. The comptroller, one Merle, drew an acerbic portrait in his annual report, at Christmas 1802:

> This service is now under the direction of a man hitherto employed in the cells of Bicêtre, who is said to be a former mental patient. He has methods and knowledge derived from long years of experience. Our own observations of his behavior, in the seven or eight months that he has been here, has in no way justified M. Pinel's opinion. . . . [Pussin] would like it known that M. Pinel only copied and wrote down his ideas, which inspired the various works published by this great physician. Anyone who can tolerate his arguments for ten minutes will be convinced of the contrary. . . . Imagine that such a man could restore their reason to persons who have lost it![53]

Perhaps even Esquirol was envious of the confidence Pinel placed in Pussin.

Beginning in the summer of 1802, the three men had daily opportunities to compare notes about theory and therapy. How could the methods elaborated at Bicêtre and in Esquirol's small, private hospital be adapted to a huge public asylum such as the Salpêtrière? Was it possible to subdivide large groups of patients into "species," as Pinel proposed, with each group separately lodged and all members of each subgroup treated according to a carefully orchestrated, purposeful policy? Might one organize lodgings, sleeping arrangements, meals, exercise, and individual freedom so as to make them conducive to the cure of groups of patients? Might the hospital thus become a "therapeutic tool," as Tenon had advocated in 1788 and Esquirol repeated thirty years later?[54] These were the crucial questions confronting the emerging psychiatric profession. The conclusions were of vital importance to the mentally ill citizen-patient, for the three men were elaborating the blueprint for Charenton, the public asylum of the future.

Blueprint for the Future: The Salpêtrière and Charenton

At the opening ceremonies of the medical faculty in 1802, Professor Hallé reported that "at the Salpêtrière, citizen Pinel has been able, this year, to give new scope to his research on mental alienation." The government had now emptied the Hôtel-Dieu of mental patients, thus raising the Salpêtrière's census of these women to 750 or 800.[55] Within a year, Citizen Pinel would publish his results.[56] The transfer of treatment for women to the Salpêtrière in 1802 overburdened Pinel at first. As soon as Pussin arrived, he turned to research and soon published three overviews. The first, presented at the public session of the Academy of sciences on 22 June 1805, and subsequently published in the *Moniteur universel,* was entitled "Research on the General Treatment of Mentally Ill Women in a Large Hospice, and Results Obtained . . . after Three Years' Experience," meaning 1802–1805.[57] He used a variety of therapeutic strategies including baths, showers, and the straitjacket, and he visited his patients at least once every day, conversing with each, often at length. Over a period of three years, about 100 out of 156 depressed patients were cured. He could do little for demented patients or idiots, but with manic patients his results were good: in three years, 224 out of 452 were sent home. Thirty-five relapsed—half of them because of premature release requested by the family, or because of new problems or distress.

Two years later, in 1807, Pinel reviewed the same evidence, again before the Academy of Sciences, but with the aim of arriving at an estimate for probability of cure.[58] He had treated 1,022 patients between April 1802 and December 1805; 604 of them were manic, 230 melancholic (and of these 38 were suicidal), 152 demented (64 of them senile), and 36 idiots. He had been greatly helped, Pinel reported, by being able to observe each category separately, and within each category those who were severely ill, improved, or ready to go home. Thus the "division into distinct species" that he advocated had been implemented and brought results. Quite honestly he often found the situation confusing because patients had been moved, according to their changing status, evidently without his knowledge. (Did Pussin overstep his bounds?)

The best remedy for the convalescent women was work, and he therefore welcomed the new sewing room. He arrived at a probability of 93 percent that patients not previously treated elsewhere would recover.[59] That, alas, was wishful thinking. "Even if the example I have set has not yet been followed," Pinel philosophically concluded his 1805 address, "I will at least have given a public accounting of my efforts and of the difficult and complex task of a hospital physician."[60] This paper, notes Gladys Swain, appeared only in the *Mémoires* of the Academy of Sciences, and not, like the first, in the widely read *Moniteur*. A third paper, extending these observations to later years, fared even less well, appearing in 1816 in the relatively obscure *Journal universel des sciences médicales*.[61]

In 1811, the situation at the Salpêtrière changed dramatically. On 7 April, Pussin died and Esquirol stepped into his role. This meant a significant upgrading of professional care for the mentally ill women, as Swain has rightly pointed out. Instead of an untutored, although talented, former inmate, the supervisor of the women's asylum would henceforth be a physician with considerable experience in the management of mentally ill patients. Psychiatry had taken another step in defining itself as a medical specialty.

◆◆◆

The choice of the Salpêtrière as the national treatment center for mentally ill women represented only a partial solution. Where to house the huge numbers of women and men in the Paris region whom treatment did not cure? One attractive possibility was the nationalized seventeenth-century Charité de Charenton, east of Paris.[62] The Convention had at first closed Charenton, on 30 June 1795, ordered families to claim their insane relatives, transferred totally indigent patients to the Petites Maisons hospice, and expelled the brothers. But soon the encouraging tone of Pinel's reports and the wish to remove mental patients from the Hôtel-Dieu induced the government to transform Charenton into a national treatment center.

A new era seemed to open for the mentally ill citizen–patient with the decree of 15 June 1797 (27 Prairial, Year V). The government's objective was to "treat madness methodically, and provide every assurance of cure." Henceforth, "all persons suffering from this kind of illness, from wherever they may come," would be treated at Charenton, which offered "the layout of buildings, the fresh air and healthfulness of the vast gardens and land, all the facilities required for the total and intensive treatment of mental illness." Payment by the rich would finance treatment for the poor; care would be identical for all. If found incurable, citizens would be transferred to Bicêtre and the Salpêtrière, as in the past. Paying guests could stay on indefinitely, at a minimum annual charge of six hundred francs.[63]

On 23 December 1797, the government appointed F. S. de Coulmiers, a former cleric and member of the Poverty Committee, as the first director, with a Dr. Gastaldy from Avignon as physician. An assistant physician, Dr. Ch. F. S. Giraudy, was added in 1804.[64] A special administrative committee of four, including Thouret and Cadet de Vaux, served as trustees.[65] De Coulmiers lost no time in sending out a prospectus, which read in part:

> [Charenton] offers double rooms, single rooms with fireplaces, and suites for those able to afford their own servant. It provides for walks on terraces in the large garden and supervised outings to the country for patients able to undertake these.
>
> There are meeting and billiard rooms, game rooms for checkers, chess, or trictrac [a form of backgammon], and a library. All kinds of entertainment and activities are organized, since isolation aggravates mental illness, whereas sociability and shared activity induce calm.
>
> The food is good: this pleasure is often the only one available to these patients. It includes soups, boiled and roasted meat and poultry, fish, pastry, vegetables, and fruit.[66]

The tradition of the Brothers of Charity had already pushed aside the democratic intentions of Revolutionary reformers: Charenton was calling for patients who could afford its amenities.

Despite de Coulmiers's blatant publicity, applications to Charenton remained discouragingly few (only ten by August 1798).[67] So the government decided to close the rival treatment facilities at the Hôtel-Dieu altogether as of 20 January 1799. But it took a long time to implement that decision; in fact, only after Chaptal visited the Hôtel-Dieu in April 1802, and was horrified by what he saw, did he insist that all mental patients be transferred out, and henceforth lodged and treated in specialized institutions. "This marks the birth of the asylum," states Gladys Swain.[68]

Before the government arrived at its definitive plan, the newly created Hospital Council of Paris had ample time to float a succession of projects. The council unsuccessfully proposed two empty monasteries at the eastern end of Paris, the Madeleine de Trenelle and the Filles de la Croix in the faubourg St. Antoine. "The council asked in vain for the two former religious houses," Camus commented sadly, imagining "the success we would have achieved if the mentally ill of each sex had been grouped in a separate establishment with a cell (not a cage) for each, with large gardens, shade trees, water, and the other commodities needed for persons whose sad state can be even worthier of sympathy than it is deplorable."[69] In the end, the decrees of 27 March and 17 June 1802 (6 Germinal and 28 Prairial, Year X) took the fateful steps that set the pattern for Paris, for France and for the future: the government chose Charenton for the treatment of mentally ill men from Paris. (In 1806 this was transferred to Bicêtre.) It also pressed Pinel into service for the treatment of women. A significant provision stipulated that a medical bulletin signed by two physicians and two witnesses must attest to the illness, while the local welfare bureau confirmed the family's indigence.[70]

Thus therapy was again mandated, again for three months, but with the doctor in the crucial new role of expert and the right of inspection granted to the hospital council. There was a new emphasis on the healing role of hospitalization, with less bleeding and purging, even though the straitjacket and violent uses of water persisted. Most important, treatment was now carried out by respected physicians, in healthful places.

De Coulmiers's directorship of Charenton was a disaster and Esquirol watched his predecessor's stewardship with dismay. He described dilapidated buildings, renovated thoughtlessly, at needless expense, and in a manner that hindered the classification of patients. Esquirol decried the lack of guidelines in the reorganization of 1797 that left the director "absolute master."[71]

In therapy, the traditional reliance on baths and showers continued under de Coulmiers. But he gave them a wicked twist: not only did he use sudden, ice cold streams of water descending on the head, but also "ascending showers," to "combat persistent constipation," and "surprise baths"—indeed, shock treatment—where a blindfolded patient, strapped into a chair, was dumped backward into six feet of cold water. A "bath of terror," comments Esquirol (years had passed since, in his thesis, he had advocated shock treatment himself). De Coulmiers tried other ingenious and ludicrous devices: wicker mannequins that left head and arms free and permitted walking about, and wooden boxes to restrain suicidal patients.

The director interpreted "psychologic treatment" (*remède moral*) to consist of dancing, plays, and musicales, with "the all-too-famous de Sade" serving as choreographer. In Esquirol's opinion:

> This spectacle was a pretense, the madmen were not playacting; rather, the director played with people's gullibility and hoodwinked the public; old and young, knowledgeable and ignorant, all wished to attend a performance given by the insane of Charenton; for several years *tout Paris* rushed in. Some were curious, others wanted to ascertain the prodigious results of this admirable therapy for the insane. The truth is: playacting cured no one.[72]

After becoming medical director, Esquirol hesitated to use theatricals for therapy, commenting: "For performances to be useful to mental patients, one would have to choose the theater, plays, music, and audience individually for each patient. The uses of psychologic influences in the treatment of mental illness must correspond to all the varieties of human feelings." He was hesitant regarding music therapy, commenting, "It does not cure, but it distracts, and therefore comforts. . . . one must therefore not reject its use."[73]

It is difficult to say exactly why patients now came to Charenton from all over France: was it the notoriety of the marquis de Sade and the startling news of musicales and plays produced by madmen? Did the news that madness was a curable illness raise widespread hope? Whatever the reason, the number of patients climbed from 202 in the first five years to 435 by 1805 and 1,007 by 1810.[74] Also, Charenton recovered wealth lost in the confiscation of 1792. In 1807, properties worth 9,315 francs of revenue reverted to the institution, and from then on the government annually allocated sizeable sums—40,000 francs in 1812–1814.[75]

Upon Gastaldy's death in 1805, A. A. Royer-Collard (1768–1825) became medical director, much to the chagrin of de Coulmiers, for he was a well-trained physician with a strong personality and connections in high political circles. The director strained to make the new physician's life difficult and his job impossible. He succeeded only too well, denying him access to patient records, budget figures, and case histories. Though Royer-Collard's "pressing and repeated protests" finally stopped the theatrical performances in July 1811, he remained powerless in patient management and hospital administration.[76] Eventually, in 1825, Esquirol succeeded Royer-Collard as medical director of Charenton.[77] He supervised large-scale architectural changes, on the basis of a U-shaped module called the "*carré isolé*." Structure was primordial to him, and so were the preeminence and power of the physician-in-chief in the asylum.[78]

◆◆◆

A historic transformation thus took place in Paris during our era, successively at Bicêtre, at Esquirol's *maison de santé,* the Salpêtrière, and at Charenton. The inspiration came from the Enlightenment belief in the natural rights of all women and men, even those whose mental faculties were defective or otherwise impaired. The transformation happened under the leadership of the medical profession, which was now ready to include mental illness in its nosology and to consider many mental patients curable. Even though this specialty began in our period, the first formal lectures by Esquirol only took place at the Salpêtrière from 1817 to 1825; the first French psychiatric journal, *Annales médico-psychologiques,* started publication in 1843; and the first chair of psychiatry was not established in Paris until

1878, at Ste. Anne Hospital, with a second chair at the Salpêtrière for Jean Martin Charcot four years later.

Essential to the early changes in the Paris region was the willingness of the Hospital Council to use its powers of triage, to reassign buildings and vote funds for their renovation and adaptation to new purposes, and to transfer Pussin to the Salpêtrière and appoint Esquirol as Pinel's assistant and as medical director of Charenton. And, finally, one is constantly aware of the strong undercurrent that pushed these changes forward, the conviction, voiced by the Poverty Committee of the National Assembly, that society indeed owed the ailing poor aid that was "prompt, free, assured, and complete."

◆◆◆

Seen in the context of the entire effort to provide the Seine Department with a rational and cost-effective health care organization, the mentally ill were the last, the most numerous, and the most complex segment of impaired citizens—compared to the deaf and the blind—that the government and its administrators, society, and the medical profession tried to assist. The Hospital Council of the Seine encouraged these initiatives and helped finance them, while the central admitting office excluded malingerers and distributed patients into the general and specialized hospitals. The administration's efforts remained focused on the patients in the twenty hospitals and hospices of the capital. Nursing care expanded under the Consulate, although the men's religious orders continued to be excluded and the women's orders found their authority in hospital wards undermined by physicians and pharmacists. Parturient women received better care from midwives, and well-trained pharmacists gradually took over everywhere. Jobs like gardening for the deaf, Braille for the blind, and therapeutic counseling for the mentally ill were so many new avenues that individual reformers pursued within the framework created by the Hospital Council. The target of the Poverty Committee's concern, sickness as a cause of indigence, was met with greater accuracy and success than under the old regime. On the negative side, this achievement unquestionably enlarged the pool of ailing and needy citizens whom the medical guardians of health care did not judge sick enough to qualify for their help.

The government's outreach in 1789–1815 to citizens with impaired hearing, sight, or mental functions was a pioneering effort to find methods of management and treatment. The centralization so typical of France enabled the minister of internal affairs and the prefect of the Seine, acting through their Hospital Council, to assign buildings, move and modify services, apportion funds, appoint personnel, set policy, and ultimately open a path for the citizen-patient. Centralization empowered the government to call on the services of physicians like Chaptal, Cabanis, Fourcroy, Pinel, Itard, and Jadelot; wealthy trustees like Delessert; dedicated administrators like Madame Lachapelle, Hombron, Alhoy, and de Sevelinges; and educators like Haüy and Sicard, and to direct them to carry out government policy. This policy called for the management of these impaired citizens of the Paris region according to available resources and to guidelines regarding order, cleanliness, thrift, and accountability. A professional as well as a political mandate propelled the Hospital Council and its policies toward culling from the mass of ailing poor those who could fulfill the duties of the citizen-patient, given health, education, and training.

◆◆◆

We have so far followed the preoccupations of the Poverty Committee and dwelt heavily on the problems of children, women, and old folk. Now we shall complete our overview by looking at the experience of several million of French men drafted into the armies, where they faced illness, privation, and other dangers to their health. We shall see how the lessons of war provided a powerful prod, preparing citizen-patients for active participation in the pursuit of public health.

V

PROSPECTS:

Hygiene and Prevention

The Citizen-Patient and the Environment

Hygiene protects from the doctor.
Motto of François-Vincent Raspail's *Manuel annuaire de la santé*, 1845

We have so far considered the citizen-patient in his own surroundings and focused on domestic health problems. But thousands
of Parisian men followed the call to arms and found themselves exposed, in the course of their military duties, to unforeseen dangers to
their health. They deserve our attention.

Calamitous news accumulated in France, beginning in the late
1790s, of the armed forces being swept by epidemics: malaria in Italy,
ophthalmia in Egypt, bubonic plague in Syria, yellow fever in the
Antilles, typhus in Germany. Thousands of soldiers battled vainly
against these communicable diseases of unknown etiology. They took
some useful precautions, such as the isolation of infected men and
increased attention to cleanliness, yet the soldiers watched many hundreds of their comrades die.

Upon returning home, Parisian medical veterans discovered a widespread interest in hygiene and public health, owing partly to a voluminous literature stimulated by the wars, partly to the highly popular
course that Jean Noël Hallé had been teaching since 1795. They learned
about the spectacular discovery of vaccination, introduced into France
in 1800. Here was a preventive measure initiated by the government,
an approach to public health that appealed to Bonaparte because he
could control it. The first consul also backed the creation of a Public
Health Council of the Seine Department in 1802. This harked back,
of course, to the Enlightenment's wish to "police" society for its
own good and to Vicq d'Azyr's emphasis on vigilance and early
intervention.

A public health movement now brought together an interdisciplinary group of experts, not only medical men such as physicians,

281

surgeons, pharmacists, and veterinarians, but also lawyers, civil engineers, architects, and administrators. They harnessed the new knowledge and defined the field of activity of a new specialist, the hygienist. It was clear to everyone that for hygiene, prevention, and sanitation to succeed, active public involvement was essential. Citizen-patients had to become the guardians of their own health.

The Ravages of Epidemic Diseases

During twenty-three years of warfare, between 1792 and 1815, France drafted 4,556,000 men.[1] At first they defended their own land from invading Prussians and Austrians, but soon they spilled across France's national boundaries and fought on unfamiliar soil, in harsh climates and unusually taxing weather, among hostile populations. They marched through the blinding sandstorms of the Egyptian desert, languished in the moist heat of the Antilles, struggled to bear the heat and drought of the Spanish mesa, and eventually endured the brutal Russian winter when thousands of men froze to death. As their supply lines stretched and broke, they became increasingly dependent on the produce of foreign lands. They faced unfamiliar foods, particularly in the Antilles and the Middle East, and water, like that of the Nile, that they hesitated to drink. They coped with dangerous animals and poisonous plants in the tropics, with fearful natural climatic phenomena. They camped in inhospitable terrain, suffered from a dearth of medicines and, in the end, straggled home hurt, maimed, or convalescing. In these hazardous situations, in dangerous environments, the soldier turned to his officers and doctors for advice. But they were as baffled as he was.

When Dominique Jean Larrey, chief surgeon of the Eastern army,[2] set foot on Egyptian soil on 1 July 1798,[3] he expected no such danger as plague. In joining the Egyptian expedition, Larrey, like other medical men, had come to assist his twenty-nine-year-old general, whom he greatly admired, in an imaginatively planned, yet grandiose, French civilizing mission. He was one of 164 health officers, in addition to 167 scientists, mathematicians, and artists among the 40,000 men who constituted Bonaparte's forces. The most eminent among them—men such as Drs. N. R. D. Desgenettes,[4] P. F. Percy,[5] and Larrey, as well as the chemist C. L. Berthollet (1748–1822) and the mathematician Gaspard Monge (1746–1818)—would constitute an Egyptian Institute, organized on the pattern of the Institut de France, to which Bonaparte had recently been elected. He soon ordered that they seek answers to a number of questions, including medical problems, particularly with regard to local remedies. The pharmacist Pierre Charles Rouyer carefully studied the Egyptians' therapeutic practices and drugs with a view to culling useful medications from what the French deemed a plethora of addictive, aphrodisiac, and useless substances favored by the indigenous population.[6]

Larrey was to act as chief surgeon, Desgenettes as physician-in-chief, Rouyer as chief pharmacist. Larrey kept a diary. At first, he wrote, "the troops were bothered only by fatigue, diarrhoea, and slight dysentery caused, it seems, by the cool nights and the excess of watermelon and not, as some doctors thought, by the Nile water, which has never bothered anyone." (In a footnote he added: "This water tastes good, is definitely safe and easy to digest. An analysis has been made that proves it of better quality than the waters of European rivers.")[7] But the men were soon attacked by "a persistent ophthalmia that made several of our soldiers absolutely desperate and many of them blind. . . . [It] spared few during the winter of 1798–1799 . . . within two and a half months more than three thousand persons had to be hospitalized."[8] A modern specialist has diagnosed this "ophthalmia" as "the very contagious but not dangerous conjunctivitis caused by the Koch-Weeks bacillus, doubtless frequently complicated by genuine trachoma."[9] The soldiers' illness furnished no clue to the etiology of these ophthalmic diseases and Larrey struggled in vain with diagnosis and therapy, blaming the sunshine refracted by the many white objects, the windblown dust, and the cool and humid nights. For remedies he advised procedures that strike us as irrelevant:

> When the ophthalmia is inflammatory, begin by bleeding at the veins of the neck, arm, or foot . . . then use leeches, applied at the temples, as close as possible to the eye. . . . later prescribe footbaths, emollient and soothing fumigations, lotions made with linseed, poppy, or oriental saffron. . . . To soothe pain at night, cover the eyes with a salve made of beaten egg-whites with a few drops of rose water and several grains of alum.[10]

This bewildered doctor, thus conjecturing wildly in an effort to be helpful to his men, was not some rank beginner, but a practitioner with ten years' experience. His diary indicates that he also diagnosed, and treated as best he could, cases of tetanus, which were often fatal; hepatitis, which he attributed to abuse of alcohol; leprosy, which he thought might be contagious; scurvy; elephantiasis; and the ever-present syphilis. Larrey and his colleague Desgenettes established hospitals wherever they went: in a Capuchin monastery near Alexandria, at Rosetta, at Gizeh.

In the winter of 1798 in Cairo, Larrey diagnosed his first case of bubonic plague. He put the patient in isolation, and when the man died, he had the body, belongings, and bedding burnt and the room fumigated. He informed only Desgenettes and addressed "a circular to all surgeons, inviting them to continue their solicitous care for these patients and at the same time take all possible precautions against the contagion."[11] The hope was that, if the word *plague* was not mentioned, panic could be avoided among the soldier-patients. In his diary Larrey noted: "One cannot deny that plague is epidemic and contagious."[12]

This became obvious to all during the spring campaign of 1799 in Syria when, during the siege of Jaffa in March, up to fifteen men died daily. Larrey advised "cleanliness, frequent ablutions with cold water and vinegar, fresh linen and clothing, exercise, and moderation."[13] Perhaps such hygienic measures were of some help, particularly if they discouraged rats. The losses—8,915 in all—were staggering: amost one-fifth of these men died of plague and among the dead were 54 of the health officers.[14]

Yellow fever in Martinique proved even more devastating than plague in Syria. The French landed on Martinique in the fall of 1802; an epidemic soon spread among them, and in the first three months over half their men succumbed. "In the hospitals almost all the doctors and surgeons died," commented Alexandre Moreau de Jonnès (1778– 1870), a widely traveled, observant, and prolific medical statistician, "we lost forty of them in succession . . . only a few aged negroes survived."[15]

Many were terror-stricken and turned superstitious, often adopting local lore. The etiology of the disease remained mysterious, not only to the French but also to the British.[16] Moreau de Jonnès suspected the weather but, despite his numerous observations, he was unable to be more specific. Mosquitoes were ubiquitous, of course, but no one understood their nefarious role. Moreau's therapy was as eclectic as his etiology. "The number and variety of remedies show only too clearly that they were useless," he concluded; "it is only through a system of public health . . . that yellow fever can be eradicated from the Antilles and prevented from invading Europe."[17] His fears were eventually confirmed, for in 1823, Spain experienced a deadly yellow fever epidemic.

Moreau de Jonnès reported mainly on Martinique. The ravages in Santo Domingo and Guadeloupe confirm his findings. In Santo Domingo over half of the French medical personnel died: six doctors, fifty-five surgeons, and nine pharmacists; in Guadeloupe, thirteen out of twenty-one medical men. In all the French lost 35,000 men during that ill-starred expedition, most of them to yellow fever, including the leader, General Leclerc, Bonaparte's brother-in-law.[18]

Disenchantment among Military Doctors

General Bonaparte handled the problem of contagion in his accustomed manner. In Egypt he decreed that plague was innocuous, and he went to great lengths to disprove its communicability. His well-known visit to the Jaffa pesthouse was a publicity stunt, immortalized in the huge canvas by Antoine Jean Gros that shows Bonaparte fearlessly touching infected patients. The soldiers were unconvinced. "Let no one think," wrote Larrey, "that our soldiers were frightened by the word *plague*. . . . They had become morally and physically toughened by the hardships they had already undergone. It would have been desirable to inform the military, at the first appearance of plague, and to explain, in a reassuring way, the true character of the disease."[19] In faraway Martinique, Moreau de Jonnès argued similarly that this lack of information frightened the soldiers most, "because they then doubted the truth of everything the men in authority told them."[20]

Not only were the men left in the dark about the etiology of yellow fever, they could not even count on a well-staffed and well-supplied medical service. Napoleon did not believe in therapeutic medicine. Beginning in 1800, and decisively after he crowned himself emperor in 1804, Napoleon imposed a military health policy congruent with the typical attitude of the professional soldier: that meant emphasis on hygiene and good morale: healthful encampments, adequate rest, solid shoes and warm clothing, sound food, fresh air, and good spirits. Typical was Napoleon's enjoinder to Marshal Davout, who commanded the German army: "If there are men who are tired in the various columns, send them to a convalescent hospital, which you can establish in Berlin, and leave them there for a week or so. This is a means of saving men and preventing sickness."[21]

Napoleon's attention to morale among combatants is legendary: the "little corporal" appeared at campfires on the eve of battle, presumably incognito, sharing stories of past victories and inspiring his men to bravery. He toured battlefields after the fighting, providing encouragement to the wounded as a temporary substitute for medical aid. As the wars spread and lasted, the foot soldier found himself abandoned to whatever impromptu medical and surgical care the doctor commanded, and to the soldier-patient's own self-reliance and ingenuity.[22]

Napoleon's contempt for medicine affected military doctors even more cruelly than the men and demoralized his medical staff. He tried to shame medical officers into bravery in the face contagious diseases. "Any health officer abandoning a first-aid station in battle,"

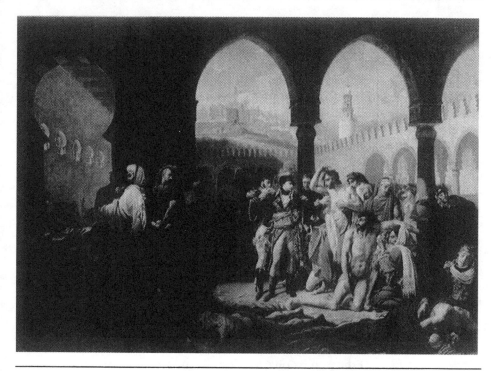

FIGURE 10.1. *General Bonaparte at the Jaffa Pesthouse*. Painting by Antoine Jean Gros. Musée de Louvre, Paris.

reads a well-known order of the day of January 1799, "or refusing to care for patients who might carry a contagious disease, shall be arrested, tried by a military tribunal, and judged according to the law dealing with deserters. Whatever his station, no Frenchman shall fear death." The general then publicly denounced a surgeon: "Citizen Boyer, surgeon at Alexandria," reads the decree, "coward enough to refuse his services to patients who had had contact with supposedly contagious cases, is unworthy of being a French citizen. He shall be dressed as a woman, paraded through the streets of Alexandria on a donkey with a sign on his back saying 'Afraid to die, unworthy of being a Frenchman.' After that, he shall be sent back to France . . . and deprived of his citizenship."[23]

Army doctors' morale sank steadily during the Republic and Empire as they struggled for acceptance by the regular officers, vainly requesting the *épaulette,* a recognizable status symbol and the sign of a permanent commission.[24] Except for a brief eight years from 1792 to 1800, army medicine was ruled by the quartermaster, subordinated to the Office of War Administration, and put on a level with the food supply, sanitation, and prisons. As late as 1872, an army surgeon still denounced "the one impediment to progress, the subordination of military medicine to the commissariat . . . contrary to all the rules of reason, truth, and justice."[25]

The well-known introduction of ambulances, a vital means of assuring prompt aid to the wounded soldier, illustrates this situation. In the Rhine army in 1792, Percy first organized the forerunners of ambulances, the "stretcher-bearers," assigning soldiers to transport casualties to a field hospital (confusingly called an "*ambulance*"). Larrey sped the process by hitching a horse to a light and maneuverable two-wheeled carriage, creating the "flying ambulance." It picked up casualties, even during battle, administered first aid and traveled quickly to the frontline "ambulant" hospital.

During the German campaign of 1799–1800, Percy devised the "*Wurst*" ("sausage"), which was longer and more cumbersome than Larrey's vehicle but could accommodate more men and supplies; up to ten doctors could bestride it and thus save their energies. Percy never received the horses to draw these wagons: "Some thought that it might have been a dangerous spectacle to see medical officers ride," commented the disappointed doctor, "since a system full of ill-will, oppression, and humiliation had long condemned them to walk and be covered with dust and dirt: they *should* walk and be miserable, otherwise, some administrators said, they would become too cocky." Percy exclaimed in disgust: "What an administration! To see the indifference and the lethargy of all those officials when one mentions hospitals, one would think that a patient or a wounded man ceases to be human when he can no longer fight."[26] Larrey had an experience similar to that of his colleague Percy; during the Syrian campaign, he had a hundred baskets made to transport wounded soldiers on camelback, but the quartermaster confiscated them.[27]

Such hostile measures foreshadowed Bonaparte's refusal to create a permanent army medical corps. The propitious moment to do so lasted from 1800 to 1804. After France defeated the Second Coalition, hundreds of medical officers, returned from the wars, could have been fashioned into a new military unit with its own schools, hospitals, and advanced battlefield stations. This would have been creative development, in line with J. F. Coste's recommendations and the pioneering efforts of Sir John Pringle in England. But in a succession of decrees issued between 1800 to 1804, the First Consul abolished the army medical schools, reduced the number of army hospitals from fifty to thirty, curtailed their staffs sharply, and reassigned their administra-

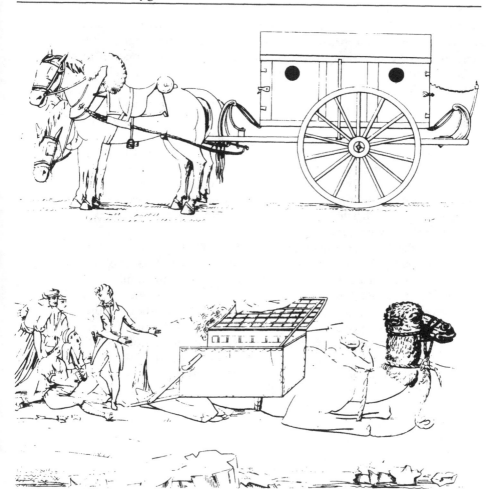

FIGURE 10.2. *Top:* D. J. Larrey's "flying ambulance." *Bottom:* Larrey's ambulance on camelback. From D. J. Larrey, *Mémoires de chirurgie militaire* (Paris: Buisson, 1812).

tion to the quartermaster. The decree of 5 January 1801 (15 Nivôse, Year IX) stated: "The army medical service is based on temporary commissions only and . . . strictly speaking, *there is no medical corps*" (emphasis added). As a result "the entire army medical corps gradually disintegrated."[28] The number of doctors declined, between 1800 and 1802, from 210 to 62 physicians, and from 1,665 to 842 surgeons; "other health personnel . . . practically no longer existed."[29] As a result, the army medical services were seething with "discouragement,

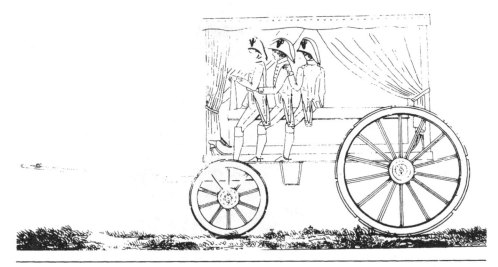

FIGURE 10.3. P. F. Percy's *"Wurst."* From D. J. Larrey, *Mémoires de chirurgie militaire* (Paris: Buisson, 1812).

rage, and revolt."[30] Napoleon, as one embittered critic put it, demoted his army doctors to the level of "the butchers and bakers"—that is, to the level of the citizen-soldier.[31]

Learning about Hygiene

Discharged and unemployed, numerous health officers who had been drafted when they were medical students now decided to go back to school and acquire an M.D. degree. If they had not done so earlier, they now registered for Jean Noël Hallé's popular lecture course on hygiene at the Paris Health School. In the summer of 1799, 571 students signed up; 649 did so in 1801, and 746 in 1802.[32] No existing amphitheater could hold all these eager youths, and the majority had to be content with copying a friend's class notes. Hallé's course alerted them to the ordinary man's needs with respect to nutrition, shelter, exercise, the environment, and protection against contagion.[33] He also discussed the soldier's problems, his food, clothing, wounds, nostalgia, and morale. Hallé analyzed the private and public aspects of his topic, traced its history since biblical and Graeco-Roman antiquity, and described the legislation, customs, and public health regulations of each epoch. He praised the writings of John Howard on prisons and of Sir John Pringle and analyzed desid-

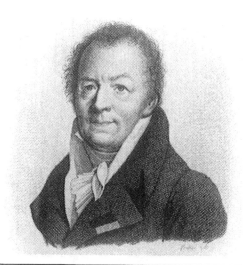

FIGURE 10.4. Jean Noël Hallé (1754–1822). Académie nationale de médecine, Paris.

erata for health maintenance in workhouses, army camps, on ships, and in the colonies. He ended by briefly mentioning health care for babies, the elderly, industrial workers, and artisans. With such a professor, a chair, a masterful definition of the subject matter, and widespread interest, one might say that "hygiene" came of age at the turn of the nineteenth century, even though a prominent journal declared in 1799: "Hygiene is still, for the majority of doctors, a very limited science."[34]

In common parlance, the term "*hygiène*" was used interchangeably with "*salubrité*," "*hygiène publique*," and "*police sanitaire*." The unsigned article on the subject in the *Encyclopédie*, written in the 1760s, is remarkable for inclusiveness, vagueness, and two dozen of those famous cross-references, ranging from "climate" and "water" to "nature" and "temperament."[35] When Hallé wrote the article "Hygiène" for the *Encyclopédie méthodique* in 1798, a quarter century after Diderot accomplished his monumental undertaking, the hygienist restricted his discussion more closely to human needs. Later he felt compelled to enlarge upon his own thought in a new article, dated 1818, for the *Dictionnaire des sciences médicales*, where he commented: "We felt that we should transpose here a rather large part of the article 'Hygiène' from the *Encyclopédie méthodique*, while making the cuts, changes, and additions that an interval of over twenty-five years allows or demands."[36] Hallé pointed out that development in hygiene was propelled by progress in chemistry, physics, physiology, comparative anatomy, electricity, and toxicology. His writings and teaching helped build a bridge from the concepts of the Enlightenment to the practical achievements and literature of the nineteenth century.

A Growing Body of Literature

In the military medical literature of the era 1792–1815, the Egyptian expedition stands out for variety and quantity of writings, particularly about the baffling problem of contagion and the soldiers' responses to the novel challenges. There were many intellectuals among the participants, who were initially filled with the expectation of adventure and optimistic about success. For a short while, the Egyptian Institute and its periodical, *La Décade égyptienne,* published health-related articles in tandem with the Institut de France at home.[37] Then, in 1800, the dramatic experience with vaccination buoyed hope that communicable diseases other than smallpox might be similarly checked, and the daily press was filled with news about the new procedure. Also, numerous participants in the Italian, Spanish, German, and Russian campaigns kept diaries and turned their notes into monographs and manuals, or into a medical thesis, as required under the licensure law of 1803.

Doctors in the military had no ready vehicle for journal articles discussing the soldiers' medical problems, given the lack of a separate military medical periodical, whereas under the old regime Richard de Hautsierck had published the *Recueil d'observations de médecine des hôpitaux militaires*[38] and Jacques De Horne had edited the *Journal de médecine, chirurgie, et pharmacie militaire,*[39] which filled seven volumes in the 1780s. Under Napoleon, the *Journal général de médecine, chirurgie et pharmacie,* the quasi-official organ of the Paris medical school, tended to publish articles by military personalities such as Desgenettes. The *Mémoires* of the Société médicale d'émulation were more open to young military talent.[40]

Toward the end of the Napoleonic era, the enterprising Parisian publisher Charles Louis Fleury Panckoucke (1780–1844) began to produce the sixty-volume *Dictionnaire des sciences médicales,* which he completed in ten years (1812–1822). Authoritative articles by the leading representatives of every aspect of medicine can be found in this monument to the medical revolution that took place in Paris at the turn of the nineteenth century. Military and naval medicine, as well as public health and hygiene, occupy important places in this compendium.

Knowledge derived from military experience passed into the civilian field not only at the young health officers' level but in the highest strata of the military establishment as well, and from there into civilian policy and down to the level of the citizen-patient. This result accrued from the long-standing French tradition (analyzed in Chapter 1 above) of appointing distinguished military medical men as inspectors of military and civilian institutions, a tradition that carried over into the nineteenth century. Seasoned by experience, they sought not only to ascertain efficiency and cost-effectiveness but also to introduce appropriate provisions for health care.[41] We know that, as early as 1772, Louis XV had appointed four outstanding and determined specialists to this position: Jean Colombier, Jean François Coste, Pierre Poissonnier, and Antoine Augustin Parmentier. Colombier died in 1789, but the others made their influences felt long into the nineteenth century through detailed reports, and eventually in their diaries and reminiscences. Under the new regime as under the old, they regularly traveled to all military and civilian installations within their sector annually, uncovering abuses and recommending changes.

Colombier and Doublet's reports on hospitals in the 1780s are a prime example of this process. We also know that, during the hearings held by Dr. Guillotin's Health Committee in 1790–1791, military experts had ample opportunity to air their views about medical education and practice and thus to influence subsequent legislation. Napoleon used a military health council too, and well into the Restoration, Coste, Desgenettes, Larrey, and Percy inspected the army; Parmentier, pharmacy; and Pierre François Keraudren,[42] the navy. The flow of military medical experience into the pool of shared civilian knowledge thus affected the medical services for the citizen-patient.

For thousands of veterans, the main medical memory of these military expeditions was of contagious disease: the men repatriated from Egypt by the British, the survivors from Santo Domingo, and the one thousand discharged medical men shared the memory and the horror of seeing their comrades die from plague and yellow fever; remitting fevers like typhoid and dysentery; intermittent fevers like malaria; and hospital, or goal, fever (typhus). Personal contact seemed a factor, but at times the disease appeared to strike from the air, which was said to be laden with "miasmata"; to arise from filth and rags; or to depend on the season or the weather. This confusion fostered "anti-contagionism"—that is, the theory that personal contact was not a necessary factor in spreading these diseases.[43] Everyone knew from observation that they were all communicable, but no one understood the mechanism of transmission. What a comfort, then, and surprise to learn that a preventive measure had been discovered against smallpox!

A Welcome Weapon: Vaccination

The public had long considered inoculation a symbol of medical enlightenment.[44] In fact, in May 1799, two professors of the Paris medical faculty, Pinel and Leroux, proposed to their colleagues that they establish a third clinical teaching service (in addition to those at the Hôtel-Dieu and the Charité) to promote this method of immunization, in the shape of an "inoculation clinic" at the Salpêtrière.[45] That summer, news of Edward Jenner's discovery reached Paris via the *Bibliothèque britannique* of Geneva, and Jenner's *Inquiry into the Causes and Effects of the Variolae Vaccinae,* published in 1798, was made available in a French translation by Antoine Aubert of Geneva the following year.[46] Aubert then traveled to Paris with vaccine from Dr. William Woodville, Jenner's assistant. He approached Pinel, and together they vaccinated three foundlings at the Salpêtrière on 16 August 1799. But the vaccine proved ineffective in this and two subsequent trials.[47]

In the meantime, the duc de La Rochefoucauld-Liancourt had returned from exile in England and the United States on 28 November 1799. He suggested to Dean Thouret the founding of a vaccination institute to be financed "in the Anglo-Saxon manner," by public subscription. The needed sum was soon raised, but Thouret evidently did not wish to leave so important a matter entirely to a public group, and he therefore submitted the project to his medical faculty. As a result, the faculty set up its own committee, on 19 January 1800, and so did the Academy of Sciences. At this point François Colon, formerly a surgeon at Bicêtre, put his country house on rue de Vaugirard at the committee's disposal, and the third (unsuccessful) clinical trial was held there.

Woodville himself now came to Paris, and on his second try, on 8 August 1800, he conducted vaccinations that proved successful.[48] His vaccine derived from several children he had immunized on his way through Boulogne, and they had been *"bien envachinés"* (so one journal put it), so that the "malady special to English cows" could now be transmitted to French children.[49]

The Paris health authorities responded to this promising innovation with speed and efficiency at the beginning of 1801. Prefect Frochot had just formed the Paris Hospital Council; three weeks later, on 7 February, he opened a "central hospice for free vaccination" near the Hôtel de Ville. Transferred in the Year XII to St. Esprit, it became the Central Vaccination Institute of Paris. Eventually the various committees merged into one prestigious and powerful support group with nine physicians, headed by Dean Thouret as chairman and including Drs. Pinel, Leroux, and Guillotin, the two physicians of the Children's

Hospital, Jadelot and Mongenot, the surgeon Parfait from the central admitting office, and physicians from the Philanthropic Society's dispensaries. For two years the committee conducted tests and met twice each *décade*. The acceptance of vaccination by the Paris medical establishment was deliberately careful and eventually wholehearted.

The government then urged departmental prefects and provincial practitioners to perform and spread this preventive measure. Addressing Napoleon Bonaparte in October 1803, the president of the Paris vaccination committee, Dr. Guillotin, declared: "There is no doubt, citizen First Consul, smallpox will be eliminated. . . . Mankind will be healthier and beautified. Your government supports vaccination: they both entered our happy land together."[50] Guillotin and his committee even obtained a special audience with Pope Pius VII in March 1805: the pope stayed on in Paris after Napoleon's coronation. The Academy of Sciences concluded in 1812 that favorable opinions regarding vaccination had by then accrued from "physicians, prefects, and public personalities from all over France and from abroad" and that "the hope of seeing this calamity disappear from civilized societies was no longer a dream."[51] This report was written by Berthollet, Percy, and Hallé, three prestigious academicians, representing science, the military, and academe. The prevention of disease had become a matter of political importance. But vaccination raised false hopes that the incidence of morbidity from communicable diseases other than smallpox could be drastically cut in a short time. Other initiatives were needed to protect and promote the public health.

The Public Health Council of Paris

When Minister of Internal Affairs Chaptal appointed the police prefect Dubois as chairman of the Public Health Council in 1802, he was heeding tradition: through Dubois the council gained the authority to "police" the town along the lines that the article "Police, jurisprudence" in the *Encyclopédie* had advised in the 1770s.[52] The police lieutenant had been a powerful figure in public health since the days of La Reynie, under Louis XIV, and his successor Lenoir, an active participant in the control of prostitution and a founder of the Vaugirard hospice for syphilitic infants. In appointing Dubois, Chaptal implied that public health was a municipal and regional concern and that he expected the police to inspect for compliance and bring offenders to justice. The capacity of Dubois, and his successors Pasquier and Anglès, to enforce the law was crucial to the success of public health policy for the citizens of Paris. Owing to Parisian influence, other

French towns adopted this new pattern for regional health protection, with important participation by the citizenry.

The men who determined policy in the Paris Public Health Council personified the humane legacy of the Enlightenment. Together with their colleagues on the Hospital Council, they now linked the pre-Revolution to the Consulate. They believed with Montesquieu that society owes the citizen a "way of life not injurious to health," and with La Rochefoucauld-Liancourt that the indigent citizen has a right to obtain free health care. The council's minutes and reports offer plentiful information on its pioneering work.

The council began modestly: Chaptal received the first suggestion from a fellow-chemist, Charles Louis Cadet de Gassicourt (1769–1821), who subsequently served as the council's secretary for nineteen years.[53] He specialized in pharmacy as it relates to food and health, interests shared by the other three initial council members, the learned veterinarian Jean Baptiste Huzard (1755–1838),[54] the tempestuous young surgeon Guillaume Dupuytren (1778–1835),[55] and the experienced chemist Nicolas Deyeux. A list of the investigations performed by Deyeux conveys an idea of the medley of items and issues that public and police submitted to the council's judgment: "contaminated containers, confiscated beverages, poisonings, invisible inks, charlatans and secret remedies; herbalists, the sale of plants in markets, mineral waters, natural and artificial public baths; merchants who sell wine, vinegar, lemonades, chocolate; the manufacture of glue, coloring substances, varnishes, mastic, oil cloth, waxed taffetas, Prussian blue, mineral acids, alums, vitriol, ammonia, soap, ink, gut for sausage casings, leathers, beer, glass, starch, sugar, liqueurs, . . . metals, soot."[56]

In 1807, a reorganized and enlarged council shifted into higher gear. With Thouret and Leroux, it added the current and future deans of the Paris Medical School; with Parmentier,[57] a link to the College of Pharmacy; with Parmentier, Cadet, Deyeux, and Huzard, it secured direct access to the Academy of Sciences.[58] The council revived the interdisciplinary approach dear to learned societies under the old régime, for it shared their interest in developments across the Channel and overseas, in military, naval, and colonial health. The councillors' comments indicate familiarity with the writings of John Howard, James Lind, Thomas Malthus, Sir John Pringle, and, of course, Edward Jenner, and with the vast military medical literature published in contemporary French and foreign journals. Thus the council members conceived of public health in international and even global terms, and as a collaborative enterprise for military and civilian experts. In their

TABLE 10.1. The Paris Public Health Council, 1802–1815

	Year Appointed	Field
Charles Louis Cadet de Gassicourt (1769–1821)	1802	pharmacy
Nicolas Deyeux (1745–1837)	1802	pharmacy
Jean Baptiste Huzard (1755–1838)	1802	veterinary medicine
Guillaume Dupuytren (1778–1835)	1802	surgery
Joseph Darcet (1777–1844)[1]	1813	pharmacy
Michel Augustin Thouret (1748–1810)	1807	medicine
Leroux des Tillets (1745–1832)	1807	medicine
Antoine Augustin Parmentier (1737–1813)	1807	pharmacy
Marc Antoine Petit (1760–1840)	1808	epidemics
Etienne Pariset (1770–1847)[2]	1808	epidemics, psychiatry
Charles C. H. Marc (1771–1841)	1815	legal medicine, psychiatry

SOURCE: Adapted from Archives de l'Assistance publique, Catalogue Fosseyeux, n.s., no. 136.
[1] Darcet replaced Parmentier
[2] Pariset succeeded Cadet as secretary in 1821

minds, public health encompassed the public and private spheres, including the citizen-patient's home and workplace. This outlook eventually resulted in the creation of social and industrial medicine. A three-pronged effort became apparent: to protect, to prevent, and to instruct in order to enlist the citizen-patient in self-help against illness.

To pursue their task, the councillors organized themselves: they elected a president—first Parmentier, then Deyeux—and a secretary—first Gassicourt, then Pariset.[59] They divided up areas of responsibility and assigned topics for comprehensive reports. The number of these rose annually, while their subject matter continued to shift:

1808	136
1811	164
1812	206
1829	270
1838	502

Council members undertook numerous inspection visits, especially to an increasing number of factories. In good eighteenth-century fashion, they listened to the reading of and commented on each other's reports at their fortnightly assemblies. Often one of them brought suspect foodstuffs, chemicals, or drugs, and one of the chemists, usually De-yeux, took these home for laboratory tests. The council had access to consultation with the French academic scientific world; sometimes Thouret sought the advice of his medical faculty and at least once, in the case of poisonous mushrooms, the famous botanist A. L. de Jus-sieu, professor at the medical faculty and the Botanical Gardens, wrote a long report.

Harnessing the New Knowledge for the Citizen-Patient

A new chapter in health protection thus opened in Paris at the turn of the nineteenth century. Reformers were now determined to use whatever tools and laws were available in order to improve the citizens' environment and thus their health. The adoption of the civil, commercial, and penal codes required that public health activity adapt to the new rules.[60] Universal standards of accuracy, measured by the new chemical quantities, the metric system, and the novel science of statistics allowed verification of public compliance with preventive and protective health measures.[61] And the gamut of interests and com-petencies among Paris Public Health Council members assured that its work would use every recent scientific and medical discovery to en-hance the population's health and the quality of their lives. These ef-forts diversified as the years rolled by.

The new law codes affected public health in multiple ways. An example is the requirement that twenty-four hours elapse before a ca-daver was buried: too many corpses had shown startling signs of life. Another example is Napoleon's attempt to curb child abandonment by establishing one turntable per department as the only legal procedure. Explicating the law codes for the purpose of the citizen's health and life was the work of F. E. Fodéré (1764–1835), professor of forensic medicine in Strasbourg from 1814 on and vice president of that city's public health council.[62] In another area, toxicology, the development of new methods to identify poisonous substances such as strychnine and arsenic allowed the ferreting out of their harmful uses. Certain murders could now be solved and the public better protected. In toxi-cology, the towering figure was M. J. B. Orfila, dean of the Paris Medical Faculty from 1831 to 1848 and a co-founder of the *Annales d'hygiène publique*.[63] In a third area, the citizen's very life could now be better defended owing to developments in psychiatry. The new con-cept of temporary insanity posited that murderers can lose command of their reason for the short period of committing that deed and thus not be responsible for their action. C. C. H. Marc (1771–1841) was the hygienist particularly interested in legal psychiatry.[64] Legal questions also preoccupied Esquirol, who became a prime advocate of the law of 1838 on confining the insane, a law that is still in force today.[65]

But the most significant direction that hygienists pursued in the early nineteenth century—significant in the sense that it affected huge numbers of poor women and men—was their investigation of the workplace—factories, mines, mills—where women and children as well as men spent long daily hours in health-damaging pollution. Thus the indefatigable Alexandre Parent-Duchâtelet investigated sewers, cesspits, and city dumps; J. H. Réveillé-Parise (1782–1852) explored the hygiene of vision; L. F. Benoiston de Châteauneuf (1776–1856) wrote on the economic and statistical aspects of hygiene; and Louis René Villermé (1782–1863) publicized the squalor and dangers of the poor man's working environment. This publicity eventually stimulated political action, but under Napoleon such activity was forbidden.

But even under the Empire citizen-patients could be involved in developments to further personal hygiene and public health, either by following the path taken by professional leaders who educated the public or through their own actions. While protective activities proliferated, the citizens' own initiatives began discreetly, constrained by the political climate. Progressive legislation to guarantee health care for a nation of citizen-patients belonged to the democratic future.

Nutrition

Providing the necessities essential to the citizen's daily life headed the Public Health Council's list of objectives: the quality and safety of foods, their efficient, swift transportation on rivers and roads, and their clean handling for sale in the markets. The councillors reasoned that cleanliness and sanitation were the crucial public measures in support of health.[66] They also knew that these goals demanded the enlightened self-interest and collaboration of the citizenry.

Among Parisians' numerous health concerns, water headed the list. They never seemed to have enough of the precious commodity for drinking and cooking, laundry and street cleaning. Nor did they find the distribution equitable throughout Paris, so that conduits needed to be laid and fountains erected. Eventually this dearth led the council to advocate construction of the Yvette canal (after Pierre Simon Girard, a civil engineer, participant in the Egyptian expedition and builder of the Ourcq canal in 1802, joined the council in 1819). Despite these efforts, the citizenry complained repeatedly about the poor quality of drinking water: early-nineteenth-century criteria of water quality were taste, smell, and purity—that is, freedom from visible particles of matter that could be filtered out, bacteria being as yet beyond the council's reach. With help from the police in bringing scofflaws to justice, the councillors were able to move factories downstream so as to reduce water pollution. They also analyzed mineral and medicinal waters for which curative powers were claimed, an activity that had taken up much of the Academy of Sciences' time in the eighteenth century. And they regulated public bathhouses on the river Seine.

Food raised endless problems—prisoners and inpatients often complained about the adulteration of bread, a commodity of enormous importance in the hospital system, which consumed some 20,000 pounds daily. The councillors not only analyzed the varieties of flour used by bakers, but also the ingredients used to cook "economic soup," and they inspected the cattle still housed within city limits, the slaughterhouses, and the meat sold in the markets. They tested a synthetic lemonade that had made some people sick (in 1809, the British blockade cut off the supply of lemons), and they took an interest in attempts at creating substitutes for other colonial products, such as sugar and coffee. They studied the properties and uses of cinchona bark, rhubarb, and ricinus oil.

The 1814 report tells of extensive tasting of wines to decide whether these had been diluted. What standards could one devise, the council asked, to detect "adulterated wines, or wines that have been mixed, tainted, or tampered with [*vins falsifiés, vins mélangés, vins altérés, vins raccommodés*]?" They added that "the wine merchants' lawyers have attacked our conclusions as too severe." But the councillors persisted and concluded that "there is need for a large-scale analysis of alcoholic beverages, but it would be difficult to do. This council could plan the work, but to prevent fraud and keep the merchants in the dark regarding the means of escaping conviction, one would have to come to an arrangement with the collector of indirect taxes, so as to arrive at a common plan."[67] Some problems are perennial.

Sanitation

Next to nutrition, sanitation headed the citizens' list of health concerns. This included waste disposal—for example, the removal of "night soil," an important commercial venture, which provided suburban fruit and vegetable farms with fertilizer. Problems of cleanliness and garbage disposal arose in slaughterhouses and horse-butchering yards, as well as with sewers and the recurrent damage resulting from inundations. In the summer of 1814, the specter of typhus came to Paris with allied occupation troops, who left their barracks "in a state of infection difficult to describe," and 3,000 dead horses "lying about in heaps."[68] Even though no one mentioned the "environment" or the "quality of life," Parisians were indeed beginning to suffer from pollution and congestion.

Smoke that darkened the air and waste water that dirtied the Seine emanated from refineries, distilleries, laundries, and tanneries that "use or produce glue, varnish, acids, salts, soap, Prussian blue, dyes, and tallow," stated the Health Council report for 1807.[69] Five years later there were fewer complaints, because "fear of costly relocation has induced the manufacturers to take the steps needed to curb harmful smoke and offensive odors."[70] The citizens had become so aggravated that they alerted the police and the council to take action.

The growth of Paris brought sanitary problems of all sorts: the population had increased from 550,800 in 1789 to 713,765, stated the council report for 1817. Traffic—including the number of horses—rose commensurately. "In 1789, there were only 900 hackney coaches, none of them with fixed stations; today there are 2,400 of them for hire. . . . [Now] the transportation of . . . merchandise calls for a prodigious number of wagons, drays, and carts in constant circulation."[71] Council reports inform us that the harsh conditions of life often drove Parisians to suicide.

The Council provided and monitored first aid equipment along the riverbanks, but its safety measures often failed: in 1817, for example, 238 corpses were recovered from the river. Richard Cobb has given us a sympathetic and dramatic account of these distraught victims' last hours.[72] The immediate question of accident? suicide? or murder? would arise—a question that involved the police. As of 1804, the police delivered corpses to the new morgue instead of the basement of the Grand Châtelet: they dredged the bodies from the Seine, gathered them from seedy hotels, and even pulled the limbs of dead babies out of the sewers. All these grisly remains would be laid out on one of ten marble tables and their clothing displayed nearby, in the hope of facilitating identification. Autopsy in suspicious deaths was mandatory, and the law called for toxicologic tests on the spot. Whether unclaimed bodies were taken to the medical school for dissection we do not know.

Autopsies served a special purpose when the cause of death was suspected to be a dangerous contagious disease: the police prefect Dubois published an ordinance on 3 July 1803 (14 Messidor, Year XI), which he had undoubtedly cleared with his Health Council, declaring inter alia: "If the symptoms of an illness suggest an epidemic or contagious disease, an autopsy may be mandated by the authorities or by the physicians or surgeons who attended the case" (art. 5). This provision reappears as Article 81 in the Civil Code of 1804.

But it was the burial of human corpses that proved most complex. Thouret's expertise on questions of interment stood the council in good stead, and they learned about the need of moving all cemeteries out of town. Although sensitive to a Catholic public's feelings about decorous ritual burial, the council believed that the traditional preference for inhumation in or near a church had to give way: they had learned of sanitary problems such as the contamination of groundwater by decomposing corpses and concluded that protection of the citizen's environment should take precedence over religious preference. It proved as complex to establish the new Père Lachaise cemetery in 1803 as it had been to open the cimetière Montmartre in 1795 and as it would be to consecrate the cimetière Montparnasse in 1826. An imperial decree of 14 June 1804 (25 Prairial, Year XII) definitively prohibited burial in or near all places of worship, ordering that "there shall be no burial in churches, temples, synagogues, hospitals, public chapels, or any enclosed building where citizens meet to celebrate their cult, or within towns and villages." Article 4 even rallied the metric system to the cause of public health and ordered that "each burial shall be in a separate grave, 1½ to 2 meters deep and 80 cm wide, subsequently filled with well-compacted soil." The decree also looked to future use of public land and added: "[After five years], the lands now used as cemeteries may be leased by the communities that own them. But they may only be seeded or planted and not dug up, nor may the foundations of buildings be constructed until further notice" (art. 9). Thus the modern state not only claimed jurisdiction over the citizen's mortal remains, but ordered their sanitary disposal and asserted its right to use the burial grounds in the future.

It also regulated the use of cadavers for teaching purposes, a task that, as we saw earlier, the old regime had shunned. While the Health Council had no jurisdiction over the delivery of cadavers for dissection, it did assume responsibility for supervising the numerous private anatomy courses that so many neighbors found objectionable. In 1813, it closed them all and the government instead authorized a new, large dissection amphitheater near the Pitié hospital.[73]

In matters involving their own bodies, the protection of their lives, food and water, and the sanitary condition of their environment, the citizens of Paris were now guarded and guided in a manner that made their health care network a model for other large cities.

Self-help

The citizen-patients' initiatives to secure the maintenance and protection of their own health can be documented in many areas. We know about the applicants who sought treatment at the Hospital Council's admitting office, 6 percent of them receiving braces and pessaries. We have seen that every year three or four thousand citizen-patients resorted to the other three busy outpatient departments at the St. Louis, Children's, and Venereal Diseases hospitals. Those who could afford a minimal payment sought admission to the "Maison Dubois" or Cullerier's private hospital; those eligible, to the "Maison de la Rochefoucauld"; and those with more means to Ste. Perinne, or, if they were mentally ill, to Esquirol's hospital on rue Buffon.

The five dispensaries of the Philanthropic Society drew up a balance sheet of their activities between 1800 and 1815. (A sixth dispensary opened in 1816.) The citizen-patients who had taken the initiative during the Consulate and Empire of getting the cards that entitled them to treatment at the dispensaries numbered 14,684; of this total, 10,770 had been cured. In addition, 1,137 parents had brought their children to be vaccinated by the dispensary doctors.[74]

Among initiatives that originated in the workers' world, the mutual aid and provident societies deserve mention. Although mutual aid in artisanal corporations has a long history, there was a new emphasis on medical care during our era. In Paris, it was again the Philanthropic Society that showed the workers the way to individual health care. In 1809, sixty-four provident societies were associated with the Philanthropic Society for the purpose of dispensary access, eighty in 1811. They collected dues and paid pensions to aged members and the medical expenses of the sick, for whom they subscribed to dispensary cards. In 1811, for example, aware of the respiratory complaints especially frequent among hatters, their Friendly Society established a prize for a more salubrious manufacturing process. In 1815, the Society for Graphic Arts sought to make wives eligible for medical care, arguing that "if a worker has to let his wife leave and send her to the hospital, that is a greater misfortune than if he himself had to go. . . . With the mother gone, there are no more rules in the house. Upon reflection one realizes more and more clearly that Dispensaries are as supportive of good habits as they are advantageous for the well-being and health of the citizenry."[75]

Finally, one might adduce the response to cost-of-living bonuses (*portion représentative*) offered by the Hospital Council to old people eligible for life in a custodial hospice. A bonus of 150–180 francs per year induced some to live with a private family instead, not necessarily

their own. This measure allowed a reduction of from 500 to 100 inmates at the Hospice des Ménages, while at Bicêtre in 1802, 120 indigents accepted the pension and left. The council's objective, of course,
was to induce relatively sturdy and self-sufficient citizen-patients to
stay out of hospice and hospital.[76]

In trying to create the new self-image of the citizen-patient, the
health care reformers eventually found allies among the Utopian Socialists, men such as Etienne Cabet (1788–1856), Ulysse Trélat (1795–
1879), and François Vincent Raspail (1794–1878), who combined their
fight for social justice with the advocacy of self-help and social medicine. "Hygiene protects from the doctor" was the motto of Raspail's
health annual, the *Manuel annuaire de la santé,* a best-seller from 1845
into the twentieth century. This innovative scientist, medical practitioner, and democratic leader preached a mixture of self-respect, hygiene, and socialism.[77] Raspail's message was that ordinary people
could lessen their dependence on expensive physicians if they practiced cleanliness and moderation in their personal habits, kept their
living quarters neatly aired and whitewashed, ate healthful food, re-
frained from polluting their environment, cared for the common enjoyment of public spaces, and obeyed the regulations of agencies such
as the Paris Public Health Council. The Utopian Socialists thus recast
the Poverty Committee's message into a social and democratic program that ordinary citizens could pursue. One can argue, without
stretching the point, that their line of reasoning derived logically from
La Rochefoucauld-Liancourt.

◆◆◆

Thus, in civilian and military life, among women as well as
men, handicapped children, the aged, and institutionalized or privately lodged patients and convalescents, multiple efforts were afoot
to pursue and realize the improvement and maintenance of the population's health. The government and the health care professions now
had a small but significant number of identifiable partners whose activities and importance would grow over time.

The Politics of Health

Useful truths are destined to outlive the circumstances that produced them.

Baron M. F. de Gérando, *De l'éducation des sourds-muets de naissance*, 1827

Medicine is . . . a social science with a social goal. It appears as one link in the great chain of social welfare institutions which we expect to find in a civilized community."

Henry E. Sigerist, in *Civilization and Disease*, 1943

This book has argued that a significant group of French reformers and doctors interpreted the Revolutionary principle of equality in a new and creative way. They believed that this principle obligated the government to provide all citizens with equal access to health care, free of charge if they were poor. Sources of this thought can be identified in the Enlightenment, when influential thinkers concerned themselves with the health of the poor and activists experimented with philanthropic establishments and small neighborhood hospitals. Reformers believed that these should replace the existing huge, degrading public institutions. A confrontation occurred in the National Constituent Assembly in 1790–1791, when the projects for national health care elaborated by the reformers of the Poverty Committee clashed with plans for modern training for doctors, pharmacists, and midwives proposed by the Health Committee. The assembly decided that the reform of medical education should have priority; however, the moral mandate to improve health care for the citizenry served as a permanent reminder of an imperative and perennial need.

It is in the civilian hospitals that the historian most clearly perceives a shift in the interrelationships among doctors, pharmacists, nurses, midwives, students, and patients during the Revolutionary and Napoleonic era. Twice daily the patient now saw the doctor on rounds and was beleaguered by a bevy of interns and students, who crowded around the bed, eager to learn. The doctor and pharmacist could now override the nurse's recommendations—she was, in fact, becoming their subordinate. Documents that analyze the new bedside medicine rarely even mention her presence. In contemporary illustrations she stands in the background, looking subservient, in contrast to her medieval model.

Whereas under the old regime women pharmacists had rivaled men in competence, privileges, and obligations, Revolutionary developments dissociated the two groups entirely, with the science of pharmacology acting as solvent. The sisters continued administering traditional "simple" medicinal substances while, in contrast, the young male pharmacist mastered the new knowledge. Women had no access to training and internships, established in 1814, and thus their competence declined, and they dropped to second-rate standing. Special training for midwives remained a qualified success: in the early nineteenth century, professional recognition for women faced social, economic, religious, and psychologic hurdles that would fall gradually, including those barring women from medical schools.

Most hospitals during the old regime were inadequate, unsanitary, overcrowded, and thus injurious to health. This situation confronted the Revolutionary physician with a dilemma: whom should he hospitalize and whom reject? was outpatient care a preferable alternative to life on a murderously deficient ward? The Hospital Council of the Seine promoted a spectrum of strategies, both old and novel, to keep patients out of the hospital. It revived the wet-nursing office and other means of infant protection, as well as home care and soup kitchens; but it also supported new initiatives, such as dispensaries, nursing homes, outpatient clinics, and infirmaries, all designed as substitutes for hospitalization. At the same time the council supervised renovation in the hospitals that would be needed despite all attempts to replace them, promoting single beds, cleanliness, orderliness, and thrift.

The inpatient now confronted many new experiences: the lack of religious symbols may have been the first shock. Then, at admission, there would be intensive interviews and, for some, selection for the small teaching wards. There, repeated visits and examinations by medical students and by the professor during teaching rounds may well have been embarrassing and frightening experiences for the citizen-patient. She, and he, then usually paid the ultimate price for free medical care: postmortem dissection.

One major purpose of these innovations was to further medical science and research, in particular the nascent specialties. Five of these—venereology, geriatrics, neonatology, pediatrics, and psychiatry—are discussed in this book in some detail, with a focus on the experience of the patient in a clinical setting. Doctors who specialized in the emerging fields were keen on seeing patients triaged according to their illnesses and assigned to specific wards—a practice that raises the question of whether physicians used the citizen-patient for their own ends. The ethical implications, so clear to us, were no issue for Revolutionary physicians. They assumed as a matter of course that the patient's services for the purpose of demonstration and research represented a fair exchange for free medical care. (Modern criticism of this early "clinic" by Michel Foucault and others is discussed in the Introduction.)

The Revolutionary reformers extended their concern to deaf and blind children and to the mentally ill. They explored innovative ways in which the handicapped could be protected and their health and abilities promoted. In 1791, the abbé Sicard secured the adoption of poor deaf children as wards of the nation and the establishment of a well-staffed school and scholarships. Logically, blind children could lay equal claim to national support, and therefore Valentin Haüy obtained a national institution, staff, and scholarships as well, later the same year.

The fate of the mentally ill also reached a turning point during this era. A new perception of the madman as a medical patient gradually gained acceptance, as did the concomitant view that mental illness may be curable. This view was promoted by Philippe Pinel, during and after his nineteen months' experience at Bicêtre, in the dramatic "Memoir on mania" read to the Society for Natural History and in the *Traité . . . sur l'alienation mentale* that became world-famous. Pinel's felicitous choice of the term "mental alienation" implied that a skilled therapist could bring an "alienated" person back to "normal" society. Pinel's clinical teaching introduced a large number of students to a psychologically sensitive approach toward the medically ill patient. The presence of a professor, academician and concerned therapist amidst the seven thousand aged women at the Salpêtrère brought them daily solace.

◆◆◆

In Chapter 10, we looked at the healthiest part of the male population, the soldiers, who were exposed, during the quarter century under review, to a gamut of exotic diseases and hitherto unknown health hazards. They became keenly aware of the dangers to health that may lurk in the environment. It is argued that the wartime experience alerted hundreds of doctors and thousands of soldiers to the urgency of hygiene and prevention. A new fraternal relationship between citizen-patients and doctors resulted from the wars, and eventually a new, respectful image of the physician found expression in French literature.

Surprisingly, the literature of French military medicine is deeply resentful of Napoleon. This is because he aggravated the soldiers' fate when he let his own prejudice against doctors determine policy regarding an army medical corps. Instead of creating such a body of experts, he discharged about 900 medical officers between 1800 and 1802. The soldier therefore faced the hazards in his environment in the company of a small number of health officers with little prestige or equipment—they confronted the challenges and dangers of war and illness as social equals.

Returning medical veterans found their new awareness reinforced by efforts at home, spearheaded by Jean Noël Hallé's teaching of a new academic subject, hygiene. And the introduction of vaccination in 1800 seemed to promise that prevention of illness could become a safe, effective, inexpensive, and universal strategy to hold communicable diseases at bay. But this required the patient's enlightened collaboration. Gradually it became clear that the role of the citizen–patient as the doctor's knowledgeable and active partner is fundamental to a nation's health.

Paris took a historic initiative with the creation of the Public Health Council of the Seine Department. Owing to the prestige of the capital, this council found imitators in the provinces and admirers abroad and should be regarded as the pioneer institution in the nineteenth-century public health movement. In 1849 it engendered the *Assistance publique à Paris* as a new branch of municipal government. One can thus perceive the outlines of what has since become a daunting reality: "prompt, free, assured, and complete" health care for all is indeed a compelling mirage, for which doctors and citizen-patients must reach together.

◆◆◆

The medical profession and the government responded imaginatively to these challenges. They created modernized, specialized teaching hospitals and they totally reformed medical training, honing the skills of interns and externs at the citizen-patient's bedside. Attention to the health of women resulted in one major Revolutionary achievement, the transfer of the maternity service from the Hôtel-Dieu to Port-Royal and the creation of an efficient establishment for childbirth and the training of midwives at the Oratory. This act of administrative efficiency orchestrated the relocation of pregnant indigent women to a transformed, healthful building, where they received prenatal care in the form of safe, quiet lodgings and good food. Nurses and administrators proceeded to a speedy triage of the babies and the transfer of the healthy ones to a country wet nurse. This complex undertaking led to a demonstrable improvement of maternal health, facilitated the regulation of wet-nursing, and accounted for a spectacular drop in infant mortality, at least in the perinatal period. This was achieved during the deeply troubled days of the Directory. But Paris's reach did not extend to the provincial foster homes, where inspection remained woefully inadequate. As a result, nine-tenths of the foster children died.

In Paris, in contrast, the medical profession was attentive to the problems of the child. A clinic for seriously ill infants and a separate hospital for children resulted from the Revolution's challenge. We have also seen that J. M. G. Itard's experience with Victor led this doctor to the serious study of otology. Only ophthalmology did not, during this era, hold out any encouraging prospects; on the other hand, the blind Louis Braille made an extraordinary contribution to enable those so afflicted to become citizen-patients.

In contrast to the successfully met challenges stands the failure to create a national health service, even though the people's needs were clear. Health Committee debates in 1790 indicate that the medical profession was uninterested, and Napoleon, for reasons of his own, chose to miss the opportunity to bring health care to his nation.

The lives of the chief planners took very different turns: Vicq d'Azyr, first physician to Queen Marie Antoinette and consulting physician to King Louis XVI and the young dauphin, attended them at the Conciergerie in 1793; one can imagine the torment of this task. Weak from overwork, delicate health, and the tragic death of his young wife, Vicq d'Azyr fell a prey to pneumonia and died in 1794, at the age of forty-six. Guillotin staggered along under the burden of guilt by association, even though he had not invented the deadly machine that bore his name, nor even baptized it. He took no more part in politics, only in work of the Academic Society of Medicine, the forerunner of the Academy of Medicine, and he actively promoted vaccination. He died in Paris in 1814.[1]

The aging Guillotin watched his rival Thouret use both the Health and the Poverty Committees' draft legislation creatively in three different ways. Thouret shaped the French medical world as dean of the Paris Health School, he helped fashion the Paris hospital world as commissioner under the Legislative Assembly and Hospital Council member under Napoleon, and he furthered public health in Paris as member of the Public Health Council.[2] A scrutiny of Thouret's sixteen-year tenure, from the Convention, where his appointment as dean originated, to his death in 1810, reveals his political skill, his fast friendships with powerful allies within and outside of medicine, his unswerving efforts to build an outstanding medical school, his concern for young students, and his lifelong support of improved care for the citizen-patient. He stands as a major figure on that bridge linking Enlightened health care reform to the accomplishments of the early nineteenth century. His life's work befits the agenda of his late father-in-law, Jean Colombier.

The man whose vision and personality were fundamental to the purpose analyzed in this book, the duc de la Rochefoucauld-Liancourt, fled France in 1792 and spent eight years in England and the United States before returning under Bonaparte's amnesty in 1799. He lived out a long life as philanthropist, promoting vaccination, agriculture, the training of artisans, the care of foundlings . . . so many aspects of the citizen-patient's health. He died at the age of eighty, in 1827. When the reactionary Bourbon monarchy purged the medical faculty of reformers in 1822, it also stripped La Rochefoucauld-Liancourt of his many functions. His response reviews his lifelong commitment to the goals discussed in this book. He wrote to the minister of internal affairs on 16 July 1823:

> I received the letter you did me the honor to write yesterday, announcing that . . . His Majesty has stripped me of the positions of general inspector of the Conservatory of Arts and Trades, member of the General Council of Prisons, of the General Council of Manufactures, of the Council of Agriculture, of the Hospital Council, and of the General Council of the Oise Department.
>
> I cannot imagine how the function of President for the Propagation of Vaccine, which I introduced into France in 1800, can have escaped Your Eminence's kindness, and I consider it my duty to bring this to Your attention.[3]

At the end of his life, as in his youth, La Rochefoucauld-Liancourt thus defied the Bourbon government in the name of the common good.

♦♦♦

This book has devoted much space to women and children in order to illustrate that recent scholarship has permanently broadened the historian's perception of the past: where "man" and mankind once subsumed everyone, we now see history peopled with men, women, and children. This awareness appropriately applies to the history of medicine as well. Also, this book has consistently emphasized health and health care rather than medicine. The purpose is to draw attention to sick women and men rather than to focus on medical research and accomplishments, in an attempt to understand the reality that the needy patient confronted in and out of the hospital.

Looking back over a fifty-year career in 1817, in the 180-page article "Hôpital" in the *Dictionnaire des sciences médicales,* Inspector Jean François Coste expressed satisfaction and even pride at French achievement, particularly in Paris. From the point of view of the citizen-patient's newfound individual importance and dignity, the number of single beds reported by Coste is significant. Our detailed knowledge now permits us to appreciate the relatively small number of 1,500 beds at the Hôtel-Dieu, all of them single, and the fact that children, incurables, the insane, and pregnant women were no longer admitted there. Even the huge numbers of inmates at Bicêtre and the Salpêtrière—2,283 and 4,369 respectively—indicate that their populations had been almost halved by 1817. On the other hand, the capacity of the Charité had more than doubled, to 300; the Children's Hospital now had 500 beds; and Coste lists four paying nursing homes, faubourg St. Jacques, faubourg St. Denis, Ste Périnne, and Montrouge, where the number of residents had risen to 150. Finally, Coste remarks that at the Venereal Diseases Hospital, "those who cannot be admitted receive advice and medications that they apply at home." By 1817, the paying patient and the outpatient had an established identity in the Paris hospital world.[4]

This book points to the paradox that interlocks medicine and democracy: our society indeed believes that it owes the suffering poor "prompt, free, assured, and complete" care. But we know, better than the duc de la Rochefoucauld-Liancourt, that, given the wonders of modern technology, we cannot afford these services for all. We are all potential medical indigents because we may need a major procedure that is available but so costly that it makes us dependent on a public subsidy. We may be forced to establish priorities and make choices that pose a moral dilemma. The alternative is that the rich continue to receive better health care than the poor, thereby defeating the democratic credo. To make matters worse, we are constantly widening the area where our society could, if it wished, intervene, owing to better understanding of nutrition, population genetics, and immunology. Our very expertise compounds the burden. Advances in medicine continually create new problems: longevity gives rise to geriatric illnesses and heroic neonatal care increases the world's ailing population. Health care has become a political problem even while the pursuit of health is a mirage. But it is a mirage that we must continue to reach for, as the French Revolutionary reformers were the first to discover.

♦♦♦

How did the plans and achievements of the Revolutionary and Napoleonic era in health care fare in the long run? The issue discussed in this book raises numerous questions regarding the subsequent history of France as well as the future of medicine. Were the reformers prescient and far-sighted or merely "powdered and sincere," as Jacques Léonard avers in *La médecine entre les pouvoirs et les savoirs*? Are reformers who pursue public health necessarily antagonists of the medical profession? And is there an inherent antithesis between preventive care and medical treatment because one intervenes before sickness strikes whereas the other applies remedies after the patient has fallen ill? What was the meaning, for French medicine and for the patient population, of the two-tier system of health care instituted by the Law of 1803 on the practice of medicine? What were the implications of Catholic disestablishment for the citizen-patient? Did women in the health professions gain or lose in status during this era? How was the citizen-patient affected by the increasing specialization that E. H. Ackerknecht so expertly analyzes in *Medicine at the Paris Hospital*? How did the nascent Industrial Revolution change the extent and quality of health care for the citizen-patient? And, finally, was the French Revolution a creative or a destructive force in the realm of health?

In parliamentary debates during the Revolution, the reformers raised health care to the rank of a constitutional right. The implications of this mandate turned out to be complex. The first national legislation concerning the health of the citizen-patient, in 1791, secured efforts of the state for the handicapped. During the Restoration, July Monarchy, and Second Empire, the citizen-patient's right did not attract much attention, except in the activities and writings of the political opposition, particularly the Utopian Socialists. Yet it was during this era, in 1838, that further national legislation was passed, governing the care of the mentally ill. When democratic governments took the helm in France, under the Second, Third, and subsequent republics, the claim of the right to health care resurfaced with the persistent urgency of a moral mandate. After a short-lived Ministry of Public Assistance of 1849, we find national health matters in the hands of the Third Republic's "Directoire," and "Conseil supérieur de l'assistance publique." Not until 1920 did France create a Ministry of Health, and even though health insurance now reaches most Frenchmen, it does not yet extend, by law, to all.[5] This reluctance is significant: taxpayers and their representatives realized what Michel Augustin Thouret had discovered as early as 1790—namely, that financing health care for the whole population is expensive. Good health for all is indeed, as René Dubos says, a compelling but elusive goal.

The seventeen doctors on the Poverty Committee realized quickly that Vicq d'Azyr's New Plan would demand sacrifices that their profession was unwilling to make. It would overload them with patients, leaving little time to take an individual history, make a careful diagnosis, and devise an appropriate therapeutic program. These constraints would pervert professional obligations and lead to superficial and often mistaken or futile therapy.

The doctors' attitude differed significantly from the hygienists' view: doctors treat sick persons after they have fallen ill; hygienists take general preventive measures on behalf of populations they have never seen. Whereas physicians balked at becoming civil servants and insisted on the individual relationship between physician and patient, hygienists envisaged preventive and therapeutic measures of broad scope that required the collaboration and power of the government. Their efforts targeted resources essential to human sustenance, such as water, that the public must learn to keep clean and sometimes to use sparingly, and they concerned themselves with sanitation. The issue points to the fundamental difference in the outlook of doctors and public health professionals: it also pits the democratic right of the citizen-patient to health care against the professional obligation of the physician to practice careful medicine in the one-to-one doctor-patient context. This issue is at the heart of the modern medical profession's opposition to socialized medicine and may be as powerful an issue as the threat to the doctors' incomes.

In this context, it is interesting to explore the temporary solution—temporary for a century—that the Law of 1803 on medical practice devised. It opened the door for all practitioners to be tested forthwith and acquire the medical degree, but it also sanctioned unlearned health officers to practice in the countryside. What an opportunity Napoleon Bonaparte missed to establish a national medical corps! Many hundreds of unemployed medics, recently discharged from the armies, were looking for work. He could have created that network of public doctors that the Royal Society of Medicine and Vicq d'Azyr called for in the New Plan of 1790. Such a system was actually tried when the enterprising prefect of Bas-Rhin, Baron Lezay-Marnésia, instituted cantonal physicians in 1810; publicly salaried rural practitioners functioned in each canton of the department until 1870.[6] But the program did not spread. Napoleon's prejudice against doctors was so fundamental that he evidently never considered this possibility. In a related field, the introduction of vaccination into France in 1800 might have served as a model for collaboration among the whole medical profession, the government, and the educated population. Here was a procedure, proven to be effective, that could bring widespread immunity. But the government's use of health officers as "vaccinators" merely underlined the contrast between two kinds of medicine, the one therapeutic, the other preventive—between what Talleyrand had called "big and little medicine." The Law of 1803 unleashed a century of competition until the health officers were finally abolished in 1892.

Most doctors welcomed the secularization of the hospital, but this political transformation brought turmoil and anxiety. In a country so deeply imbued with Catholic values, where daily habits and familiar practices often express centuries-old traditions, the nationalization of hospital buildings and confiscation of Catholic property signaled an upheaval. When religious buildings became available for medical uses, architects not only patched and adapted old monastic structures, but could now envisage bold interventions to accommodate the needs of the new medicine. There is no more dramatic symbol of medical revolution than the transformation, around 1800, of the Brothers of Charity's chapel into Corvisart's clinical school. And perhaps it was with malice aforethought that the architect Clavareau chose the brothers' former dormitory as the ward for women patients at the new Charité Hospital. Elsewhere in Paris we find the administrator of the Foundlings' Home wondering whether his sedentary wet nurses, now located in the former Jansenist cells at the Port-Royal Maternity Hospice, were not doing God's work better than the contemplative nuns, because they saved young lives.

The most controversial aspect of medical secularization involved the female nursing orders. By common agreement of doctors and administrators, they were irreplaceable. But the Revolutionary reformers could not tolerate their presence because they were so stubbornly Catholic—not necessarily "Papist," but determined to protect priests who would say mass for them. No attempt was made during this whole era to replace them with well-trained lay nursing personnel. Napoleon failed to bully the nursing orders into nationalization, and Chaptal called the sisters back and allowed them to follow their own traditional regulations. Now subordinated to physician and pharmacist in the hospital wards, it is understandable that their religious orthodoxy stiffened. Their ranks multiplied under the Restoration, but the requirement that they undergo scientific training only became law under the Third Republic.

The best-trained professional women during this era, not only nurses, but pharmacists and midwives, have not received sufficient attention from qualified historians. Colin Jones's current work helps refine our picture of the Sisters of Charity, showing us well-trained and closely supervised professional personnel. It is likely, judging from the brief references by Marcel Fosseyeux and Maurice Bouvet, that similar results would emerge from a study of women pharmacists active in hospitals under the old regime. As for women volunteers, they were obviously active at the welfare centers and soup kitchens and in delivering home care, but, given their anonymity and the minimal acknowledgement they received in the contemporary literature, their contributions are difficult to assess. The best-trained professional women in the lay world were the midwives: the learned and widely appreciated treatises written by Marie Louise Lachapelle and Marie Anne Victoire Boivin leave no doubt that practical experience and even a professional education were accessible to determined and well-connected women in that field. Nina Gelbart is at work on a biography of Madame Du Coudray, the eighteenth-century midwife, that will shed new light on this profession.

But on the whole, the Revolution affected women health professionals adversely, closing off hospital pharmacies, which were now reserved for men with modern training, enhancing the power of male physicians and pharmacists in the hospital ward, and promoting the learning and authority of the obstetrician at the expense of the midwife. Like the Civil Code, early-nineteenth-century organized medicine assigned women to an inferior station. We have no information as to how the demotion of the nurse may have affected the hospitalized citizen-patient; one is left to speculate that they drew closer to each other, remembering their common humble origins.

We have identified a group of influential hospital administrators, in addition to leaders with medical credentials, political power, or the authority of a headmaster, who were committed to the welfare of the unfortunate. Their lifelong work endowed the world of Paris hospital administration with stability over time. Several Sisters of Charity, Hombron and his son-in-law Hucherard, Pussin and his wife Marguerite Jubline, and members of the administrative commission for the hospitals such as Alhoy and Duchanoy belong to this group. So do certain trustee members of the Hospital Council of the Seine—for example, A. C. Camus, the trustee in charge of the Maternity Hospice, who cared deeply about the young mothers and about the many hundreds of babies lost every year. And Pinel's gratitude to Richard d'Aubigny, the trustee supervising the Salpêtrière, is also on record. Much credit is due the administrators who publicized the issues of health care, thus educating the public.

In fact, education and learning theory form a most interesting part of the debate. The reformers reaped some rich but challenging rewards from their attention to individual boys. Jean Massieu taught the abbé Sicard French sign language, but Sicard unfortunately stifled a debate about methodology that is still not settled. He argued that the deaf should learn to fingerspell, write and lip-read; others contended that they should learn to talk. Only recently have teachers of the deaf gone back to the brilliant deaf youngster who taught Sicard that the deaf have a language of their own. Modern advocates argue that it behooves the majority to learn it.

Then, in 1800, another "wild" child was brought to the abbé's institution and an equally interesting new controversy erupted: could an "uncivilized" human being be socialized? The Society of the Observers of Man debated these questions, and one of its members, the physician J. M. G. Itard, convinced that Victor was retarded rather than defective and could therefore be educated, developed a detailed method to teach young children—a method that influenced Maria Montessori. Sicard's school attracted Thomas Hopkins Gallaudet from the United States, and a teacher at Sicard's school, Laurent Clerc, followed Gallaudet to Hartford, Connecticut, and the first American Asylum for the Deaf.

Logically, the nation's blind children should have profited from similar benefits, and the National Assembly indeed granted them. But their teacher, Valentin Haüy, was no skilled politician like the abbé Sicard, albeit a brilliant rebel. While he developed their minds and native gifts, he gave no thought to their physical welfare and chose narrow quarters for his school, with neither fresh air nor sunshine. And he wasted his strength on political activities that eventually led to his exile in Russia. The children survived miserably; yet it was at Valentin Haüy's school that a brilliant young man, Louis Braille, eventually found a way for the blind of the whole world to communicate.

In fact, new challenges for the education of the handicapped were but one aspect of the innovations of the French Revolution that were left for subsequent generations to complete. The elaboration of new standards applicable to health form a part of this legacy. Mention has been made of how the introduction of the metric system and of the Napoleonic codes standardized pharmacology and the regulation and supervision of drugs, foodstuffs, the water supply, and burials. The new fields of toxicology and forensic medicine empowered scientists and lawyers to pursue the protection of the citizen with new weapons. We have seen how the administrative structure created by the Law of 16 Vendémiaire, Year V, used the municipal hospital council as its managerial brain and executor. The council could channel national funds to local projects, while at the same time stimulating local volunteerism. Hospital councils could conveniently dovetail their activities with those of the new municipal public health institutions, and we have explored the multifaceted creative and regulatory interventions of these councils in the Seine department during the Napoleonic era. The Law of 16 Vendémiaire, Year V, became the "predecessor and model of hospital legislation for the whole country," according to Jean Imbert, and a paradigm for much of Europe.[7] It influenced the dimensions and direction of twentieth-century French ministries concerned with hygiene, assistance, the family, work, the environment, and the "quality of life."

In early nineteenth-century France, the Industrial Revolution began profoundly to affect the living conditions of the poor, intensifying the need for sanitation, prevention, and public health measures. Out of the thought and preliminary work of the Revolutionary and Napoleonic era grew the pioneering French public health movement. Men such as Villermé, Parent-Duchâtelet, and Benoiston de Châteauneuf studied and condemned the health hazards facing French factory workers, the threats of substandard housing, the abject existence of Paris prostitutes, the hecatombs of newborns. Clearly these hygienists carried the Revolutionary message into the nineteenth century.

Hygienists reached into the citizen's home and workplace and helped evolve a *social* medicine to cope with the impact of overcrowding, bad housing, poor food, and occupational hazards to health.[8] The advocates of this new medicine soon realized that health care would not progress significantly until citizen-patients became the doctors' partners and recognized that they had duties as well as rights. The reformers conceived of attention to one's individual health as a symbol of self-respect, self-confidence, and pride. They believed it was impossible to dictate attention to cleanliness or moderation in food and drink; but they thought such behavior could be learned, and that the poor would take an important step toward securing their rights as "men" if they practiced a hygienic physical regimen. Attention to personal hygiene, the reformers believed, also influenced interpersonal relations; it made women and men more respectful of others and thus acted as a spur to democratic political behavior. Further, they believed, such attitudes aided in strengthening marriages and restraining parents from abandoning their babies to public care. Children, of course, best learned the rules of health maintenance in the home.

The Paris Public Health Council's long-range influence would be considerable: in 1829 it "fathered" the most important public health journal in nineteenth-century France, the *Annales d'hygiène publique et de médecine légale,* which continued publication for over a century;[9] council members constituted two-thirds of the editorial board.[10] It spurred the creation of similar councils in other large French towns;[11]

stimulated public health activity among lawyers, chemists, civil engineers, architects, and administrators (as well as among physicians, surgeons, pharmacists, veterinarians, and, soon, "hygienists"); and led to the creation of a consultative bureau for hygiene in the Ministry of Commerce in 1830. In the 1840s, the focus of its interests shifted to industrial health, an area in which Britain was fast outpacing France. Ann LaBerge argues that, for this reason, leadership in *hygiène publique* then passed from France across the Channel.[12] British leaders appreciated France's role as the pioneer in public health: witness comments from key personalities such as Edwin Chadwick and Florence Nightingale.[13]

The activities of the Paris Public Health Council thus proliferated, and it was not long before they provoked rivalry and opposition. The mere attempt to collect information beyond the departmental boundaries brought outcries of protest. In its annual report for 1817, for example, the council stated that it had sought to become "a national center for health information." But the prefect "has not found it advisable—for reasons we fail to grasp—to view this idea with favor."[14] In contrast, the 1828 report claimed that published annual reports had "helped mayors, prison inspectors, hospital administrators to improve the lot of inmates and of the indigent classes in general." Furthermore, it noted, "economists and knowledgeable physicians have, in the past nine years, published a great number of studies on these subjects, and well-edited journals have appeared, worthy of public support."[15] There is thus no doubt that by the early nineteenth century, the health of the citizen-patient had become a major public preoccupation. Hygienists knew that the public powers could do no more than provide healthful resources, issue guidelines, and attempt to educate: it was the citizens' task to maintain individual and family health, follow their doctor's orders, come to clinic or dispensary when scheduled, alert the authorities to the appearance of suspect or alarming symptoms of illness, and observe preventive measures and therapeutic guidelines. The advocates of public health and social medicine looked to a citizen who undertook significant responsibilities for her or his own health and for the protection of the environment.

This new image of the citizen should be complemented with a new image of the doctor, the result of his dedicated service in the Revolutionary and Napoleonic campaigns. In the memories and stories of the common soldier, the citizen-patient in uniform, the doctor was a respected comrade who had marched with him into battle, treated his wounds, and comforted his dying companions. Gone from French literature are Molière's caricatures of expensive and outrageous charlatans; they are replaced with Balzac's humane practitioners.

◆◆◆

The French Revolution thus leaves us with a triple heritage and a paradox. The legacy lies, first, in the spectacular achievements of the Paris Clinical School in scientific investigation, hospital medicine, and the therapy of illness after the patient is stricken; second, in the imperative of health maintenance and preventive care, to which, according to the French Revolutionary reformers, the citizen-patient is entitled. And thirdly, these reformers even envisioned compensatory social and medical services for citizens shortchanged by nature. Theirs was a democratic vision of citizen-patients with equal access to equally good care. They could not yet imagine the modern paradox where medical science, in saving endangered lives, increases longevity, sustains marginal existences, and creates new illnesses as it cures others. The ruinous economic implications of the Revolutionary reformers' plans did not discourage them from arguing in this manner even though, when it came to achieving practical results, they—like ourselves—found their projects curtailed by shortages of funds and manpower: the debate between Thouret's Poverty Committee and Guillotin's Health Committee continues.

Together they created the new concept of citizens who take their social responsibilities as patients seriously and expect the same of others. When they fall ill, they have equal access to decent care, free of charge for the indigent. In return for these services, such patients will act as intelligent partners in the therapeutic regimen prescribed by the doctor; as frugal consumers of hospital resources, including food and medications; as quiet and helpful companions to other hospitalized citizens; as careful users of appliances and expendable supplies. From Tenon to Coste, that is the model of the citizen-patient designed for us by the medical reformers of the French Revolution and Napoleonic era. To be sure, these reformers were "powdered and sincere." But just as certainly they were responsible for the striking contrasts between single beds and six patients to a bed, medical therapy and indiscriminate charity, a centralized municipal hospital system rather than duplication of services, and, most important of all, initiatives all over town by citizen-patients making their own decisions regarding their health.

The final dilemma is how to motivate patients to act as citizens. The Poverty Committee applied the pedagogy of the Enlightenment and prescribed conduct, expecting that rational, responsible persons would comply. They expected citizen-patients to teach by example. They envisioned partnership between patient and physician as the only dignified and democratic basis on which the physician may recommend, but not impose, treatment. Their debates, projects, achievements, and shortcomings foreshadow our own recognition that the health of the nation ultimately depends on the judgment and decisions of the citizen-patient.

Appendix A

Legislative Proposals

Fourth Report of the Poverty Committee: Assistance to Paupers at Different Ages and in Diverse Circumstances of Life*

TITLE I: AID TO PATIENTS

Chapter 1: In the Countryside

i. Indigent patients shall be treated free of charge, in their homes, by surgeons or doctors established in the countryside.

ii. These doctors or surgeons shall be assigned by canton.

iii. The administration of the canton shall annually provide them with a list of indigents eligible for free treatment.

iv. They shall care for these families in their homes speedily, treating their infirmities, illnesses, or wounds. They shall supervise the health of foundlings, wet nurses, and other wards of public assistance. At regular intervals, they shall inoculate children and other registered paupers free of charge. In the case of serious illnesses, whether slow or acute in onset, and at the beginning of epidemics, they shall inform the district relief agencies and ask for the advice of their consulting physicians. They shall provide the district directory with an annual report containing their comments on the climate and soil of the canton, on epidemic diseases and their treatment, and a comparative overview of births, marriages, and deaths.

v. Doctors and surgeons shall not be in charge of dispensing drugs; in each canton a centrally located drug depository shall be established.

vi. Cantonal doctors or surgeons shall receive an annual salary of 500 livres.

vii. Doctors and surgeons shall be appointed by the departments upon nomination by the district and departmental relief agencies. Only capable, well-trained, and legally approved candidates shall be eligible.

*This report was read to the National Assembly on 31 January 1791 by the duc de la Rochefoucauld-Liancourt. The original French text may be found in C. Bloch and A. Tuetey, eds., *Procès-verbaux et rapports du Comité de mendicité de la Constituante, 1790–1791* (Paris: Imprimerie nationale, 1911). For "Secours aux malades," see 399–402; for "Secours à donner aux enfants," see 407–410; for "Secours aux vieillards et infirmes," see 424–426.

viii. If the majority of cantonal municipalities should complain about the physician's or surgeon's bad conduct, negligence, or incapacity, the district shall investigate and report to the department. The doctor will thereupon have every opportunity to present a defense. If this is unsatisfactory, he may be dismissed.

ix. A list of resident midwives shall be established in each canton. These must be approved by the departmental health agency. They will be paid from public funds for each delivery and for care given to women registered on the poor list.

x. For the distribution of free food and drugs, each canton shall heed the advice of the district and the decision of the department, and take measures appropriate to the locality and circumstances, while observing a strict economy.

Chapter 2: In Towns

i. Indigent patients residing in towns shall receive free medical care at home.

ii. Towns with populations under 4,000 will share health services with the adjacent countryside.

iii. Towns with populations between 4- and 12,000 will have one doctor for the poor.

iv. In more populous towns doctors shall be assigned by arrondissement or borough. . . .

v. Apart from home care, towns of over 4,000 will have communal houses for the sick, or hospitals, for patients who cannot be cared for at home.

vi. Towns under 16,000 shall have one hospital. . . .

vii. Communities may, on the decision of their council, consolidate the patients from several arrondissements in one hospital, provided the number of patients does not exceed 500.

viii. The duties and functions of municipal and cantonal physicians shall be identical.

ix. Municipal physicians shall be appointed by the department upon nomination by the communal council, with the concurrence of the departmental and district relief agencies. These physicians can be dismissed under the same conditions and rules as cantonal doctors; their salary shall also be 500 livres.

x. A drug depository shall be established in the capital of every borough or arrondissement.

xi. The preparation and distribution of medications and of free food and soup shall be the task of persons chosen for this work by the communities.

xii–xiii. . . .

xiv. The provisions for municipal midwives shall follow those for cantonal midwives.

xv. In addition to communal hospitals, large towns shall have general hospitals for homeless patients, illnesses requiring special treatment, contagious and venereal diseases, curable mental illness, major surgical operations and deliveries. According to the size of towns, one or several hospitals may be required.

xvi. These hospitals shall have appropriate numbers of physicians and surgeons.

xvii–xxi [on hospital administration]

TITLE II: AID TO CHILDREN

i. Abandoned children shall be brought to the municipal building or to a specially indicated place.

ii. The municipal officers shall immediately provide for their nourishment.

iii. The chief justice of the commune, always the ex-officio guardian of foundings, shall provide for the registration of their baptismal name, and all the information that can identify a child and confirm its civil status. He shall record the name of the person who brought the child, if known, and ask for a signature.

iv. . . . .

v. If a reputedly legitimate child be abandoned by his parents, the justice of the peace shall inquire whether there are known relatives in the department. If so, he shall . . . ask whether they can and wish to care for the child. If they refuse, they shall choose a tutor acceptable to the justice of the peace. He shall safeguard the interests of the child who remains a public ward.

vi. . . . .

vii. Cantonal surgeons shall visit all children who are public wards and provide for their health care.

viii. They shall render a monthly account of these children's condition to the community responsible for them and to the district relief agency.

ix. If one of these children should die, the death certificate shall be filed with the municipality. . . .

x. When the children are weaned, the directory of the district shall entrust them to families who are willing and able to care for them well. These families shall receive a stipulated sum until the girls reach 14, the boys 15 years of age.

xi. This sum may not exceed 90 livres for the first year, 40 livres for the second year, and shall be fixed every two years by the department. The working day salary prevailing in the department shall provide the baseline, the highest pay being 20 sols.

xii. Foster families shall agree to inform the municipality three months before they wish to cease their care.

xiii–xiv. . . . .

xv. [The royal commissioners of the district and the cantonal justice of the peace] shall . . . provide for children with congenital infirmities for whom no foster parents can be found.

xvi. The same officials . . . shall make sure that foundlings profit from public education and receive all the training appropriate to assure their future livelihood and turn them into good citizens useful to the state; at the required age their names shall be entered in the civil register.

xvii. At the age of 18 . . . these children shall be free to work on their own. . . .

xviii–xxii. . . .

xxiii. A legitimate or illegitimate child claimed by its parents on sufficient proof shall be returned free of charge if they are welfare clients. If not, they shall pay 30 livres for each year the child has been supported by the department.

xxiv. Children abandoned in one department shall not be taken into another, and those abandoned outside the kingdom shall under no condition be brought in, lest penalties provided by the police code become operative.

xxv. Public officials charged with the supervision of foundlings shall render detailed accounts every six months. . . .

xxvi. . . .

xxvii. Paupers who can prove their inability to provide for their children shall receive a small pension for child support at home under public supervision. . . .

TITLE III: AID TO THE AGED AND INFIRM

i. There shall be two kinds of aid for the aged and infirm: home care and support in public asylums.

ii. Home care shall consist of the usual assistance. Support in public asylums shall be available only to individuals unable to receive it at home, either because they have no family or because their serious infirmities require special care or for similar reasons.

iii. Home care shall begin gradually . . . at age sixty. In public asylums, support shall begin at seventy, for the aged without serious and certified infirmities.

iv. Infirm, mutilated, or accidentally disfigured paupers may nevertheless be admitted to public hospitals at any age.

v. Increase in home care shall compensate for decreases in the working capacity of the recipient.

vi. This gradation shall correspond to ¼, ½, ¾ of the total. On the advice of the district attorney and the cantonal surgeon, the municipal officials and cantonal judges of the peace shall determine the amount in each case.

vii. Pensions shall be evaluated every two years by the department. They shall never exceed 120 livres. . . .

viii–x. [Those who refuse to support their aged relatives shall be publicly denounced.]

xi. Exempt from this judgment are children and relatives whose aged parents suffer from infirmities requiring care that cannot be given in the home.

xii. A pensioner shall have the right to live with any family in the canton, district, or department if he has the misfortune not to want to live with his own.

xiii. Persons of 70 shall only be admitted to the public hospital on the decision of the district directory following a request by the justice of the peace and the municipal officials of their canton.

xiv. The infirm, admissible to the public hospital at any age, shall be admitted on the same basis as 70-year-olds, but shall also require a certificate of the patient's communal surgeon, verified by the relief agency.

xv. Infirm children under 16 unacceptable to any foster family shall be admitted to the public hospital on the request of their tutor or guardian following similar conditions and formalities.

xvi. The hospitalized aged and infirm shall receive their pensions partly in kind, partly in money, according to special regulations.

xvii. These aged and infirm shall be provided with work appropriate to their abilities and be allowed to keep the pay.

xviii. Those aged and infirm admitted to public hospitals who prefer to receive their pension at home may claim it if they can prove the agreement of the family with whom they will live.

xix–xxii. . . .

Health Committee Draft Legislation: A Plan for National Health Care*

TITLE IX: RELIEF AND HEALTH CARE AGENCY

1. In the capital of each department a Relief and Health Care Agency shall be established composed of nine persons, namely, four doctors, one pharmacist, and four laymen.

2. The members of the Relief and Health Care Agency shall be appointed by the general council of the department.

3. To be eligible, physicians and pharmacists must have practiced in the department for three years.

4.–5. [administrative details]

6. The Agency shall hold weekly meetings . . . at a fixed time.

7. Each year, the Agency shall establish an alphabetic list of all departmental health personnel: physicians, pharmacists, and midwives. The list shall include the year when the person was certified, the home address, any public medical position that person has occupied, such as cantonal physician, member of the Agency, etc. These lists shall be printed, distributed to all tribunals and government agencies and sent to the National Institute in Paris.

8. The Agency's responsibilities include the examination of foodstuffs of all kinds, solid and liquid, drinking water, wines, etc.; supervision of aid in outbreaks of epidemic, contagious, endemic, and epizootic diseases, and first aid to drowning and asphyxiated persons; inspection of all matters regarding mineral waters, the sale and distribution of drugs and medicines by pharma-

---

*For the original of this plan for national health care, see H. Ingrand, *Le comité de salubrité de l'Assemblée nationale constituante (1790–1791): Un essai de réforme de l'enseignement médical des services d'hygiène, et de protection de la santé publique* (Thèse médecine, Paris, 1934), 157–165. Critical comparison with the preceding report by the Poverty Committee on "Assistance to Paupers at Different Ages and in Diverse Circumstances of Life" will confirm the conclusion reached in Chapter 3 that the two legislative proposals were complementary. La Rochefoucauld-Liancourt and Vicq d'Azyr collaborated in constructing a national health-care network.

cists and druggists, the application of the relevant laws, and particularly those forbidding secret remedies. The Agency shall urge tribunals to apply these laws and pursue the destruction of charlatanism in every possible way.

The Agency shall regulate public establishments that relate to the citizens' health, such as land used for cemeteries and the precautions to observe in burials, etc. The Agency shall supervise mines and ore-bearing areas, the reclamation of swamps, drainage ditches, garbage dumps, the disposal of sewage, sewers, etc.; butcher shops, slaughterhouses, and the trades of all those who deal in animal or mineral extracts and those who mass-produce fermented liquors. The Agency shall establish precautions to be introduced into those trades, and into all others for the preservation of the workers.

The Agency shall regulate the location, construction, and siting of correctional institutions, prisons, hospitals, and hospices; see to the optimal use and distribution of water, air, and heat to render these institutions healthful and administer them efficiently to keep them clean, regulate the food, and the use of medical, surgical, and pharmaceutical remedies. The Agency shall conduct the correspondence regarding all matters that concern the hospitals and the establishments that collaborate with them.

9. When an epidemic or epizootic disease occurs in a town, municipality or canton of the department, the Agency shall immediately hold a special meeting and decide on the speediest aid. The Agency shall inform the department which will take appropriate measures.

10. The Agency shall supervise the laws concerning the healing art in the entire department. Every time it learns of an infraction, the Agency shall alert the administration or the courts. They shall take speedy action.

11. [The Agency nominates candidates for cantonal doctor or midwife.]

12. The Agency shall offer advice and counsel when requested by administrative or municipal bodies and correspond with all health officers and departmental officials regarding matters of health and public welfare.

TITLE X: MEDICAL HOME CARE *

1. Each canton shall provide for a physician who shall care for poor patients in their homes free of charge.

2. Towns with fewer than 4,000 inhabitants shall share all health care support with the surrounding countryside.

3. [Every town] with a population of 4,000 to 12,000 inhabitants shall have its own doctor for the poor.

4. In larger towns, doctors for the poor shall be appointed [proportionately to size of population].

4. To qualify as cantonal or district physician, a doctor must (1) be legally certified; (2) submit a certificate of good conduct issued by the municipality where he lives; (3) have practiced medicine for three years since his graduation or worked for two years as medical assistant in a hospital, before or after graduation.

5. These doctors are appointed for life, but [appointment is] revokable on

*This section was drafted in collaboration with the Poverty Committee.

complaints of objectionable conduct or negligence brought by the majority of cantonal municipalities and sent to the Agency. The case shall be referred to the department and the accused shall have every opportunity to defend himself. On the documented advice of the Agency the department shall keep or dismiss the doctor.

7. The salary of cantonal or district doctors shall be 500 livres annually, with a retirement annuity of 250 livres after twenty years of practice and of 500 livres after thirty years.

8. A list of eligible poor families in each district shall be established annually at the cantonal or municipal capital. This list shall establish the free services the doctors shall provide.

9. These doctors shall provide care to all those families. The doctors shall visit the sick in their homes as soon as asked or informed and treat their infirmities, illnesses or wounds.

The doctors shall supervise the health of foundlings and wet nurses, and of all persons eligible for public assistance. At fixed dates and upon request, they shall inoculate children and persons on the poor lists free of charge. Finally, they shall provide the departmental Relief and Health Agency with annual observations on the climate and soil of the canton, on endemic, epidemic, and epizootic diseases and their treatment, on births, marriages, and mortality.

10. Every cantonal or municipal physician shall be the ex officio inspector in all aspects of health throughout his sector. He shall refer all infractions of health regulations to the legal authorities and involve the Agency in all matters that demand its participation or intervention.

11. . . . [administrative details].

12. The physician of the poor shall not be responsible for dispensing drugs. A depot shall be established at the most central location in the canton.

13. Midwives approved by the departmental agency and living in each canton shall be paid with public funds for the care given to pregnant women registered on the poor list. They shall receive a fixed sum for each delivery.

14. As for the free distribution of food, soup, and medications, each canton shall, according to departmental decision and after consulting the Agency, take the measures that seem most suitable, helpful and economical under the circumstances.

Appendix B

Concordance of the Republican and Gregorian Calendars

	Year II[a] 1793–1794	Year III 1794–1795	Year IV 1795–1796
1 Vendémiaire	22 Sept. 1793	22 Sept. 1794	23 Sept. 1795
1 Brumaire	22 Oct.	22 Oct.	23 Oct.
1 Frimaire	21 Nov.	21 Nov.	22 Nov.
1 Nivôse	21 Dec.	21 Dec.	22 Dec.
1 Pluviôse	20 Jan. 1794	20 Jan. 1795	21 Jan. 1796
1 Ventôse	19 Feb.	19 Feb.	20 Feb.
1 Germinal	21 Mar.	21 Mar.	21 Mar.
1 Floréal	20 Apr.	20 Apr.	20 Apr.
1 Prairial	20 May	20 May	20 May
1 Messidor	19 June	19 June	19 June
1 Thermidor	19 July	19 July	19 July
1 Fructidor	18 Aug.	18 Aug.	18 Aug.
Sans-Culottides	17–21 Sept.	17–22 Sept.	17–21 Sept.

	Year V 1796–1797	Year VI 1797–1798	Year VII 1798–1799
1 Vendémiaire	22 Sept. 1796	22 Sept. 1797	23 Sept. 1798
1 Brumaire	22 Oct.	22 Oct.	22 Oct.
1 Frimaire	21 Nov.	21 Nov.	21 Nov.
1 Nivôse	21 Dec.	21 Dec.	21 Dec.
1 Pluviôse	20 Jan. 1797	20 Jan. 1798	20 Jan. 1799
1 Ventôse	19 Feb.	19 Feb.	19 Feb.
1 Germinal	21 Mar.	21 Mar.	21 Mar.
1 Floréal	20 Apr.	20 Apr.	20 Apr.
1 Prairial	20 May	20 May	20 May
1 Messidor	19 June	19 June	19 June
1 Thermidor	19 July	19 July	19 July
1 Fructidor	18 Aug.	18 Aug.	18 Aug.
Sans-Culottides	17–21 Sept.	17–21 Sept.	17–22 Sept.

	Year VIII 1799–1800	Year IX 1800–1801	Year X 1801–1802
1 Vendémiaire	23 Sept. 1799	23 Sept. 1800	23 Sept. 1801
1 Brumaire	23 Oct.	23 Oct.	23 Oct.
1 Frimaire	22 Nov.	22 Nov.	22 Nov.
1 Nivôse	22 Dec.	22 Dec.	22 Dec.
1 Pluviôse	21 Jan. 1800	21 Jan. 1801	21 Jan. 1802
1 Ventôse	20 Feb.	20 Feb.	20 Feb.
1 Germinal	22 Mar.	22 Mar.	22 Mar.
1 Floréal	21 Apr.	21 Apr.	21 Apr.
1 Prairial	21 May	21 May	21 May
1 Messidor	20 June	20 June	20 June
1 Thermidor	20 July	20 July	20 July
1 Fructidor	19 Aug.	19 Aug.	19 Aug.
Sans-Culottides	18–22 Sept.	18–22 Sept.	18–22 Sept.

	Year XI 1802–1803	Year XII 1803–1804	Year XIII 1804–1805	Year XIV 1805
1 Vendémiaire	23 Sept. 1802	24 Sept. 1803	23 Sept. 1804	23 Sept. 1805
1 Brumaire	23 Oct.	24 Oct.	23 Oct.	23 Oct.
1 Frimaire	22 Nov.	23 Nov.	22 Nov.	22 Nov.
1 Nivôse	22 Dec.	23 Dec.	22 Dec.	22 Dec.
1 Pluviôse	21 Jan. 1803	22 Jan. 1804	21 Jan. 1805	
1 Ventôse	20 Feb.	21 Feb.	20 Feb.	
1 Germinal	22 Mar.	22 Mar.	22 Mar.	
1 Floréal	21 Apr.	21 Apr.	21 Apr.	
1 Prairial	21 May	21 May	21 May	
1 Messidor	20 June	20 June	20 June	
1 Thermidor	20 July	20 July	20 July	
1 Fructidor	19 Aug.	19 Aug.	19 Aug.	
Sans-Culottides	18–22 Sept.	18–22 Sept.	18–22 Sept.	

SOURCE: R. B. Holtman, *The Napoleonic Revolution* (Baton Rouge: Louisiana State University Press, 1967), 218–219.

ᵃThe Republican calendar went into effect only with Year II; documents of the preceding year were redated from Gregorian to Republican. The first day of the Republican calendar coincided with the fall equinox.

Appendix C

Supplementary Tables

TABLE C.1 Growth of the National Midwifery School under the First Empire

Year	Number of Students
1803	46
1804	30
1805	83
1806	89
1807	59
1808	81
1809	121
1810	129
1811	125
1812	142
1813	161
1814	131

SOURCES: Adapted from Seine, CGAHHCP, *Rapports au conseil général des hospices sur les hôpitaux et hospices, les secours à domicile, et la direction des nourrices* (Paris: Imprimerie des hospices civils, An XI [1803]), 153, and H. Carrier, *Origines de la Maternité de Paris: Les maîtresses sages-femmes et l'Office des accouchées de l'ancien Hôtel-Dieu, 1378–1796* (Paris: Steinheil, 1888), 260.

TABLE C.2 Emergency Admissions as a Percentage of Total Admissions, Necker Hospital and Hôtel-Dieu

	1806	1809	1812
Necker Hospital			
All admissions	1,039	1,036	1,335
Emergency admissions	801 (77%)	845 (82%)	1,001 (76%)
Hôtel-Dieu			
All admissions	11,536	9,320	11,007
Emergency admissions	3,001 (26%)	3,535 (31%)	2,173 (20%)

SOURCE: Adapted from Seine, CGAHHCP, *Rapport fait au conseil général des hospices par un de ses membres sur l'état des hôpitaux, des hospices, et des secours à domicile, à Paris, depuis le 1er janvier 1804 jusqu'au 1er janvier 1814* (Paris: Imprimerie de Mme Huzard, 1816), table 3, p. 232.

TABLE C.3. Number of Patients Admitted to Paris Hospitals and Hospices

Year	Total	Processed by the Admitting Office	
		Number	Percentage
1806	28,225	18,622	66
1807	29,982	22,070	74
1808	31,359	17,119	54
1809	31,878	18,530	59
1810	33,210	18,209	55
1811	32,506	20,444	63
1812	37,667	20,620	55
1813	35,211	16,704	48

SOURCE: Adapted from Pastoret's report, Seine, CGAHHCP, *Rapport fait au conseil général des hospices par un de ses membres sur l'état des hôpitaux, des hospices, et des secours à domicile, à Paris, depuis le 1er janvier 1804 jusqu'au 1er janvier 1814* (Paris: Imprimerie de Mme Huzard, 1816), table 3, p. 232.

TABLE C.4 Stillbirths at the Hôtel-Dieu Maternity Service

Year	All births	Stillbirths	
		Number	Percentage
1776	1,534	121	7.8
1777	1,549	114	7.4
1778	1,558	119	7.6
1779	1,552	136	8.7
1780	1,566	138	8.8
1781	1,528	124	8.1
1782	1,479	106	7.2
1783	1,413	122	8.6
1784	1,428	126	8.8
1785	1,482	119	8.0
1786	1,440	122	7.7

SOURCE: Jacques Tenon, *Mémoires sur les hôpitaux de Paris* (Paris: Pierres, 1788), 261–266.

TABLE C.5 Stillbirths at the New Maternity Hospice

Year	All births	Stillbirths	
		Number	Percentage
1804	1,624	75	4.6
1805	1,701	75	4.4
1806	1,642	76	4.6
1807	1,695	92	5.4
1808	1,690	68	4.0
1809	1,795	93	5.2
1810	1,814	72	3.9
1811	2,395	111	4.6
1812	2,450	106	4.3
1813	2,228	97	4.3

SOURCE: Adapted from Seine, CGAHHCP, *Rapport fait au conseil général des hospices par un de ses membres sur l'état des hôpitaux, des hospices, et des secours à domicile, à Paris, depuis le 1er janvier 1804 jusqu'au 1er janvier 1814* (Paris: Imprimerie de Mme Huzard, 1816), 100–103.

Bibliographic Essay

Part I of this essay inventories and analyzes the archival documentation used for this book, the primary printed sources, the most useful reference works, the main serial publications, and the relevant secondary printed works that span the Revolution and Empire thematically.

Part II contains the bibliographic references found most informative or thought-provoking. This part is subdivided according to the subject matter discussed in the book's ten chapters. The essay ranges far beyond the work actually quoted in the book, particularly as regards French source material.

This bibliography does not pretend to be exhaustive, but scholars may find it useful.

Part I

ARCHIVES

Paris possesses inexhaustible archival holdings dealing with the multifaceted subject of health care in the Revolutionary and imperial period. These archives are difficult to use in a methodical manner because they are fragmented and incomplete. A devastating fire during in Commune in 1871 caused huge losses and is blamed for whatever seems hard to find. The lack of adequate inventories frequently makes scholars dependent on local archivists, printed references, time, and luck to extract the needed documentation. Grateful acknowledgement is owed to the staffs of the Archives nationales, the Archives de l'Assistance publique, the Bibliothèque interuniversitaire de médecine, and the Académie de médecine, as well as to M. J. Imbault-Huart for sharing her personal notes in "Sources de l'histoire de la médecine aux Archives nationales de 1750 à 1822," *Revue d'histoire des sciences et de leurs applications,* 1972, *25*: 45–53.

The **Archives de l'Assistance publique à Paris** served as headquarters for research about the nineteenth-century part of this book. They house the papers of the Conseil général administratif des hôpitaux et hospices civils de la Seine, a rich though idiosyncratic card catalogue, a good library, and collection of reference works. This fine resource is the work of a dedicated *conservateur,* the late Marcel Candille, who spurred his staff to complete the typewritten "Inventaire analytique des délibérations du conseil des hospices" from

333

1801 to our day. This was achieved according to the method of classification used by Marcel Fosseyeux in *Catalogue des manuscrits des Archives de l'Assistance publique*, n.s. (1913). The result is what the present *conservateur*, Mme Valérie Poinsotte, calls a "marvelous collection of odds and ends." She is now rationalizing the inventory according to the system that the Archives nationales uses for "Archives hospitalières" (see V. Poinsotte, "Les archives révolutionnaires de l'Assistance publique à Paris," *Bulletin de la société française d'histoire des hôpitaux*, 1989, *59*: 25–39; also Florence Castaigne Greffe, "Le Conseil général des hospices civils de Paris et les secours publics, 1801–1830" [Thèse Ecole des Chartes, Paris, 1975], which has remained in manuscript).

The **Archives nationales** hold inexhaustible documentary riches, which are difficult to use for similar reasons. Most rewarding for this study was the "F" series, pertaining to Internal Affairs and other ministries. "F[15]: Hospitals and Assistance" consists of over 4,250 cartons of documents, of which only 276 have been inventoried. Thanks are owed to one archivist, Madame Devos, who generously shared her handwritten survey. Several other series provided documentation, especially "F[7]: General Police," "F[8]: Sanitary Police," and "F[17]: Public Instruction." The Archives nationales also contain special collections, such as "AJ[2]: Charenton"; "AJ[15]: Muséum d'histoire naturelle," with information about the teaching of chemistry and botany; and "AJ[16]: Académie de Paris," with rich evidence pertaining to the Paris Health School. These holdings were transferred from the Bibliothèque de l'Ecole de médecine a few years ago: it appears that other documentation was lost in the move, and that some was left behind. Furthermore, the **Minutier central** now makes available the legal documents of all Parisian notaries, up to the time limit set by the law, in the new C.A.R.A.N. building (Centre d'accueil et de recherches des Archives nationales). Valuable information about individual leaders was culled from that collection, supplemented by the **Etat civil reconstitué**, where information lost in the fire of 1871 is being reassembled from notarial acts and private sources.

The **Archives de la Seine** furnished dossiers concerning abandoned children, foundlings and orphans. The **Archives de la Prefecture de police, Paris** (APPP), hold the manuscript "Procès-verbaux" and "Rapports" of the Public Health Council. (The council's working papers were in all likelihood destroyed in the fire of 1871.) See APPP, "Organisation du conseil de salubrité, documents 1802–1899" (MS folio); "Procès-verbaux des séances du conseil de salubrité, 7 novembre 1807–21 mars 1823" (MS folio); and "Rapports du conseil de salubrité" (4 vols., MS folio).

The **Bibliothèque historique de la ville de Paris** retains its own archives, where some letters and manuscripts were located—for example, those pertaining to deaf and blind children educated in Paris. At the **Institut de France,** each of the five academies houses its own papers. The archives of the **Académie des sciences** were particularly helpful regarding certain of its members involved in shaping the reform of public health and of medical education. Readers need to know that for each session this academy keeps an envelope where relevant documents can be found. Also, the **Bibliotheque de l'Institut** houses archives of its own.

The **Academie nationale de médecine** owns the papers of the Société royale de médecine, which are essential for information about the reform of health care from 1776 until the society's dissolution in 1793. An inventory of the society's enormous collection of documents has been prepared, but it is not in publishable form. The documents fill over two hundred boxes. The importance of this archival collection was first publicized by J. Meyer in "Une enquête de l'Académie de médecine sur les épidémies, 1774–1794," *Annales: Economies, sociétés, civilisations,* 1966, *21*: 729–749; see also D. B. Weiner, "Le droit de l'homme à la santé: Une belle idée devant l'assemblée constituante," *Clio medica,* 1970, *5*: 209–233. The Académie de médecine also houses the papers of other medical societies, such as the Procès-verbaux de la Société académique de médecine. In addition, there are archival dossiers for all the members of the academy, beginning in 1820.

Most Paris libraries have their own archives, beginning with those in the **Département des manuscrits, Bibliothèque nationale.** The papers of Jacques Tenon were an outstanding source used for this book. They consist of seven folio volumes of his correspondence on the subject of hospitals. Ten more volumes contain Tenon's exhaustive studies on hospitals and prisons. Finally, archival documentation was found in the **Archives de l'Archevêché de Paris;** and the **Museum national d'histoire naturelle** (see "Procès-verbaux de la Société d'histoire naturelle" [MS 464]). It was also well worth exploring the holdings of museums such as the **Musée Carnavalet,** which specializes in the history of Paris, and especially the **Musée de l'Assistance publique,** and of private societies such as the **Société philanthropique de Paris.** See Société philanthropique de Paris, *Rapports et comptes-rendus* (published annually, beginning in the Year XI, first by Everat and subsequently, from 1815 on, by Baron; complete sets can be found at the society's headquarters in Paris and at the Bibliothèque de l'Institut de France but are unavailable at the Bibliothèque nationale and in the United States).

The novel questions pursued here led the author into archival collections that were quite untouched. The inquiry into hospital nursing led to the **Religious Augustinian Nurses of the Hôtel-Dieu of Paris** (now lodged at Notre-Dame du Bon Secours, rue des Plantes), whose archivist, the late sister St. Scholastica, turned out to be a wonderful source of historic documents, as well as of stories. See "Constitutions faites en 1652 pour les religieuses de l'Hôtel-Dieu de Paris, leur Supérieur, et revues en 1725" (folio, 486 pp.); "Décès de 1793 à 1877" (folio register); "Extrait des naissances de 1783 à 1860"; "Histoire des religieuses Augustines hospitalières de l'Hôtel-Dieu, 8ème au 20ème siècle, St. Landry, fondateur (1919)" (typescript, bound in four fascicles of 256 pp., 187 pp., 175 pp., and 60 pp., folio); "Extraits de naissance, 1748–1787. Registre pour enregistrer les novices entrées depuis le 6 juillet 1748. Notes et souvenirs" (folio MS, 742 pp.); "Petites notices concernant l'Hôtel-Dieu de Paris et l'abrégé de la vie de quelques religieuses" (folio; 245 pp.); and "Procès-verbaux des chapitres de 1792 à 1884" (MSS of various sizes, bound in one folio volume).

Equally valuable were the collections of Father Chalumeau, archivist of the **Lazarists** in Paris (who, as confessors to the **Sisters of Charity,** are the keepers of their documents). Sister Stanislas Kostka, archivist of the **Ladies of St. Thomas de Villeneuve** at Neuilly, also proved an invaluable collaborator. May they all here receive my thanks.

Uncharted paths led to documentation about the handicapped: the **Institution nationale des jeunes aveugles,** 56, boulevard des Invalides, preserves little about its founder, Valentin Haüy, and a *"fonds"* of material in St. Petersburg, where he lived in exile, has remained inaccessible. But the private **Institution Valentin Haüy pour le bien des aveugles** owns letters and documents in raised print (Haüy's specialty) and in Braille.

There are some treasures, including the thirteenth-century charter, in the dungeonlike archives of the **Hospice des Quinze-Vingts,** rue de Charenton (see M. Robinet, *Inventaire général des archives des Quinze-Vingts* [Paris: Hôpital des Quinze-Vingts, 1962]; M. Battelle, *Notice historique et statistique sur l'Hôpital royal des Quinze-Vingts* [Paris: Chapelet, 1856]). The richest documentation in the Quinze-Vingts archives for the period 1801–1815 is in series B 109, dossiers 6,715–6,722, and a few additional documents may be found at the Institution nationale des jeunes aveugles.

Access to the labyrinthine cellars of the **Institution nationale des jeunes sourds** was finally obtained on a fourth attempt in 1978 owing to the kindness of a new director, M. Louis Dessaint. The plentiful, possibly complete, documentation of the institution's history was quickly located. It has already resulted in a Ph.D. thesis (A. Karakostas, "L'institution nationale des sourds-muets de Paris de 1790 à 1800: Histoire d'un corps à corps" [Thèse de médecine, Paris, 1981]) and has yielded materials for a museum (see the catalogue of an exhibition held in the Sorbonne chapel in the winter of 1989 in connection with the Bicentennial of the Revolution).

Finally, the records of the **Enfants trouvés** (the Paris Foundlings' Hospice) have now become accessible to researchers interested in the approximately four thousand infants abandoned annually during the Revolutionary and Napoleonic era. Owing to the kind help of the curator, Madame Demeulenaere-Douyère (now the archivist of the Académie des sciences), many cartons of documents relating to the 5 percent of infants who survived were graciously made available. These can be consulted at the Archives de la Seine, boulevard Serrurier.

In conclusion, it may be worth mentioning that documents turn up in unlikely places. Thus a visit to the église St. Louis at Salpêtrière Hospital, and the kindness of the almoner, led to a walk around the roof (affording a wonderful view) and access to the attic, where rough-hewn shelves house not only sheaves of early X-ray records but the account books of the Paris hospital service, from its inception, in over fifty manuscript folio volumes. There has been no explanation of so strange a choice of storage place.

PRIMARY PRINTED SOURCES

Given the problems with orderly manuscript documentation for the twenty-five years reviewed in this book, the excellent printed primary source material is especially precious. For the old regime, see Jacques Tenon's *Mémoires sur les hôpitaux de Paris* (henceforth *TM*) (Paris: Pierres, 1788; see also D. B. Weiner, ed. and int., *Jacques Tenon's Memoirs on Paris Hospitals* [Canton, Mass.: Science History Publications, forthcoming]); on the work of the Société royale de médecine (*Histoire et mémoires de médecine et de physique médicale* [10 vols.; Paris: Pierres, 1776–1789]); and on M. Möring, C. Quentin, and L. Brièle, eds., *Délibérations de l'ancien Hôtel-Dieu*, vols. 1 and 2 of *Collection de documents pour servir à l'histoire des hôpitaux de Paris* (4 vols.; Paris: Imprimerie nationale, 1881–1887).

The sections of this book devoted to the debates and policies of the Revolutionary assemblies on health care make abundant use of the minutes and reports of the Comité de mendicité (Poverty Committee) found in France, Ministère de l'instruction publique, *Procès-verbaux et rapports du comité de mendicité de la Constituante, 1790–1791* (henceforth *PVR*), ed. C. Bloch and A. Tuetey (Paris: Imprimerie nationale, 1911). Discussions concerning medical education can be found in H. Ingrand, *Le Comité de salubrité de l'Assemblée nationale constituante (1790–1791): Un essai de réforme de l'enseignement médical, des services d'hygiène, et de protection de la santé publique* (Thèse médecine, Paris, 1934). These debates constantly lead the scholar back to collections such as S. Lacroix, ed., *Actes de la Commune de Paris pendant la révolution* (7 vols.; Paris: Cerf & Noblet, 1894–1909), and A. Tuetey, ed., *L'Assistance publique à Paris pendant la révolution* (henceforth *TA*) (4 vols.; Paris: Imprimerie nationale, 1895–1987). This documentation is very helpful for the history of the first three Revolutionary assemblies but thins out during the Directory.

The eighteenth-century reports reflect the views of medical men like Tenon and Thouret and of aristocratic liberals like Liancourt. The Consulate and Empire, on the other hand, promoted the views of scholarly politicians adept at conciliating new and traditional structures, texts, rules, techniques, and persons, and here this book relies heavily on two lengthy printed reports of the Paris Hospital Council's work: Seine, Conseil général d'administration des hôpitaux et hospices civils de Paris (henceforth Seine, CGAHHCP), *Rapports au conseil général des hospices sur les hôpitaux et hospices, les secours à domicile, et la direction des nourrices* (Paris: Imprimerie des hospices civils, An XI [1803]), and id., *Rapport fait au conseil général des hospices par un de ses membres sur l'état des hôpitaux, des hospices, et des secours à domicile, à Paris, depuis le 1er janvier 1804 jusqu'au 1er janvier 1814* (Paris: Imprimerie de Mme Huzard, 1816). In the first of these reports, A. G. Camus gives a well-documented and detailed accounting of the finances, achievements, and shortcomings of hospital policy up to 1803; this includes home care, foundlings, and wet-nursing, all of which were under the council's jurisdiction. Count C. E. J. P. Pastoret brings the account up to 1815. Camus conveys dedicated, not to say passionate, concern, whereas Pastoret assumed the more distant stance of the legislator and often uses older sources such as Tenon.

The reports of the Hospital Council are complemented by its accounts and the reports of the central admitting office. The accounts may be found in Seine, CGAHHCP, *Comptes généraux des hôpitaux et hospices civils, enfants aban-*

donnés, secours à domicile, et direction des nourrices de la ville de Paris: Recette, Dépense, Population (6 vols. in folio; Paris: Imprimerie des hospices, 1805–1813). These were published as follows:

AN XI in 1805
An XII in 1808
An XIII in 1808
An XIV in 1808
1808 in 1808
1810 in 1813

The remaining figures for the Empire can be found in Pastoret's report of 1816.

For the reports of the central admitting office from 22 March 1802 to 24 September 1803, see Seine, CGAHHCP, *Rapport sur les opérations du bureau central d'admission dans les hôpitaux pendant les six derniers mois de l'An X et l'An XI* (Paris: Imprimerie des hospices civils, An XII [1803–1804]). This is continued by *Rapport . . . An XIII* (Paris: An XIV [1805–1806]) and *Rapport . . . An XIV et 1806* (Paris: 1809). All these reports have numerous invaluable tables.

Two documents essential for understanding the workings of the maternity service at Port-Royal and of the Foundlings' Hospice are Seine, CGAHHCP, *Mémoire historique et instructif sur l'Hospice de la maternité* (Paris: Imprimerie des hospices civils, 1808), which derives in large part from Seine, CGAHHCP, *Rapports au conseil général* (1803), 131–183, but adds much personal comment by Jacques Benoît Hucherard, the administrator; and Seine, CGAHHCP, *Code spécial de la maternité* (Paris: Imprimerie des sourds-muets, An X [1801–1802]), which gives details regarding training in midwifery.

There is a rare example of a French initiative seeking inspiration elsewhere than in England: France, Ministère de l'intérieur, *Recueil de mémoires sur les établissements d'humanité traduits de l'allemand et de l'anglais, publiés par ordre du ministre de l'intérieur* [N. L. François de Neufchâteau], ed. A. C. Duquesnoy (18 vols. in 7; Paris: Agasse, An VII–VIII [1799–1800]). The collection contains translations, not only of John Aiken's *Thoughts on Hospitals* and of material about Bedlam and Bridewell, but also of documents about health care in Bern, Hamburg, Barcelona, Berlin, Madrid, and Copenhagen.

Finally, the published record of the Public Health Council of Paris was edited by V. de Moléon, *Rapports généraux sur la salubrité publique rédigés par les conseils ou les administrations établies en France et dans les autres parties de l'Europe. 2ème partie officielle: Rapports généraux sur les travaux du Conseil de salubrité de Paris et du département de la Seine exécutés depuis l'année 1802 jusqu'à l'année 1826 inclusivement (25 ans)* (Paris: Au bureau du Recueil industriel, 1828).

OUTSTANDING REFERENCE WORKS

The *Almanach (royal–national–impérial–royal)* served as a basic source of information. Another useful aid was France, Ministère de l'Instruction publique et des Beaux-arts, *Enquêtes et documents relatifs à l'enseignement supérieur*, ed. A.

de Beauchamps, vols. 37–38, *Médecine et pharmacie: Projets de lois* (Paris: Imprimerie nationale, 1888–1890); id., *Tables générales de la législation sanitaire française, 1790–1955*, 3 vols. (Paris: Imprimerie nationale, 1957); and Seine, CGAHHCP, *Table alphabétique, chronologique et analytique des règlements relatifs à l'administration générale des hôpitaux, hospices, enfants-trouvés et secours de la ville de Paris* (Paris: Huzard, 1815).

Dictionaries and encyclopedias, all modeled on Denis Diderot's *Encyclopédie ou Dictionnaire raisonné des sciences, des arts, et des métiers* (35 vols.; Lausanne & Berne: Chez les sociétés typographiques, 1782), served as the primary compendia of knowledge from the Enlightenment to the early nineteenth century. The most useful for the purposes of this book was the 60-volume *Dictionnaire des sciences médicales* assembled by the enterprising Charles Louis Fleury Panckoucke between 1812 and 1822, "a kind of museum," he says in his Preface, "filled with riches, . . . so attractive because it contains the most complete and faithful image of a medical epoch." In 1782 Panckoucke's father, Charles Joseph, had begun publication of the *Encyclopédie méthodique ou par ordre des matières* (its 194 volumes were not completed until 1832). Its 13-volume section on medicine, edited by F. Vicq d'Azyr, was used here. These works were supplemented in due course by similar undertakings, of which the following have been consulted: Amédée Dechambre's *Dictionnaire encyclopédique des sciences médicales* (100 vols.; Paris: Asselin & Masson, 1854–1889); the *Encyclopædia Britannica*, 11th ed.; and the *Dictionary of Scientific Biography*, ed. C. C. Gillispie (16 vols.; New York: Scribner's, 1970).

A number of **specialized reference works** proved very helpful in areas obvious from their titles: J. W. Estes, *Dictionary of Protopharmacology: Therapeutic Practices, 1700–1850* (Canton, Mass.: Science History Publications, 1990); *Gallaudet's Encyclopedia of Deaf People and Deafness*, ed. J. V. Van Cleve (New York: McGraw-Hill, 1987); M. Marion *Dictionnaire des institutions de la France aux 17ème et 18ème siècles* (Paris: Picard, 1972); C. Molette, *Guide des sources de l'histoire des congrégations féminines françaises de vie active* (Paris: Editions de Paris, (1974); A. Robert, *Dictionnaire des parlementaires français, comprenant tous les membres des assemblées françaises et tous les ministres français depuis le 1er mai 1789 jusqu'au 1er mai 1889, avec leurs noms, état civil, états de service, actes politiques, votes parlementaires* (5 vols.; Paris: Bourloton, 1891); Baron A. de Watteville, ed., *Législation charitable et Recueil des lois arrêtés, décrets, ordonnances royales, avis du Conseil d'état, circulaires, décisions et instructions des Ministres de l'Intérieur et des Finances, arrêts de la Cour des comptes, etc. qui régissent les établissements de bienfaisance, mise en ordre et annotée* (Paris: Hévis, 1843); and R. E. Zupko, *French Weights and Measures before the Revolution* (Bloomington: Indiana University Press, 1978).

An outstanding international (although mostly French) **bibliography** on health-related topics was begun in 1957 by Marcel Candille in the *Revue de l'Assistance publique à Paris*; it was first continued by *L'Hôpital et l'aide sociale à Paris* and is now published in the *Bulletin de la Société française d'histoire des hôpitaux*. See also M. Tourneux, *Bibliographie de l'histoire de Paris pendant la révolution française* (5 vols.; Paris: Imprimerie nouvelle, 1900).

SERIALS

Among the one hundred **serial publications** cited in this book, some stand out for importance or special significance. The *Archives parlementaires, ou Moniteur universel de 1787 à 1860*, ed. J. Mavidal and E. Laurent (87 vols.; Paris: Dupont, 1862–1914), is essential.

Academies and learned societies usually published both minutes and papers by their members. For the old regime, see France, Académie royale des sciences, *Histoire et mémoires*, and, after 1795, France, Institut national, Académie des sciences, *Procès-verbaux et rapports*, as well as *Histoire et mémoires*. Before the creation of the Académie de médecine in 1820, the Paris medical faculty sponsored the quasi-official *Recueil périodique de la société de santé (médecine) de Paris* (15 vols., 1796–1802), later titled the *Journal général de médecine, chirurgie et pharmacie* (46 vols., 1802–1830). A society created by outstanding students in 1796 published the *Mémoires de la Société médicale d'émulation* (9 vols., Year V [1796–1797]–1826). Significantly, these *Mémoires* ran to five volumes in seven years under the Republic, but to only two volumes in eleven years under the Empire.

Among **medical and scientific journals of the old regime**, the most significant for this study were the *Journal de médecine, de chirurgie, et de pharmacie;* two military medical publications (*Journal de médecine, chirurgie, et pharmacie militaire* (7 vols., 1782–1789) published by Jacques de Horne, and *Recueil d'observations de médecine des hôpitaux militaires* (2 vols., 1766, 1772) edited by F. M. C. Richard de Hautsierck; and publications launched by enterprising enlightened individuals, such as the abbé Rozier's *Observations sur l'histoire naturelle, sur la physique, et sur les arts*, continued as the *Journal de physique* (1773–1802).

Among the host of publications during the Revolution, the most important for this book were the Ideologues' *La décade philosophique, littéraire, et politique, par une Société de républicains* [later *gens de lettres*] (Paris: An II [1793–1794]–1807]) and the short-lived venture of the physician-chemist Antoine Fourcroy, *La médecine éclairée par les sciences physiques, ou Journal des découvertes relatives aux différentes parties de l'art de guérir* (1791–1792). And as a source of information and local color, one should not forget the gossips: the *Journal de Paris* (1777–1792); L. P. de Bachaumont, *Mémoires secrets pour servir à l'histoire de la république des lettres en France depuis 1762 jusqu'à nos jours* (36 vols.; London: Adamson, 1783–1789); and Sebastien Mercier, *Tableau de Paris* (12 vols.; Amsterdam: n.p., 1783).

Several publications kept Frenchmen informed of **foreign developments** in medicine and public health. Foremost among these was the *Bibliothèque britannique* of Geneva (1796–1815), which brought Frenchmen medical news of the British Isles. (On the important function of the Genevan *Bibliothèque britannique* as translator and mediator of British scientific and medical thought during this era, see M. A. Barblan, "La santé publique vue par les rédacteurs de la *Bibliothèque britannique*, 1796–1815," *Gesnerus*, 1975, *22*: 129–146, and id., *Journalisme médical et échanges intellectuels au tournant du 18ème siècle: Le cas de la Bibliothèque britannique, 1796–1815*, in *Archives des sciences* (Geneva), 1977,

30: 283–398. Another important conduit of foreign medical news was the *Bibliothèque germanique médico-chirurgicale,* or *Traductions des meilleurs auteurs allemands qui ont écrit sur l'art de guérir* (8 vols., 1798–1802).

Among nineteenth-century serials of special significance, one stands out for its interest in the problems of public health and social medicine that the Napoleonic era had formulated, the *Annales d'hygiène publique et de médecine légale.* Begun in 1829 and published until World War II, it gave birth in 1921 to *Annales de médecine légale, de criminologie et de police scientifique,* and in 1923 it turned into *Annales d'hygiène publique, industrielle et sociale.*

SECONDARY PUBLICATIONS

This book is meant to complement the pioneering work of Erwin H. Ackerknecht, Pierre Huard, and George Rosen. In an indispensable paper on "Hygiene in France, 1815–1848," *Bulletin of the History of Medicine* (henceforth cited as *BHM*), 1948, *22*: 117–155, Ackerknecht pointed to the "odd gap" usually left by scholars between the acknowledged contributions of the late-eighteenth-century French philosophes and the practical achievements of mid-nineteenth-century Englishmen. In that paper, Ackerknecht proceeded to fill this gap, but, oddly, he begins in 1815, thus leaving a smaller but still significant opening for 1789–1815. He provided further guidance in "Die Therapie der Pariser Kliniker zwischen 1795 und 1840," *Gesnerus,* 1958, *15*: 151–163, and "Die Pariser Spitäler als Ausgangspunkt einer neuen Medizin," *Ciba Symposia,* 1959, *7*: 98–105. His work ultimately resulted in what has remained a reference work for this era, *Medicine at the Paris Hospital, 1794–1848* (Baltimore: Johns Hopkins Press, 1967), tr. by F. Blateau as *La médecine hospitalière à Paris (1794–1848)* (Paris: Payot, 1984).

Equally important are the numerous articles (often published in collaboration with M. J. Imbault-Huart) by Pierre Huard and that author's *Sciences, médecine, pharmacie, de la révolution à l'empire* (Paris: Dacosta, 1970), a work outstanding by reason of its iconography. Huard's practical experience as a military doctor and as an administrator is perceptible throughout his writings.

The influence of the late George Rosen pervades the relevant literature. Rosen separated out the concept of "cameralism"—that is, enlightened, though despotic, rule by royal decree—and its medical application as "*Medizinalpolizei,*" prevalent in German-speaking countries. See his "Cameralism and the Concept of Medical Police," *BHM,* 1953, *27*: 21–42, and "The Fate of the Concept of Medical Police, 1780–1815," *Centaurus,* 1957, *5*: 97–113. Rosen applied the concept of medical police to France in "Mercantilism and Health Policy in Eighteenth-Century France," *Medical History,* 1959, *3*: 259–277. He also spelled out important elements explored in this book in "Hospitals, Medical Care and Social Policy in the French Revolution," *BHM,* 1956, *30*: 124–149, and in "The Philosophy of Ideology and the Emergence of Modern Medicine in France," *BHM,* 1946, *20*: 328–339.

See R. Valléry-Radot, *Paris d'autrefois, ses vieux hôpitaux Deux siècles d'histoire hospitalière* (2 vols.; Paris: Dupont, 1947). This book does not, however, recount the exploits of the medical profession, as was done recently by

J. C. Sournia in *La médecine révolutionnaire, 1789–1799* (Paris: Payot, 1989), and in Liliane Pariente and Philippe Deville in *Les médecins pendent la révolution* (Paris: Editions Louis Pariente, 1989).

While the present book acknowledges poverty as a cause of illness, it does not study poverty per se. In probing that theme, older works dwelled on religious charity or lay welfare. Many of these works remain valuable for background and reference, especially C. Bloch, *L'assistance et l'état en France à la veille de la révolution, 1764–1790* (Paris: Picard, 1908); M. Bouchet *L'Assistance publique en France pendant la révolution* (Paris: Jouve, 1908); L. Lallemand, *Histoire de la charité*, vol. 4, *Les temps modernes* (Paris: Picard, 1910); A. L. de Lanzac de Laborie, *Assistance et bienfaisance*, vol. 5 of *Paris sous Napoleon* (5 vols.; Paris: Plon, 1908); S. T. McCloy, *Government Assistance in Eighteenth-Century France* (Durham, N.C.: Duke University Press, 1946); and L. Parturier, *L'assistance à Paris sous l'ancien régime et pendant la révolution* (Paris: Larose, 1897). The following more recent discussions are outstanding: M. Rochaix, *Essai sur l'evolution des questions hospitalières de la fin de l'ancien régime à nos jours* (Paris: Fédération hospitalière de France, 1959); Isser Woloch, "From Charity to Welfare in Revolutionary Paris," *Journal of Modern History*, 1986, *58*: 779–812; and M. Candille, "Evolution des principes d'assistance hospitalière," *Revue d'assistance publique*, 1958, *9*: 43–51, and "Les soins en France au 19ème siècle," *Bulletin de la société française d'histoire des hôpitaux*, 1973, *28*: 33–77.

Scholars now tend to focus on the lives and needs of the poor themselves. Discussion of contemporary perceptions of the poor as resourceful copers, as dangerous elements, and as expendable individuals was pioneered, respectively, by O. Hufton, *The Poor of Eighteenth-Century France, 1750–1789* (New York: Oxford University Press, 1975), L. Chevalier, *Classes laborieuses et classes dangereuses à Paris pendant la première moitié du 19ème siècle* (Paris: Plon, 1958), and Richard Cobb, *Death in Paris: The Records of the Basse-Geôle de la Seine, October 1795–September 1801, Vendémiaire Year IV–Fructidor Year IX* (New York: Oxford University Press, 1978).

Alan Forrest focuses on the poor in the provinces in *The French Revolution and the Poor* (New York: Oxford University Press, 1981), but many other scholars concentrate their attention on one significant town: see, for example, C. Fairchilds, *Poverty and Charity in Aix-en-Provence, 1640–1789* (Baltimore: Johns Hopkins University Press, 1976); J. P. Gutton, *La société et les pauvres: L'exemple de la généralité de Lyon, 1534–1789* (Paris: Les belles lettres, 1971); C. Jones, *Charity and bienfaisance: The Treatment of the Poor in the Montpellier Region, 1740–1815* (Cambridge: Cambridge University Press, 1982); and K. Norberg, *Rich and Poor in Grenoble, 1600–1814* (Berkeley and Los Angeles: University of California Press, 1985). Others have looked at solutions from "below," such as begging: T. M. Adams, *Bureaucrats and Beggars: French Social Policy in the Age of Enlightenment* (New York: Oxford University Press, 1990), or from "above," such as policing: R. B. Schwartz, *Policing the Poor in Eighteenth-century France* (Chapel Hill: University of North Carolina Press, 1988). Jean Imbert has recently published a collaborative volume, with chapters by other distinguished historians, such as Louis Trénard, Guy Thuillier, and Jean Tulard, entitled *La protection sociale sous la révolution française* (Paris: Association pour l'étude de l'histoire de la sécurité sociale, 1990). These authors share the historical perspective of the present book. They regard the Enlightenment as the fertile soil in which Revolutionary principles grew and believe that the Revolution definitively established the principle of the poor person's right to public support. They adduce evidence from all over France to discuss the legal, administrative, political, and economic aspects of social protection. Imbert views the Directory as the most creative period in hospital legislation. *La protection sociale* does not focus on the recipients of aid, it pays little attention to women, and it does not discuss the efforts of physicians, pharmacists, midwives, and nurses in any detail. However, it complements the present volume in important ways.

This book remains focused on the impact of poverty on health and on the experience of citizen-patients and their changing relationships with the health professions and the administrative powers, in the light of evolving cultural, economic, and social conditions and of the contemporary revolution in medicine and health care. Outstanding, from this point of view, are the writings of our late regretted colleague William Coleman, especially *Death Is a Social Disease: Public Health and Political Economy in Early Industrial France* (Madison: University of Wisconsin Press, 1982). Matthew Ramsey's *Professional and Popular Medicine in France, 1770–1830: The Social World of Medical Practice* (New York: Cambridge University Press, 1988), which analyzes popular medicine as a valid alternative to its professional counterpart, is a most revealing work, pointing to the resourcefulness of the poor and the many alternatives to an expensive doctor. J. Léonard's *La médecine entre les pouvoirs et les savoirs* (Paris: Aubier Montaigne, 1981) is helpful on the subject of medicine's political parameters in France. And the analyses of this book, particularly those of Chapter 10, are carried forward in Ann F. LaBerge's *Mission and Method: The Early Nineteenth-Century French Public Health Movement* (New York: Cambridge University Press, 1992).

Numerous scholars have raised specific important points related to health care, hygiene, and public health. Jean Imbert stands alone in dealing with the legal and legislative aspects of the subject, his lifelong concern. Imbert's *Le droit hospitalier de la révolution et de l'empire* (Paris: Sirey, 1954) remains indispensable, and he is also the co-author of a recent brief, but comprehensive, survey of the scholarly and medical problems involved, J. P. Gutton and J. Imbert, "Les hôpitaux français sous la révolution," *Bulletin de la société française des hôpitaux*, 1989, *58*. The rising importance of surgeons is documented in T. Gelfand, *Professionalizing Modern Medicine: Paris Surgeons and Medical Science and Institutions in the Eighteenth Century* (Westport, Conn.: Greenwood Press, 1980), and M. J. Imbault-Huart, *L'école pratique de dissection de Paris de 1750 à 1822, ou l'influence du concept de médecine pratique et de médecine d'observation dans l'enseignement médical au dix-huitième siècle et du début du 19ème siècle* (Lille: Service de reproduction de thèses, 1975). Others have turned their attention to epidemics: see J. Meyer, "Une enquête de l'académie de médecine sur les épidémies, 1774–1794," *Annales: Economies, sociétés, civilisations*, 1966, *21*: 729–749, and J. P. Desaive et al., *Médecins, climat, et épidémies à la fin du dix-huitième siècle* (Paris: Mouton, 1972). An interest in diet is shown in

R. Mandrou and J. P. Aron, "Un problème de diététique à l'Hôtel-Dieu de Paris à la veille de la révolution," in *Actes du 93ème congrès national des sociétés savantes* [Tours, 1968] (3 vols.; Paris: Bibliothèque nationale, 1971), vol. 1, 125–137, and id., *Essai sur la sensibilité alimentaire à Paris au 19ème siècle*, Cahiers des *Annales*, 25(Paris: Armand Colin, 1967). Finally, scholars have raised problems about the appropriate nosology and taxonomy to use for diseases of the eighteenth century that we can only know in an indirect way: see, for example, J. P. Peter, "Une enquête de la société royale de médecine, 1774–1794: Malades et maladies à la fin du dix-huitième siècle," *Annales: Economies, sociétés, civilisations*, 1967, *22*: 711–751; id., "Les mots et les objets de la maladie," *Revue historique*, 1971, *499*: 13–38; and id., "Le corps du délit," *Nouvelle revue de psychanalyse*, 1971, *3*: 71–108.

Thus there is now a broad basis of scholarly involvement in the social history of medicine in eighteenth- and nineteenth-century France; witness, for example, the nineteenth Congrès national des sociétés savantes at Nantes in 1972, which provided the substance for "Médecins, médecine et société en France aux 18ème et 19ème siècles," *Annales: Economies, sociétés, civilisations*, 1977, *32*, tr. as vol. 6 of *Medicine and Society in France: Selections from the "Annales,"* ed. R. Forster and O. Ranum (Baltimore: Johns Hopkins University Press, 1980), which contains articles on industrial health (A. Farge, "Les artisans malades de leur travail"); popular medicine (J. P. Goubert, "L'art de guérir: Médecine savante et médecine populaire dans la France de 1790"); hospital administration (M. Joerger, "La structure hospitalière de la France sous l'ancien régime"); midwifery (J. Gélis, "Sages-femmes et accoucheurs: L'obstétrique populaire au 17ème et 18ème siècles," and M. Laget, "La naissance aux siècles classiques: Pratique des accouchements et attitudes collectives en France au 17ème et 18ème siècles"); the nursing orders (J. Léonard, "Femmes, religion et médecine: Les religieuses qui soignent, en France au 19ème siècle"); wet-nursing (M. F. Morel, "Ville et campagne dans le discours médical sur la petite enfance au 18ème siècle"); and the medical profession (D. Roche, "Talents, raison et sacrifice: L'image du médecin des lumières d'après les éloges de la société royale de médecine").

New journals such as *Social History of Medicine* and *History of Psychiatry* and new societies such as the European Association for the History of Medicine and Health and the European Association for the History of Psychiatry indicate the active involvement of scholars in issues that were quite novel a generation ago. This book is the result of that involvement.

Part II

I. ENLIGHTENED INNOVATION

The involvement of philosophes and scientists in health care reform is discussed in M. Candille, "Commentaires autour du chapitre de l'*Esprit des lois* relatif aux hôpitaux," *Revue de l'Assistance publique à Paris*, 1953, *22*: 315–323, C. C. Gillispie, *Science and Polity in France at the End of the Old Regime* (Princeton: Princeton University Press, 1980), and numerous articles by L. S. Greenbaum, such as "The Humanitarianism of Antoine Laurent Lavoisier," *Studies on Voltaire and the Eighteenth Century*, 1972, *88*: 651–675; "Health Care and Hospital Building in Eighteenth-Century France: Reform Proposals of Dupont de Nemours and Condorcet," ibid., 1976, *152*: 895–930; "Tempest in the Academy: Jean Baptiste Le Roy, the Paris Academy of Sciences, and the Project of a new Hôtel-Dieu," *Archives internationales d'histoire des sciences*, 1974, *24*: 122–140; "'Measure of Civilization': The Hospital Thought of Jacques Tenon on the Eve of the French Revolution," *BHM*, 1975, *49*: 43–56; "Jean Sylvain Bailly, the Baron de Breteuil, and the 'Four New Hospitals' of Paris," *Clio medica*, 1973, *8*: 261–284; "Jacques Necker and the Reform of the Paris Hospitals on the Eve of the French Revolution," ibid., 1984, *19*: 216–230; and "Jacques Necker's Enquête of the Paris Hospital (1777)," Consortium on Revolutionary Europe, *Proceedings*, 1984: 26–40.

On the ideologues, see George Rosen, "The Philosophy of Ideology and the Emergence of Modern Medicine in France," *BHM*, 1946, *20*: 328–339. In the vast literature on Ideology, the following have special bearing on health: G. Gusdorf, *La conscience révolutionnaire: Les idéologues* (Paris: Payot, 1978); B. W. Head, "The Origins of 'La science sociale' in France, 1770–1800," *Australian Journal of French Studies*, 1982, 19: 125–126; C. B. Welch, *Liberty and Utility: The French Ideologues and the Transformation of Liberalism* (New York: Columbia University Press, 1984); and M. Regaldo, *Un milieu intellectuel: La Décade philosophique, 1794–1807* (5 vols.; Paris: Champion, 1976). From the voluminous work of Sergio Moravia on Ideology, see especially *La scienza dell'uomo nel settecento* (Bari: Laterza, 1970); *Il pensiero degli Idéologues: Scienza e filosofia in Francia, 1780–1815* (Florence: La nuova Italia, 1974); "The Capture of the Invisible: For a (Pre)History of Psychology in Eighteenth-Century France," *Journal of the History of the Behavioral Sciences*, 1983, *19*: 370–378; "The Enlightenment and the Sciences of Man," *History of Science*, 1980, *18*: 246–268; "From 'homme machine' to 'homme sensible': Changing Eighteenth-Century Models of Man's Image," *Journal of the History of Ideas*, 1978, *39*: 45–60; "Les idéologues et l'âge des lumières," *Studies on Voltaire and the Eighteenth Century*, 1976, *154*: 1465–1486; and "Philosophie et médecine en France à la fin du 18ème siècle," ibid., 1972, *89*: 1089–1151.

On **Cabanis,** see M. S. Staum, *Cabanis: Enlightenment and Medical Philosophy in the French Revolution* (Princeton: Princeton University Press, 1980), and the review by T. E. Kaiser in *JHM*, 1982, *54*: 121–123. See also A. Cadet de Gassicourt, "Un médecin au Panthéon: P. J. G. Cabanis, 1757–1808," *Histoire de la médecine*, 1953, 29–36; F. Colonna d'Istria, "La logique de la médecine d'après Cabanis," *Revue de métaphysique et de morale*, 1917, *24*.: 59–73; H. Durand, *Cabanis: Sa vie et son oeuvre médicale* (Paris: Jouve, 1939); A. Guillois, *Le salon de Madame Helvétius: Cabanis et les idéologues* (Paris: Calmann Lévy, 1894); E. Lesky, "Cabanis und die Gewissheit der Heilkunde," *Gesnerus*, 1954, *2*: 152–182; S. Moravia, "'Moral'–'Physique': Genesis and Evolution of a 'Rapport,'" in *Enlightenment Studies in Honor of Lester Crocker*, ed. J. Bingham and V. W. Topazio (Oxford: Voltaire Foundation, 1979), 163–174; C. A. Pierson, *Georges Cabanis, psycho-physiologiste et sénateur: Un précurseur de la réforme des études médicales au lendemain de la révolution française*

(Paris: Maloine, 1946); F. Thurot, "Lettres sur divers mémoires du citoyen Cabanis," *Décade philosophique,* 1800, *25:* 262–270, 461–468, 521–528; and A. Vartanian, "Cabanis and La Mettrie," *Studies on Voltaire and the Eighteenth Century,* 1976, *155:* 2149–2166. I wish to thank Dr. Alain Segal of Rheims, France, for making available a number of manuscript documents relating to Cabanis's doctoral thesis in Rheims, where he graduated in 1783.

There is no full-length biography of **Vicq d'Azyr** except for the out-of-date A. Dufresne, *Notes sur la vie et les oeuvres de Vicq d'Azyr, 1748–1794: Histoire de la fondation de l'Académie de médecine* (*sic;* the book discusses the Royal Society of Medicine) (Bordeaux: Cassignol, 1906). The best biographical sketches are: P. J. G. Cabanis, "Eloge," in *Oeuvres complètes* (5 vols.; Paris: Bossange, 1825), *5:* 177–216; Pierre Huard and M. J. Imbault-Huart, "Vicq d'Azyr," in the *Dictionary of Scientific Biography;* J. M. Moreau de la Sarthe, ed., "Eloge," in *Oeuvres de Vicq d'Azyr* (8 vols.; Paris: Duprat-Duverger, 1805), vol. 1, 1–88; J. Noir, "Vicq d'Azyr," *Concours médical,* April 6, 1927, 927–929; and C. A. de Sainte-Beuve, "Notice sur Vicq d'Azyr," *Union médicale,* 1854, *8:* 355–356, 359–361, 371–372. . Vicq d'Azyr's illegible handwriting may well preclude a definitive, well-documented biography.

The work of the Société royale de médecine has been analyzed by C. C. Hannaway in "Medicine, Public Welfare, and the State in Eighteenth-Century France" (Ph.D. diss., Johns Hopkins University, 1974). She has further pursued various aspects of the society's work in articles such as "The Société royale de médecine and epidemics in the ancien régime," *BHM,* 1972, *46:* 257–273; and id., "Veterinary Medicine and Rural Health Care in Pre-Revolutionary France," *BHM,* 1977, *51:* 431–447. On that favorite pursuit of Vicq d'Azyr's, see also H. Hours, *La lutte contre les épizooties et l'école vétérinaire de Lyon au dix-huitième siècle* (Paris: Presses Universitaires, 1957), and A. Railliet and L. Maulé, *Histoire de l'école d'Alfort* (Paris: Asselin & Houseau, 1908).

Some information about the royal remedy boxes and regulation of remedies can be found in T. Gelfand, "Public Medicine and Medical Careers," in "Proceedings of the 28th International Congress of the History of Medicine" (Paris, 1980), *Histoire des sciences médicales,* 1982, *17:* numéro special, vol. 2, 103–108, and particularly in C. C. Hannaway, "The Regulation of Remedies in Eighteenth-Century France," in ibid., 265–269. Eighteenth-century doctors seem to have been unappreciative of this royal largesse. See the *cahier* of the physicians of Rheims quoted in J. P. Goubert and D. Lorillot, eds., *Les cahiers de doléances des médecins, chirurgiens et apothicaires, 1789: Le corps médical et le changement* (Toulouse: Privat, 1984).

The best books on **Necker Hospital** are R. Gervais, *Histoire de l'Hôpital Necker* (Thèse médecine, Paris, 1885), and J. Cotinat, *Hospice de Charité (Necker): La fondation et les débuts de l'Hospice Necker à Paris* (Thèse médecine, Paris, 1972). See also C. Neauport, *L'Hospice de Charité des paroisses St. Sulpice et du Gros Caillou (1778–1789)* (Thèse lettres, Paris, 1970), and M. Poisvert, "Les débuts de l'Hôpital Necker," *Histoire des sciences médicales,* 1973, *7:* 315–326. See also Ministère de l'instruction publique, *Procès-verbaux et rapports du comité de mendicité de la Constituante, 1790–1791,* ed. C. Bloch and

A. Tuetey (Paris: Imprimerie nationale, 1911) (henceforth cited as *PVR*), 660–663; Jacques Tenon, *Mémoires sur les hôpitaux de Paris* (Paris: Pierres, 1788), 55–59; and Valléry-Radot, *Deux siècles*, 137–145.

On the postgraduate hospital (*hospice de perfectionnement*), see A. Corlieu, *L'Hôpital des cliniques de la Faculté de médecine de Paris* (Paris: Delahaye, 1878); T. Gelfand, "The Hospice of the Paris College of Surgery (1774–1793), 'A Unique and Valuable Institution,'" *BHM*, 1973, 47: 375–393, and "Les caractères originaux d'un hospice parisien à la fin de l'ancien régime," in *Mensch und Gesundheit in der Geschichte*, ed. A. E. Imhof, Abhandlungen zur Geschichte der Medizin und der Naturwissenschaften, 39 (Husum, Germany: Matthiesen, 1980), 339–356.

On **eighteenth-century surgery,** see Gelfand, *Professionalizing Modern Medicine;* id., "A Clinical Ideal: Paris 1789," *BHM*, 1977, *51*: 397–411; id., "Deux cultures, une profession: Les chirurgiens français au 18ème siècle," *Revue d'histoire moderne et contemporaine*, 1980, 27: 468–484; id., "Empiricism and Eighteenth-Century French Surgery," *BHM*, 1970, 44: 40–53; id., "The Gestation of the Clinic," in *Actes du 25ème congrès international d'histoire de la médecine* [Québec] (3 vols.; 1976), 2: 680–698; and id., "From Guild to Profession: The Surgeons of France in the 18th Century," in *Texas Reports on Biology and Medicine*, 1974, *32*: 121–134. See also Pierre Huard and M. J. Imbault-Huart, "De l'hospice de perfectionnement de l'Académie royale de chirurgie à l'Hôpital des cliniques de la Faculté de médecine de Paris (1775–1876)," *Bulletin de la Société française d'histoire des hôpitaux*, 1972, 27: 37–47; Imbault-Huart, *L'école pratique;* O. Temkin, "The Role of Surgery in the Rise of Modern Medical Thought," *BHM*, 1951, *25*: 248–259; and J. D. Thompson and Grace Goldin, *The Hospital: A Social and Architectural History* (New Haven: Yale University Press, 1975), 139.

On the question of transferring or rebuilding the Hôtel-Dieu of Paris, see M. Candille, "Les projets de translation de l'Hôtel-Dieu de Paris hors de la Cité," *Revue de l'Assistance publique à Paris*, 1956, 7: 743–752, 1957, 8: 239–263, 343–359, 433–449. See also D. B. Weiner, ed., *Jacques Tenon's Memoirs on Paris Hospitals* (Canton, Mass.: Science History Publications, forthcoming), particularly the introduction, "Surgical Procedure: Jacques Tenon (1724–1816), Hospital Reform, and the French Enlightenment," and bibliography. See also M. Fosseyeux, *L'Hôtel-Dieu de Paris au 17ème et 18ème siècles* (Paris: Berger-Levrault, 1912); M. D. Iberti, *Observations générales sur les hôpitaux, suivies d'un projet d'hôpital* (London: n.p., 1788) and D. Jetter, "Frankreich's Bemühen um bessere Hospitäler," *Sudhoff's Archiv für Geschichte der Medizin,* 1965, *49*: 147–169.

2. THE PUBLIC HOSPITAL

The history of the hospital in the eighteenth and early nineteenth centuries, particularly in Paris, is well documented. See L. MacAuliffe, *La révolution et les hôpitaux, Années 1789, 1790, 1791* (Paris: Bellais, 1901); P. Valléry-Radot, *Paris d'autrefois, ses vieux hôpitaux: Deux siècles d'histoire hospitalière* (Paris: Dupont, 1947); A. Bonde, *Le domaine des hospices de Paris, 1789–1870* (Paris:

Berger-Levrault, 1906); and M. C. R. Gillett, "Hospital Reform in the French Revolution" (Ph.D. diss., American University, 1978).

On the **Hôtel-Dieu of Paris,** see M. Fosseyeux, *L'Hôtel-Dieu de Paris au 17ème et 18ème siècles* (Paris: Berger-Levrault, 1912).

There are two interesting studies of **Bicêtre,** namely, P. Bru, *Histoire de Bicêtre: Hospice, prison, asile* (Paris: Progrès médical, 1890), which is not very scholarly but reprints documents, and E. Richard, *Histoire de l'hôpital de Bicêtre (1250–1791)* (Thèse médecine, Paris, 1889), which is detailed, well-documented, and has good references. All the other studies known to me are useless.

Two strange documents have special relevance: the first, not germane to medical history, but passionate and picturesque, stems from the pen of the comte de Mirabeau, who knew prisons from the inside: *Observations d'un voyageur anglais sur la maison de force appelée Bicêtre, suivies de réflexions sur les effets de la sévérité des peines et sur la législation criminelle de la Grande Bretagne; imité de l'anglais, par le comte de Mirabeau, avec une lettre de M. Benjamin Franklin* (Paris: n.p. 1788). The *voyageur anglais* is Sir Samuel Romilly, who furnished material for the work. See the *Dictionary of National Biography*, s.v. "Romilly." The second document is the account of a contemporary employee at Bicêtre: see L. Boulle, ed., *Les souvenirs du Père Richard* (forthcoming).

On the **Salpêtrière,** the best historical studies are R. Gasco, "La Salpêtrière, 1789–1794" (Diplôme d'études supérieures d'histoire, M. Reinhard, dir., Paris, 1969), and M. Henry, *La Salpêtrière sous l'ancien règime: Les origines de l'élimination des antisociaux et de l'assistance aux aliénés chroniques* (Thèse médecine, Paris, 1922). An interesting monographic study is L. Hautecoeur, "L'Architecture hospitalière et la Salpêtrière," *Médecine de France*, 1958, *96*: 21–36.

On the history of **St. Louis Hospital,** see M. Dogny, *Histoire de l'Hôpital St. Louis depuis sa fondation jusqu'au 19ème siècle* (Thèse médecine, Paris, 1911); P. Hardy, "Documents pour servir à l'histoire de l'Hôpital St. Louis au commencement de ce siècle: Alibert, Biett, Lugol, Manry, Emery," *Annales de dermatologie et de syphiligraphie*, 2d ser., 1885, *6*: 629–638; Pierre Huard and M. J. Imbault-Huart, "L'Ecole dermatologique de St. Louis," *Histoire des sciences médicales*, 1974, *8*: 703–720; and R. Sabouraud, *L'Hôpital St. Louis* (Lyon: Ciba, 1937).

On the survival and health of **foundlings,** see L. Lallemand, *Histoire des enfants abandonnés et délaissés* (Paris: Picard, 1885), and J. Dehaussy, *L'assistance publique à l'enfance: Les enfants abandonnés* (Paris: Sirey, 1951). For a scholarly view of the problem in provincial France during the Revolution, see Forrest, *French Revolution and the Poor*, ch. 7; for an excellent recent overview, though without bibliography or notes, see J. Sandrin, *Enfants trouvés, enfants ouvriers, 17ème–19ème siècles* (Paris: Aubier, 1982), and for the period after the Revolution, see R. Fuchs, *Abandoned Children: Foundlings and Child Welfare in 19th-Century France* (Albany, N.Y.: SUNY Press, 1983).

A recent book suggests some contrasts between Paris and London: see R. K. McClure, *Coram's Children: The London Foundling Hospital in the Eighteenth Century* (New Haven: Yale University Press, 1981). Founded in 1741, and financed and administered by private donors, with intermittent help from Parliament, this hospital admitted only as many infants as it could afford to maintain. In comparison to the Parisian annual census of 5,000, the London numbers pale: a total of 15,000 admitted in twenty years, from 1741 to 1760 (ibid., p. 261). The Londoners also farmed their foundlings out to wet nurses for pay but prevailed upon local clergy, gentry, and tradesmen to act as inspectors (ibid., p. 88). The Londoners also fostered apprenticeships, which averaged 400 a year in the 1760s, but they favored enlistment in the navy (ibid., p. 132). They arranged for their charges' medical care by the best physicians and surgeons in London, including Dr. William Cadogan, the author of an *Essay on Nursing* (1749). The institution's endowment profited from a famous art collection featuring the work of William Hogarth, a patron, and from annual performances of *The Messiah,* personally conducted by another patron, Georg Friedrich Handel.

3. CITIZEN-PATIENTS AND CITIZEN-DOCTORS

The best biographic studies of Guillotin are A. Chéreau, *Guillotin et la guillotine* (Paris: Union médicale, 1870) and the more comprehensive and equally inaccessible E. J. Guérin, "Le docteur Joseph Ignace Guillotin," *Revue d'Aunis et de Saintonge,* 1908, *28*: 101–128, 183–192, 224–245, 288–313. See also D. B. Weiner, "The Real Doctor Guillotin," *J.A.M.A. Annual Book Number,* 1972, *200*: 85–89.

Guillotin's papers seem to be in private hands, in the Aisne Department, according to information received from the Private Archives section of the Archives nationales. There are bits of his correspondence in the Manuscript Section of the Bibliothèque nationale (NAF 14,478 and 23,006) and in the archives of the Société royale de médecine, at the Paris Academy of Medicine. The French National Archives own a small collection of letters and documents connection with Guillotin's life as a public official during the French Revolution (D XVI 14, F⁷ 3303 and 4736, and F¹7 1240ᴬ· 3679, and 3680). In addition there is a slim folder of Guillotin papers at the Bibliothèque historique de la Ville de Paris.

Jean Gabriel Gallot had obtained one of the Royal Society's prizes for an essay on the "Medical Topography of Poitou." His "Vues générales" cover the same subject matter as Vicq d'Azyr's New Plan and present the same ideas. He attended as many meetings of the Royal Society as his parliamentary duties allowed, and he transmitted its views to the Health Committee. His major manuscripts are to be found in box 189 of the archives of the Royal Society of Medicine, National Academy of Medicine, Paris.

Jean François Coste wrote a pharmacopoeia for his troops, *Compendium pharmaceuticum militaribus gallorum nosocomiis in orbe novo boreali adscriptum* (Newport, R.I.: Barber, 1780), and on the occasion of his honorary appointment to the University of Virginia in 1782 he gave a speech in Latin, "De antiqua medica philosophia orbi novo adaptanda." His major work is *Du service des hôpitaux militaires rappelés aux vrais principes* (Paris: Croullebois, 1790) and the authoritative article "Hospital" for the famous *Dictionnaire des sciences médicales.* In 1796, Coste became physician-in-chief of the Hôtel des Invalides, and in 1803, of the Grand Army. On Coste, see M. Bihan, "Prétexte à quelques questions sur la biographie de J. F. Coste, médecin pendant les révolutions du 18ème et 19ème siècles," in *Atti del XXI congresso internazionale di storia della medicina* (Siena, 1968), 1415–1419.

On the ways of the eighteenth-century French poor in managing illness, see Goubert, "L'art de guérir"; M. Ramsay, "Repression of Unauthorized Medical Practice in Eighteenth-Century France," *Eighteenth-Century Life*, 1982, *7*: 118–135; and H. Mitchell, "Rationality and Control in French Eighteenth-Century Medical Views of the Peasantry," *Comparative Studies in Society and History*, 1979, *21*: 82–112.

4. THE CARING PROFESSIONS

There is as yet no overall treatment of **nursing** during the French Revolution. Documents in the Archives nationales are generally to be found in the Series S VII, or in the huge, uninventoried collection of papers of the Ministry for Internal Affairs, F 15.

On the Augustinian nurses, see D. B. Weiner, "The French Revolution, Napoleon, and the Nursing Profession," *BHM*, 1972, *46*: 274–305; L. S. Greenbaum, "Nurses and Doctors in Conflict: Piety and Medicine in the Paris Hôtel-Dieu on the Eve of the French Revolution," *Clio medica*, 198, *13*: 247–267; and id., "Science, Medicine, Religion: Three Views of Health Care in France on the Eve of the French Revolution," *Studies in Eighteenth-Century Culture*, ed. H. C. Payne 1981, *10*: 373–391.

For the period up to 15 April 1791, it is useful to consult *AP* and M. Möring et al., *Délibérations*. For the Revolutionary decade, see J. Boussoulade, *Moniales et hospitalières dans la tourmente révolutionnaire: Les communautés de religieuses de l'ancien diocèse de Paris de 1789 à 1801* (Paris: Letouzey & Ané, 1962). Despite its obvious bias and poor organization, this book contains much valuable information and many archival documents not otherwise available. On the Lazarists, confessors of the Sisters of Charity, see J. W. Carven, *Napoleon and the Lazarists* (The Hague: Nijhoff, 1972), and the abbé Molette's *Guide des sources de l'histoire des congrégations féminines françaises de vie active*.

The partisan Catholic literature has little scholarly value, but often provides unique documents and typical stories. To this group belong A. Tenneson, *Les Religieuses Augustines de l'Hôtel-Dieu de Paris, 7ème au 20ème siècle* (Paris: Religieuses Augustines, 1953); G. Bernoville, *Les Religieuses de Saint-Thomas de Villeneuve, 1661–1953* (Paris: Grasset, 1953); and A. Chevalier, *L'Hôtel-Dieu de Paris et les soeurs Augustines, 650-1810* (Paris: Champion, 1901).

Two recent theses are disappointing with regard to nursing care. B. Plongeron, *Les réguliers de Paris devant le serment constitutionnel: Sens et conséquences d'une option* (Paris: Vrin, 1964), ignores women altogether, and C. Langlois, *Le catholicisme au féminin: Les congrégations françaises à supérieure générale au 19ème siècle* (Paris: Cerf, 1984) presents nurses as mere servants.

In *The Charitable Imperative: Hospitals and Nursing in Ancien Regime and Revolutionary France* (New York: Routledge, 1989), Colin Jones suggests that the traditional image of the public hospital as a *"mouroir"* is wrong, and that the Sisters of Charity were well-trained professionals.

On the reemergence of the religious nurses during the Consulate, the most important source is J. A. Chaptal, comte de Chanteloup, *Mes souvenirs sur Napoleon* (Paris: Plon Nourrit, 1893). On Chaptal, see M. Peronnet, *Chaptal* (Toulouse: Privat, 1989); J. Pigeire, *La vie et l'oeuvre de Chaptal* (Paris: Donat-Montchrétien, 1932); and M. Crosland, *The Society of Arcueil: A View of French Science at the Time of Napoleon I* (Cambridge, Mass.: Harvard University Press, 1967).

On the Brothers of Charity, the most recent article, with a detailed international bibliography, is D. B. Weiner, "The Brothers of Charity and the Mentally Ill in Pre-Revolutionary France," *Social History of Medicine*, 1989, *2*: 321–337. See also P. Sérieux, "Le parlement de Paris et la surveillance des maisons d'aliénés et de correctionnaires au 17ème et 18ème siècles," *Revue historique du droit français et étranger*, 1938, *83*: 404–459, and id., "Le traitement des maladies mentales dans les maisons d'aliénés du 18ème siècle," *Archives internationales de neurologie*, 1924, *43* (2): 97–119, 145–154, 191–203; 1925, *44* (1): 21–31, 50–63, 90–104, 121–133(see especially *44*: 100–101).

On **pharmacy** during this era, the following books by M. Bouvet are essential: *Histoire de la pharmacie en France des origines à nos jours* (Paris: Occitania, 1937); *Les origines de la pharmacie hospitalière à Paris: L'Hôpital général des origines à 1789* (Poitiers: Imprimerie française, 1938); *Les origines de la pharmacie hospitalière à Paris avant 1789: L'Hôtel-Dieu et ses annexes* (Poitiers: Imprimerie moderne, 1935); *La pharmacie dans les hôpitaux de paroisse et les établissements privés de Paris avant 1789* (Toulouse: Ménard, 1943); *La pharmacie hospitalière à Paris de 1789 à 1815* (Paris: Société d'histoire de la pharmacie, 1943); and *La pharmacie hospitalière à Paris avant 1789: Le Grand bureau des pauvres* (Toulouse: Ménard, 1947).

Many important historical facts about professional hospital pharmacy are recorded in *La pharmacie à l'hôpital*, special issue of the journal *L'hôpital et l'aide sociale à Paris*, 1963, *4* (24). The first effort by Paris pharmacists to define their substances and quantities in French was *Formules médicales de l'Hôtel-Dieu ou Pharmacopée* (1753), which was followed in 1767 by *Formules de médicaments, usitées dans les différents hôpitaux de la ville de Paris*. Nomenclature and dosages still varied, even from one hospital to another and proprietary recipes were the jealously guarded rule. To gain some idea of the confusion still prevalent in Lavoisier's time, one has but to scan the inventory of substances in the back of his *Elements of Chemistry* (1789): he lists eight kinds of gold, six kinds of silver, seven sorts of water.

The vitality of the profession is attested to by the founding of a "Free Society of Paris Pharmacists" in 1796, followed by an official society in 1803, with a *Bulletin,* beginning in 1809. Eventually a new section was added to the Academy of Medicine: surgery had been section two; pharmacy became section three in 1825 and eventually blossomed into an independent Academy of Pharmacy in 1946. The archives of all of these establishments and publications are deposited at the Bibliothèque interuniversitaire de Pharmacie in Paris. See (anon.,) "Les archives conservées à la Bibliothèque interuniversitaire de pharmacie de Paris," *Revue d'histoire de la pharmacie,* 1981, *28*: 248–254.

Just as authoritative as French scholarship are a number of articles by A. Berman, an American: "The Cadet Circle: Representatives of an Era in French Pharmacy," *BHM,* 1966, *40*: 101–111; "Conflict and Anomaly in the Scientific Orientation of French Pharmacy, 1800–1873," *BHM,* 1963, *37*: 440–462; "The Pharmaceutical Component of 19th-Century French Public Health and Hygiene," *Pharmacy in History,* 1969, *11*: 5–10; and "The Scientific Tradition in French Hospital Pharmacy," *American Journal of Hospital Pharmacy,* 1961, *1*: 110–119.

For a general introduction to the subject of **Midwifery,** see Paul Delaunay, *La Maternité de Paris. Port-Royal. Port-Libre. L'hospice de la Maternité. L'Ecole des sages-femmes et ses origines (1625–1907)* (Paris: Rousset, 1909). Three well-known treatises by midwives of this era are Madame Le Boursier du Coudray, *Abrégé de l'art des accouchements, dans lequel on donne les préceptes nécessaires pour le mettre heureusement en pratique. On y a joint plusieurs observations intéressantes sur des cas singuliers. Ouvrage très utile aux jeunes sages-femmes et généralement à tous les élèves en cet art, qui désirent de s'y rendre habiles* (Châlons-sur-Marne: Bouchard, 1773); M. L. Lachapelle, née Dugès, *Pratique des accouchements, ou Mémoires ou observations choisies sur les points les plus importants de l'art* (Paris: Baillière, 1821; 2d ed., 1825); and M. A. V. Boivin, *Mémorial de l'art des accouchements, suivi 1) des Aphorismes de Mauriceau, 2) de ceux l'Orazio Valota, 3) d'une série de 136 gravures représentant le mécanisme de toutes les espèces d'accouchements, tant naturels qu'artificiels . . .* (Paris: Méquignon, 1813; 2d ed. 1817).

For biographies of famous midwives, see A. Delacoux, *Biographies de sages-femmes célèbres, anciennes, modernes, et contemporaines* (Paris: Trinquart, 1833); G. J. A. Witkowski, *Accoucheurs et sages-femmes célèbres: Esquisses biographiques* (Paris: Steilheil, 1891); and H. Carrier, *Origines de la Maternité de Paris: Les maîtresses sages-femmes et l'Office des accouchées de l'ancien Hôtel-Dieu, 1378–1796* (Paris: Steinheil, 1888). A biography of Madame Le Coudray by Nina Gelbart is forthcoming. See also J. Gélis, "La formation des accoucheurs et des sages-femmes aux 17ème et 18ème siècles: Evolution d'un matériel et d'une pédagogie," in *Annales de démographie historique* (Paris and The Hague: Mouton, 1977), 153–180. For a historical overview, see J. Gélis, M. Laget, and M. F. Morel, *Entrer dans la vie: Naissances et enfances dans la France traditionnelle* (Paris: Gallimard, 1978), and M. Laget, *Naissances: L'accouchement avant l'âge de la clinique* (Paris: Seuil, 1982).

Training for midwives was also offered in an academic setting. The most famous course taught by an accoucheur was that of J. L. Baudelocque; see his *Principes sur l'art des accouchements par demandes et réponses en faveur des sages-femmes de la campagne* (Paris: Méquignon, 1775; 2d ed., 1787). This is an adaptation of his *L'art des accouchements* (2 vols.; Paris: Méquignon, 1781), which was republished in 1789, 1796, 1807, 1815, 1822, and 1833. These small in-12 volumes of over 500 pages are detailed practical handbooks adapted for women, whose "mind, memory, and judgment" Baudelocque found "uncultivated and undisposed toward study" (Baudelocque, *Principes,* vii.) His text was dubbed a "catechism" because of its question-and-answer style. On Baudelocque, see F. Chaussier, "Notice sur la vie et les ouvrages de M. Baudelocque: Discours lu à la séance publique de l'Hospice de la Maternité, le 20 juin 1810," in J. L. Baudelocque, *L'art des accouchements,* 5th ed. (2 vols.; Paris: Mequignon, 1815), vol. 1, 8–16, and J. J. Leroux, "Discours prononcé sur la tombe de M. Baudelocque le 3 mai 1810," in ibid., 1–7.

5. THE OUTPATIENT

See Forrest, *French Revolution and the Poor,* Gillett, "Hospital Reform in the French Revolution," and MacAuliffe, *La révolution et les hôpitaux.* The classic treatment of legal issues is Imbert, *Le droit hospitalier.* See also S. Woolf, "The Société de charité maternelle," in J. Barry and C. Jones, eds., *Medicine and Charity before the Welfare State* (London: Routledge, 1991), 98–112.

On Nicolas **Frochot,** see L. Passy, *Frochot, préfet de la Seine* (Evreux: Herissey, 1867), and M. Candille, "Un grand commis de l'administration française, Nicolas Frochot, 1761–1828," *L'Hôpital et l'aide sociale à Paris,* 1961, *2:* 605–609. Less helpful is J. Riche, "Frochot, préfet de la Seine sous le premier empire, sa carrière, pendant l'époque révolutionnaire," Société pour l'histoire du droit et des institutions des anciens pays bourguignons, comtais et romands, *Mémoires,* 1960, *21:* 43–62.

Interest in the **history of infancy and childhood** has been lively ever since Philippe Ariès aroused the attention of historians, forty years ago. The books and articles most helpful for the present study are A. Bideau, "L'envoi des jeunes enfants en nourrice: L'exemple d'une petite ville, Thoissy-en-Dombes, 1740–1840," *Sur la population française au 18ème et au 19ème siècles: Hommage à Marcel Reinhard* (Paris: Société de démographie historique, 1973), 48–58; T. G. H. Drake, "Infant Welfare Laws in France in the Eighteenth Century," *Annals of Medical History,* 1935, *7:* 49–61; M. Fosseyeux, "Sages-femmes et nourrices à Paris au 17ème siècle," *Revue de Paris,* 1921, *28:* 535–554; and P. Galliano, "Le fonctionnement du bureau parisien des nourrices à la fin du 18ème siècle," in *Actes du 93ème congrès national des sociétés savantes* [Tours, 1968] (3 vols.; Paris: Bibliothèque nationale, 1971), vol. 2, 67–93.

Information about the **welfare centers** can be derived from Woloch, "From Charity to Welfare." The richest older source is M. Fosseyeux, "Les comités de bienfaisance de Paris sous la révolution," *Annales révolutionnaires,* 1912, *5:* 192–205, 344–358; and see also id., "Les comités de bienfaisance des sections du Finistère et du Panthéon," *La révolution française,* 1911, *40:* 505–535, and J. Boussoulade, "Soeurs de charité et comités de bienfaisance des faubourgs St. Marcel et St. Antoine," *Annales historiques de la révolution française,* 1970, *42:* 350–374.

The **dispensaries** of the Philanthropic Society of Paris are discussed in D. B. Weiner, "The Role of the Doctor in Welfare Work: The Example of the Philanthropic Society of Paris, 1780–1815," *Historical Reflections / Réflexions historiques,* 1982 9 (1 & 2): 279–304; see also J. F. Payen, *Notice historique sur la société philanthropique de Paris, fondée en 1780* (Batignolles: Hennuyer, 1846), and M. P. Péan de St. Gilles, *La maison philanthropique de Paris* (Paris: Lemerre, 1892). Details about physicians and pharmacies collaborating with the dispensaries can be found in J. P. Goubert and R. Rey, eds., *Médecine et santé*, vol. 7 of *Atlas de la révolution française* (Paris: Ecole des hautes études en sciences sociales, forthcoming).

On dispensaries in general, see H. R. Ruser's excellent, although brief, "Wandlung des Dispensairegedankens," *Zeitschrift zur gesammten Hygiene*, 1977, *23*: 766–768; Z. Cope, "The History of the Dispensary Movement," in F. N. L. Poynter, ed., *The Evolution of Hospitals in Britain* (London: Pitman, 1964), 73–76; I. S. L. Loudon, "The Origin and Growth of the Dispensary Movement in England," *BHM*, 1981, *55*: 322–342; and U. Tröhler, "The Doctor as Naturalist: The Idea and Practice of Clinical Teaching and Research in British Policlinics, 1770–1850," in *Clinical Teaching, Past and Present* (symposium, University of Leiden), *Clio medica*, 1987–1988, vol. 21, 21–34.

Information on outpatient clinics, soup kitchens, nursing homes, and home care does not seem to be available in monographic work for the area under study in this book. It has to be culled from the primary and archival literature.

6. THE INPATIENT

Hospital architecture received considerable attention during this era, when the Seine Department employed the architects Nicolas Etienne Clavareau, Charles François Viel, and Jacques Gondoin. See N. E. Clavareau, *Mémoires sur les hôpitaux civils de Paris* (Paris: Prault, 1805); C. F. Viel, *Des anciennes études de l'architecture, de la nécessité de les remettre en vigueur, et de leur utilité pour l'administration des bâtiments civils* (Paris: Tilliard, 1807); id., *Principes de l'ordonnance et de la construction des bâtiments: Notices sur divers hôpitaux, et autres édifices publics et particuliers* (Paris: Tilliard, 1812); id., *Le grand égout de Bicêtre, ordonné par le roi Louis XVI: Plans, élévations, coupes, et profils* (Paris: Tilliard, 1817); and J. Gondoin, *Description des Ecoles de chirurgie* (Paris: Cellot & Gombert, 1780).

The earliest-known example of **clinical teaching** in a hospital ward, by Giovanni da Monte (1498–1552), occurred in Padua. Herman Boerhaave (1668–1738) re-"discovered" the method at Leiden, Gerhard van Swieten (1700–1772) took it to Vienna, and S. A. Tissot (1728–1797) to Pavia. See C. D. O'Malley, ed., *History of Medical Education: An International Symposium* (Berkeley and Los Angeles: University of California Press, 1970). A detailed analysis of teaching at Edinburgh is found in G. B. Risse, *Hospital Life in Enlightenment Scotland: Care and Teaching at the Royal Infirmary of Edinburgh* (Cambridge: Cambridge University Press, 1986).

The importance of the numerical method, and of incipient medical statistics have recently been pointed out in the following works: Coleman, *Death Is a Social Disease;* O. Keel, "The Politics of Health and the Institutionalisation of Clinical Practices in Europe in the Second Half of the Eighteenth Century," in W. F. Bynum and R. Porter, eds. *William Hunter and the Eighteenth-Century Medical World* (Cambridge: Cambridge University Press, 1985), 207–258; and U. Tröhler, "Britische Spitäler und Polikliniken als Heil- und Forschungsstätten," *Gesnerus*, 1982, *39*: 115–131.

On **G. L. Bayle**, see A. Rousseau, "Gaspard Laurent Bayle, le théoricien de l'Ecole de Paris," *Clio medica,* 1971, *5*: 205–211, and Pierre Huard and M. J. Imbault-Huart, "Gaspard Laurent Bayle, ou la méthodologie de la médecine anatomo-clinique, 1774–1816," *Gazette médicale de France,* 1974, *81*: 4943–4949.

On **Laënnec,** see Jacalyn M. Duffin, "The Medical Philosophy of R. T. H. Laënnec (1781–1826)," *History and Philosophy of the Life Sciences,* 1986, *8*: 195–219; id., "Vitalism and Organicism in the Philosophy of R. T. H. Laënnec," *BHM,* 1988, *62*: 525–545; and id., "The Cardiology of R. T. H. Laënnec," *Medical History,* 1989, *33*: 42–71.

On the persistent problem of securing **cadavers,** see M. Fosseyeux, "Le prix des cadavres à Paris aux 17ème et 18ème siècles," *Aesculape,* February 1913, 52–56; M. Genty, "La dissection à Paris sous la révolution et l'empire," *Progrès médical, supplément illustré,* 1932, *3*: 19–24; D. Trenel, "Bichat, voleur de cadavres," *Bull. soc. française hist. med.,* 1932, *26*: 97–106; and M. J. Imbault-Huart, *L'école pratique de dissection,* 225–239.

On Parent-Duchâtelet, see F. Leuret, "Notice historique sur A. J. B. Parent-Duchâtelet," *AHPML,* 1836, *16*: v–xxi, and Ann F. LaBerge, "Parent-Duchâtelet: Hygienist of Paris, 1821–1836," *Clio medica,* 1977, *12*: 279–301. On prostitution in Paris, see also *AP,* vol. 4, 51–61, and J. Harsin, *Policing Prostitution in 19th-Century Paris* (Princeton: Princeton University Press, 1985).

On R. J. H. Bertin, see A. Lellouch and R. Rullière, "René Joseph Hyacinthe Bertin, vénérologue," *Histoire des sciences médicales,* 1980, *14*: 325–336. See also M. J. Cullerier, "Observations sur la contagion syphilitique, dans les rapports des nourrices avec les nourrissons," *Journal général de médecine, de chirurgie, et de pharmacie,* 1816, *55*: 32–45.

On the **Venereal Diseases Hospital,** see M. J. Cullerier, *Notes historiques sur les hôpitaux établis à Paris, pour traiter la maladie vénérienne* (Paris: n.p., An XI [1802–1803]); A. Pignot, *L'Hôpital du Midi et ses origines: Recherche sur l'histoire médicale et sociale de la syphilis à Paris* (Paris: Dupont, 1885), which is largely based on the above and other published documents; and C. Berthollier, *La population de l'Hospice des vénériens entre 1792 et 1794: Situation antérieure et évolution de l'hospitalisation* (Paris: Mémoire de maîtrise, 1974). See also Valléry-Radot, *Paris d'autrefois, ses vieux hôpitaux,* 171–176; *PVR,* 610; and CGAHHCP, *Rapports au conseil général* (1803), 67–69.

On the history of **dermatology** in France, see F. Ebneter, *Die Dermatologie in Paris von 1800 bis 1850* (Zürich: Juris, 1964), and P. Hardy, "Documents pour servir à l'histoire de l'Hôpital St. Louis au commencement de ce siècle: Alibert, Biett, Lugol, Manry, Emery," *Annales de dermatologie et de syphiligraphie,* 1885, 2d ser., *6*: 629–638. On the general history of dermatology, see P. Richter, *Geschichte der Dermatologie,* vol. 14, pt. 2 of J. Jadassohn, *Handbuch der Haut- und Geschlechtskrankheiten* (Berlin: Springer, 1928), and W. Schonfeld, *Kurze Geschichte der Dermatologie und Venerologie* (Hannover: Oppermann, 1954).

J. L. Alibert was building on an important French tradition in dermatology, his chief forerunners being the two Montpellerian physicians Jean Astruc (1684–1766) and A. C. Lorry (1726–1783). The latter's *Tractatus de morbis cutaneis* (1777) ranked as the French classic. Alibert's student L. T. Biett

(1781–1840), who trained in England, became converted to the dermatologic classification taught by Robert Willan (1757–1812), which he adopted at St. Louis in preference to Alibert's system. Willan based his classification on the teaching of the Austrian J. J. Plenck (1738–1807), professor of chemistry, botany, surgery, anatomy, and obstetrics in Vienna. His major work was *Doctrina de morbis cutaneis* (1776). Biett taught from 1815 on, followed by his student P. A. Cazenave (1795–1877). Alibert's major writings were: *Nouveaux éléments de thérapeutique et de matière médicale* (Paris: Crapart, 1804), *Description des maladies de la peau observées à l'Hôpital St. Louis* (Paris: Barrois, 1808–1814), and *Physiologie des passions* (Paris: Béchet, 1825). On Alibert, see A. Alfaric, J. L. *Alibert, fondateur de la dermatologie en France: Sa vie, son oeuvre* (Paris: Baillière, 1917); L. Brodier, *J. L. Alibert, médecin de l'Hôpital St. Louis* (Paris: Maloine, 1923); and P. E. Becher's brief *Jean Louis Alibert, One of the Founders of French Dermatology* (New York: Medical Journal and Record, 1932).

7. CHILDREN AT RISK

On child abandonment, see the section on **Foundlings** in Bib. Ess., 2. The Public Hospital," above.

In addition to the relevant sections of the 1803 and 1816 reports by the Paris Hospital Council, two official publications are essential for understanding how the maternity service and the Foundlings' Hospice functioned: Seine, CGAHHCP, *Memoire historique et instructif sur l'Hospice de la maternité* and *Code spécial de la maternité*, listed under Primary Printed Sources above.

On the **Foundlings' Hospice** of the Maternité at Port-Royal, see also the authoritative A. Dupoux, *Sur les pas de Monsieur Vincent: Trois cents ans d'histoire parisienne de l'enfance abandonnée* (Paris: Revue de l'Assistance publique, 1958), written after the author retired as director of the former Paris Foundlings' Hospice, now called the Hôpital-Hospice Saint Vincent de Paul pour les enfants assistés. He had access to records that no one had used before, some of which have now been deposited in the Archives de la Seine, but much appears to have been discarded as useless trash that took up valuable space. But see also Poirot, *Notice sur l'Hospice de la Maternité* (Paris: Renaudière, An IX [1800–1801]), the stridently critical voice in a generally laudatory chorus. He calls himself "*préposé-en-chef*" at the Maternité, but cannot be found on the employees' roster.

There is a considerable literature on **wet-nursing.** Among the best studies are T. G. H. Drake, "The Wet-Nurse in France in the Eighteenth-Century," *BHM,* 1940, 7: 934–948 (old-fashioned, but good documentation); and G. D. Sussman, *Selling Mothers' Milk: The Wet-Nursing Business in France, 1715–1914* (Urbana: University of Illinois Press, 1982). Sussman concentrates on the middle class and artisans, rather than foundlings.

Much of the literature focuses on **morbidity and mortality** among wet nurses and babies, especially foundlings. See P. Baron, *Dissertation sur l'hygiène des nourrices* (Thèse médecine, Paris, 1818), a dissertation directed by Pinel; D. Risler, *Nourrices et meneurs à Paris au 18ème siècle* (Thèse Lettres, Nanterre, 1971); and F. Brochard, *De la mortalité des nourrissons en France, spécialement dans l'arrondissement de Nogent-le-Rontrou (Eure-et-Loir)* (Paris: Baillière, 1866). Brochard argues that artificial feeding does not work and also objects to vaccinating infants who are one day old: they arrive in the country with a fever, will not suck, and die (p. 8); the panacea he proposes is breast-feeding by the mother.

The debate over **infant feeding** continued throughout the nineteenth century. See, for example, I. G. Wickes, "A History of Infant Feeding," *Archives of Disease in Childhood,* 1953, *28:* 151–158, 232–240, 343–350, 416–421, 494–501; L. A. Barnes, "History of Infant Feeding Practices," *Amer. J. Clin. Nutr.,* 1987, *46* (suppl.), 168–170; M. A. Gendron, "Note sur la création d'un dépôt d'enfants-trouvés de Paris placé dans l'arrondissement de Vendôme (Loir-et-Cher), et sur les avantages et les inconvénients respectifs de l'allaitement naturel et de l'allaitement artificiel dans ce pays," *AHPML,* 1831, *6:* 80–88; and N. Senior, "Aspects of Infant Feeding in Eighteenth-Century France," *Eighteenth-Century Studies,* 1983, *16:* 367–388.

8. THE DEAF AND BLIND

For general discussion, political background, and detailed documentation, see D. B. Weiner, "Les handicapés et la révolution française: Aspects de médecine sociale," *Clio medica,* 1977, *12:* 97–109; id., "Three Champions of the Handicapped in Revolutionary France," in *From Parnassus: Essays in Honor of Jacques Barzun,* ed. D. B. Weiner and W. R. Keylor (New York: Harper & Row, 1976), 161–176; and id., "The Blind Man and the French Revolution," *BHM,* 1974, *48:* 60–89. Additional detailed bibliographic information can be found in these articles. See also R. Heller, "Educating the Blind in the Age of Enlightenment: Growing Points of a Social Service," *Medical History,* 1979, *23:* 392–403.

Deafness has recently received sensitive scholarly treatment from Harlan Lane, *The Deaf Experience: Classics in Language and Education* (Cambridge, Mass.: Harvard University Press, 1984), and *When the Mind Hears: A History of the Deaf* (New York: Random House, 1984). See also Oliver Sacks, *Seeing Voices: A Journey into the World of the Deaf* (Berkeley and Los Angeles: University of California Press, 1989). I wish to acknowledge Harlan Lane's help in understanding the key issues in the education the deaf. He was most generous both with his time and in lending me copies of his work-in-progress.

The mixture of therapeutic interest in the deaf and the blind is apparent, for example, in the useful bibliography by C. Guyot and R. T. Guyot, *Liste littéraire philocophe, ou Catalogue d'étude de ce qui a été publié jusqu'à nos jours sur les sourds-muets; sur l'oreille, l'ouïe, la voix le langage, la mimique, les aveugles, etc.* (Groningen: Oomkens, 1842). See also P. A. Dufau, "Aveugles et sourds-muets," in *Réunion internationale de charité, Annales de la charité,* 1855, *11:* 583–598, R. A. H. Bébian, *Journal de l'instruction des sourds-muets et des aveugles* (2 vols.; Paris: Au bureau du journal, 1826–1827), Ch. L. Carton wrote a *Mémoire sur l'éducation des sourds-muets mise à la portée des instituteurs primaires et des parents* (Brussels: Goemaere, 1856) and edited the journal *Le sourd-muet et l'aveugle: Journal mensuel* (Bruges: Vandercasteele-Werbrouk, 1837–1841).

The classic early texts regarding the education of the deaf in the French conte.·ᵗ are Abbé C. M. de l'Epée, *La véritable maniere d'instruire les sourds-*

muets, confirmée par une longue experience (Paris: Nyon, 1784), and Abbé R. A C. Sicard, *Cours d'instruction d'un sourd-muet de naissance, pour servir à l'éducation des sourds-muets et qui peut être utile à celle de ceux qui entendent et qui parlent* (Paris: Le Clerc, An VIII [1799–1800]).

For an elucidation of "manualist" versus "oralist" arguments, see C. R. Garnett, Jr., *The Exchange of Letters between Samuel Heinicke and Abbé Charles Michel de l'Epée: A Monograph on the Oralist and Manualist Methods of Instructing the Deaf in the Eighteenth Century, Including the Reproduction in English of Salient Portions of Each Letter* (New York: Vantage Press, 1968). On the abbé de l'Epée, see F. Berthier, *L'abbé de l'Epée: Sa vie, son apostolat, ses travaux, sa lutte et ses succès, avec l'historique des monuments élevés à sa mémoire à Paris et à Versailles* (Paris: Michel Lévy, 1852). For historical perspective, see M. F. de Gérando in *De l'éducation des sourds-muets de naissance* (2 vols.; Paris: Méquignon, 1827), and on teaching the deaf how to communicate, see especially J. P. Siegel, "The Enlightenment and the Evolution of a Language of Signs in France and England," *J. Hist. Ideas,* 1969, *30*: 96–115; H. Peet, "Memoir on the Origin and Early History of the Art of Instructing the Deaf and Dumb," *Am. Annals for the Deaf and Dumb,* 1850–1851, *3*: 126–160; and Ferdinand Berthier, *Essai sur les sourds-muets et sur le langage naturel ou Introduction à une classification naturelle des idées avec leurs signes propres* (Paris: Dentu, 1817). Berthier was an advocate of signing and later headed an institution at Rouen. See also E. Fournié, *Physiologie et instruction du sourd-muet d'après la physiologie des divers langages* (Paris: Delahaye, 1868), and Th. Denis, *Notice sur l'institution nationale des sourds-muets de Paris depuis son origine jusqu'à nos jours, 1760–1896, accompagnée de documents concernant l'enseignement scolaire, l'enseignement professionnel, conditions d'admission des élèves, etc., et suivie du catalogue du Musée universel des sourds-muets* (Paris: Institution nationale, 1896). A recent scholarly thesis provides new insights, as well as a collection of documents; see Alexis Karakostas, "L'institution nationale des sourds-muets de Paris de 1790 à 1800: Histoire d'un corps à corps" (Thèse de médecine, Paris, 1981). Karakostas is also rescuing instructive artefacts to be exhibited at the institution.

Blindness: The classic statement on educating the blind, in the French context, is V. Haüy, *Essai sur l'éducation des aveugles, ou Exposé de differents moyens vérifies par l'expérience pour les mettre en état de lire à l'aide du tact, d'imprimer des livres dans lesquels ils puissent prendre des connaissances de langues, d'histoire, de géographie, de musique, etc., d'exécuter differents travaux aux métiers, etc.* (Paris: Imprimé par les enfants aveugles, 1786). To this should be added an essay that was possibly published in St. Petersburg in 1810, and which shows extraordinary prescience: V. Haüy, "Moyens nouveaux, propres, si l'on ne s'abuse, à étendre et peut-être même à perfectionner le service du télégraphe."

P. A. Dufau, *Notice sur Valentin Haüy, créateur des procédés spéciaux d'enseignement à l'usage des aveugles* (Paris: Fain & Thenot, 1844); H. Maître, "Valentin Haüy et ses fonctions d'interprète," *Correspondance historique et archéologique,* 1901, *8*: 242–247, 258–263, the best short biography of Haüy; P. Henri, *Valentin Haüy, premier instituteur des aveugles* (Paris: Association Valentin Haüy, 1967). For an overview, see P. Henri, *La vie des aveugles,* Collection Que sais-je? (Paris: Presses universitaires de France, 1969), and id., *Les aveugles et la société: Contribution à la psychologie sociale de la cécité* (Paris: Presses universitaires de France, 1958)

On the Quinze-Vingts Hospice, see M. Battelle, *Notice historique et statistique sur l'Hôpital royal des Quinze-Vingts* (Paris: Chapelet, 1856); L. Le Grand, "Les Quinze-Vingts depuis leur fondation jusqu'à leur translation au faubourg St. Antoine, 13ème au 18ème siècles," in Société de l'histoire de Paris et de l'île de France, *Mémoires,* 1886: *13*: 107–260, 1887, *14*: 1–208; and F. G. Riffard-St. Martin, *Rapport sur l'Hôpital des Quinze-Vingts* (Paris:Imprimerie nationale, 1792).

See also P. A. Dufau, *Essai sur l'état physique, moral et intellectuel des aveugles-nés, avec un nouveau plan pour l'amélioration de leur condition sociale* (Paris: Imprimerie royale, 1837), and Dr. S. Guillié, *Essai sur l'instruction des aveugles, ou Exposé analytique des procédés pour les instruire* (Paris: Imprimé par les aveugles, 1817). The latter *Essai* was reissued twice, in 1819 and 1820; it was translated into English by R. Philips (London: 1819). J. G. Knie, the director of the school for the blind at Breslau, translated Dufau's *Essai* as *Versuch über den leiblichen, sittlichen und geistigen Zustand der Blindgeborenen* (Berlin: Nicolai, 1839), and he translated Guillé's *Essai* as *Versuch über den Unterricht der Blinden* (Breslau: 1820). And see, too, J. Guadet, *L'institution des jeunes aveugles de Paris, son histoire et ses procédés d'enseignement* (Paris: Thunot, 1849), and E. Guilbeau, *Histoire de l'Institution nationale des jeunes aveugles* (Paris: Belin, 1907). The breakthrough for the blind came with Louis Braille's invention of the six-dot cell used to represent all letters of the alphabet and all numerals. See L. Braille, *Procédé pour écrire les paroles, la musique, et le plain-chant au moyen de points, à l'usage des aveugles et disposés pour eux* (Paris: Imprimé à l'Institution des aveugles, 1829).

9. THE MENTAL PATIENT

Quite apart from the **"anti-psychiatric" movement** which has been spearheaded by Michel Foucault (see pp. 14–15), the recent literature on the emergence of psychiatry in France is substantial. The most innovative recent contribution is the French psychiatrist Gladys Swain's *Le sujet de la folie: Naissance de la psychiatrie* (Toulouse: Privat, 1977). See also id. and M. Gauchet, *La pratique de l'esprit humain: L'institution asilaire et la révolution démocratique* (Paris: Gallimard, 1980). Jan Goldstein's recent *Console and Classify: The French Psychiatric Profession in the Nineteenth Century* (New York: Cambridge University Press, 1987) is a work of impressive scholarship. Goldstein views the beginnings of psychiatry from the vantage point indicated in her subtitle and dismisses the earlier period as "charlatanism"—an opinion worthy of a detailed refutation. French developments have recently been explored in J. Postel and C. Quétel, eds., *Nouvelle histoire de la psychiatrie* (Toulouse: Privat, 1983); see specifically the contributions to chs. 3–5 by Michel Gourévitch, Pierre Morel, Jackie Pigeaud, Jacques Postel, and Claude Quétel. Unfortunately, the bibliographic apparatus in this volume is minimal.

For the **British context,** see R. Porter, *Mind-Forg'd Manacles: A History of Madness in England from the Restoration to the Regency* (London: Athlone, 1987); G. S. Rousseau, "Psychology," in id. and R. Porter, eds., *The Ferment* of Knowledge: Studies in the Historiography of Eighteenth-Century Science (Cambridge, England: Cambridge University Press, 1980), 143–210; R. Porter, W. Bynum, and M. Shepherd, eds., The Anatomy of Madness (3 vols.; New York: Methuen, 1984–1990); A. Scull, Museums of Madness: The Social Organization of Insanity in 19th-Century England (New York: St. Martin's Press, 1979); id., Madhouses, Mad-Doctors and Madmen: The Social History of Psychiatry in the Victorian Era (Philadelphia: University of Pennsylvania Press, 1981); and id., Social Order / Mental Disorder: Anglo American Psychiatry in Historical Perspective (Berkeley and Los Angeles: University of California Press, 1989).

For the **German context,** see M. Schrenk, Über den Umgang mit Geisteskranken: Die Entwicklung der psychiatrischen Therapie vom "moralischen Regime" in England und Frankreich zu den "psychischen Curmethoden" in Deutschland (New York and Heidelberg: Springer, 1973); K. Dörner, Madmen and the Bourgeoisie: A Social History of Insanity (Oxford: Basil Blackwell, 1981), a translation of Bürger und Irre: zur Sozialgeschichte und Wissenschaftssoziologie der Psychiatrie (Frankfurt: Europäische Verlangsanstalt, 1969); and certain aspects of a recent thesis, Ute Frevert, Krankheit als politisches Problem, 1770–1880 (Göttingen: Vandenhoek & Ruprecht, 1984).

Medieval attitudes toward the mentally ill are at last being studied seriously. See, for example, J. Kroll, "A Reappraisal of Psychiatry in the Middle Ages," Archives of General Psychiatry, 1973, 29: 276–283; J. Kroll and B. Bachrach, "Sin and Mental Illness in the Middle-Ages," Psychological Medicine, 1984, 14: 507–514; R. Neugebauer, "Treatment of the Mentally Ill in Medieval and Early Modern England: A Reappraisal," Journal of the History of the Behavioral Sciences, 1978, 14: 158–169; and id., "Diagnosis, Guardianship and Residential Care of the Mentally Ill in Medieval and Early Modern England," American Journal of Psychiatry, 1989, 146: 1580–1584. See also George Rosen, "Western and Central Europe during the late Middle Ages and the Renaissance" and "Irrationality and Madness in Seventeenth- and Eighteenth-Century Europe," in Madness in Society: Chapters in the Historical Sociology of Mental Illness (London: Routledge & Kegan Paul, 1968).

On **hysteria,** see H. Trillat, Histoire de l'hystérie (Paris: Seghers, 1986), and I. Veith, Hysteria: The History of a Disease (Chicago: Chicago University Press, 1965). On witchcraft, see J. S. Neaman, Suggestions of the Devil: The Origins of Madness (Garden City, N.Y.: Doubleday, Anchor Books, 1975).

On the varieties of shelters for real or presumed mental patients, see E. H. Ackerknecht, "Political Prisoners in French Mental Institutions," Medical History, 1975, 19: 250–255, and "Wechselnde Formen der Unterbringung von Geisteskranken," Schweizer Medizinische Wochenschrift, 1964, 93: 1541–1546.

On workhouses, see P. Sérieux, Le quartier d'aliénés du dépôt de mendicité de Soissons au 18ème siècle d'après des documents inédits (Soissons: Acrosse, 1934); Adams, Bureaucrats and Beggars; and H. Mitchell, "Politics in the Service of Knowledge: The Debate over the Administration of Medicine and Welfare in Late Eighteenth-Century France," Social History, 1981, 6: 185–207.

On interdiction, see the authoritative article by F. E. F. Fodéré in Dictionnaire des sciences médicales, 1818, 25: 469–481.

The secondary literature on leaders other than Pinel is fairly sparse. On

Daquin, see C. Caron, *Joseph Daquin et les malades mentaux en Savoie à la fin du 18ème siècle* (Thèse médecine, Lyon, 1964); id., "Les malades mentaux en Savoie à la fin du 18ème siècle," *Information psychiatrique,* 1975, *51:* 887–896; and J. R. Nyffeler, *Joseph Daquin und seine "Philosophie de la folie"* (Zürich: Juris, 1961). The expert on Vincenzo Chiarugi is George Mora, who has supervised translation of *Della pazzia in genere ed in specie* into English as *On Insanity and Its Classification* (Canton, Mass.: Science History Publications, 1987). Mora's Introduction is the best summary of Chiarugi's work. On Switzerland, see also W. Morgenthaler, *Bernisches Irrenwesen, von den Anfängen bis zur Eröffnung des Tollhauses, 1749* (Bern: Grunau, 1915).

On Philippe Pinel's origins and education, see P. Chabbert, "Les années d'étude de Philippe Pinel: Lavaur, Toulouse, Montpellier," *Monspeliensis Hippocrates,* 1960, *3:* 15–23, and D. B. Weiner, "Philippe Pinel, clerc tonsuré," *Annales medico-psychologiques,* 1991, *149:* 169–173.

A governmental decree should be listed first among the **primary sources** that document the **rise of psychiatry** in modern France. It is Jean Colombier and François Doublet, "Observations faites dans le département des hôpitaux civils; Instructions sur la manière de gouverner les insensés, et de travailler à leur guérison dans les asiles qui leur sont destinés," *Journal de médecine, chirurgie et pharmacie,* 1785, *64:* 529–583. Next in importance rank the guidelines followed by the supervisor of the mentally ill men at Bicêtre Hospice; for an English translation see D. B. Weiner, "The Apprenticeship of Philippe Pinel: 'Observations of Citizen Pinel on the Insane,' " *American Journal of Psychiatry,* 1979, *136:* 1128–1134 (the original manuscript is in Archives nationales, 27 AP, dossier 8). For the earliest—and fundamental—paper by Pinel on the subject, see D. B. Weiner, "Philippe Pinel's 'Memoir on Madness' of 11 December 1794: A Fundamental Text of Modern Psychiatry," *American Journal of Psychiatry,* 1992, *149* (6): 725–732 (the original manuscript is in the privately held Fonds Semelaigue.)

Philippe Pinel should be considered as the founder of psychiatry in France. He published three books, of which only the *Traité* was translated into English. See: Philippe Pinel, *Nosographie philosophique, ou Méthode de l'analyse appliquée à la médecine* (Paris: Brosson, 1798; 2d ed., 3 vols., 1802–1803; 3d ed., 1807; 4th ed., 1810; 5th ed., 1813; 6th ed., 1818). A student named Chaude wrote a résumé in Latin of the 5th edition, *Nosographiae compendium* (Paris, 1816).

Id., *Traité médico-philosophique sur l'aliénation mentale ou la manie* (Paris: Caille et Ravier, An VIII [1799–1800]). A second, revised and enlarged edition of the *Traité* was published in 1809 as *Traité médico-philosophique sur l'aliénation mentale, edition entièrement refondue et très augmentée* (Paris: Caille et Ravier, 1800), with the ambiguous phrase "*ou la manie*" dropped from the title. The book was translated into German, Spanish, English, and Italian (in this order): into German by the Hungarian physician Michael Wagner as *Philosophisch-medizinische Abhandlung über Geistesverirrungen oder Manie* (Vienna: Schaumburg, 1801); into Spanish by Dr. Guarnerio y Allavena, *Tratado medico-filosófico de la enagenación del alma or mania* (Madrid: Imprenta real, 1804); into English by Dr. D. D. Davis, under the unsatisfactory title *A Treatise on Insanity* (London: Cadell & Davies, 1806); and into Italian by Dr. C. Vaghi as *Trattato medico-filosofico sopra l'alienazione mentale* (Lodi: Orcasi, 1830).

Id., *La médecine clinique rendue plus précise et plus exacte par l'application de l'analyse, ou Recueil et résultats d'observations sur les maladies aigües, faites à la Salpêtrière* (Paris: Brosson, 1802; 2d ed., 1804; 3d ed., 1815).

On Pinel as a clinical teacher, see Philippe Pinel, *The Clinical Training of Doctors: An Essay of 1793,* ed. and tr. D. B. Weiner (Baltimore: Johns Hopkins University Press, 1980).

The documentation regarding relations between doctors and the government that concern the rise of psychiatry can be found in an appendix entitled "Documents pour servir à l'histoire de la naissance de l'asile, 1797–1811" in M. Gauchet and G. Swain, eds., *Des passions considérées comme causes, symptômes, et moyens curatifs de l'aliénation mentale par D. Esquirol* (Paris: Librairie des deux-mondes, 1980), and the whole period is analyzed in Jacques Postel, *Genèse de la psychiatrie: Les premiers écrits du Philippe Pinel* (Paris: Le sycomore, 1981).

The early activities of J. .E. D. Esquirol are also of great importance in bringing about reform: see his report on a national inquiry entitled *Des établissements des aliénés en France* (Paris: Huzard, 1819), and his "Mémoire historique et statistique sur la maison royale de Charenton," *AHPML,* 1835, *13:* 5–192.

Further primary source material, as well as the secondary literature on Pinel and on Esquirol, can be found in comprehensive bio-bibliographic Notes in D. B. Weiner, "Mind and Body in the Clinic: Philippe Pinel, Alexander Crichton, Dominique Esquirol and the Birth of Psychiatry," in G. S. Rousseau, ed., *The Languages of Psyche: Mind and Body in Enlightenment Thought* (Berkeley and Los Angeles: University of California Press, 1990), 331–402, and in D. B. Weiner, "Philippe Pinel, the Chain-Breaker: History of a Psychiatric Myth," in M. S. Micale and R. Porter, eds., *Discovering the History of Psychiatry* (New York: Oxford University Press, 1993). A comprehensive study, tentatively entitled "Observe and Heal: Philippe Pinel and the Rise of a Humane Public Medicine in Revolutionary and Imperial Paris," will be forthcoming.

10. THE CITIZEN-PATIENT AND THE ENVIRONMENT

Military historians have long ignored medical problems. One searches in vain in the pages of H. Lachouque's *Napoleon's Battles* (London: Allen & Unwin, 1964), for example, or in the 1,170 pages of D. Chandler's *Campaigns of Napoleon* (London: Weidenfeld & Nicolson, 1967) or Alan Forrest's *The Soldiers of the French Revolution* (Durham, N.C.: Duke University Press, 1990) for an informed discussion of medical care as it affected the lives and health of soldiers. On the other hand, some medical historians have dealt with military developments during the French Revolution and under the Empire. Pierre Huard's *Sciences, médecine, pharmacie de la révolution à l'empire,* which reflects the author's own military experience and abounds in charts, inventories, illustrations, capsule biographies, and has a good bibliography, is outstanding. Less ambitious but more focused is R. L. Blanco's *Wellington's Surgeon Gen-*

eral: Sir James McGrigor (Durham, N.C.: Duke University Press, 1974), which, even though it deals with events on the other side of the battle line, treats similar conditions and identical medical problems. D. M. Vess's *Medical Revolution in France, 1789–1796* (Gainesville: University Presses of Florida, 1975) is less satisfactory because it deals only with part of the story; but it draws heavily on military medical sources.

Several members of the French Army Medical Corps outlined its history long ago. See L. J. Bégin, *Etudes sur le service de santé militaire en France* (Paris: Baillière, 1849); Brice and Bottet, *Le corps de santé militaire en France: Son évolution, ses campagnes, 1708–1882* (Paris: Berger-Levrault, 1907); J. des Cilleuls, "Le service de santé militaire des origines à nos jours," *Revue internationale des services de santé des armées de terre, de mer et de l'air,* 1951, *24:* 1–130; P. J. Gama, *Esquisse historique du service de santé militaire en général et spécialement du service chirurgical depuis l'établissement des hôpitaux militaires en France* (Paris: Baillière, 1841). See also S. L. L. Kouchnir, *Considérations sur l'évolution du service de santé militaire de 1789 à 1814* (Thèse médecine, Paris, 1955).

Isser Woloch, *The French Veteran from the Revolution to the Restoration* (Chapel Hill: University of North Carolina Press, 1979), illuminates the health problems of the ailing, maimed, and aging soldier and the financial problems of his widow.

In contrast to the lack of overall accounts, the literature by participants, with details about specific campaigns, diseases, or incidents is very large. The **commanding medical officers** made important contributions to this literature. D. J. Larrey's main writings are "Les rapports originaux de Larrey à l'armée d'Orient," in *Mémoires de l'Institut d'Egypte: Relation historique et chirurgicale de l'expédition de l'armée d'Orient en Egypte et en Syrie* (Paris: Demonville, 1803); *Clinique chirurgicale, 1792–1829* (5 vols.; Paris: Gabon, 1829–1836); and *Mémoires de chirurgie militaire, 1812–1817* (4 vols.; Paris: Buisson, 1812). The principal writings of N. R. D. Desgenettes include *Histoire médicale de l'armée d'orient* (Paris: Crouillebois, 1802; 2d ed., Firmin Didot, 1830). P. F. Percy's major writings are *Journal des campagnes du baron Percy, chirurgien-en-chef de la grande armée (1745–1825)* (Paris: Plon, 1904). P. F. Keraudren wrote *Mémoire sur les causes des maladies des marins et sur les soins à prendre pour conserver leur santé dans les ports et à la mer* (Paris: Imprimerie royale, 1817; 2d ed., 1824) and *De la fièvre jaune observée aux Antilles et sur les vaissaux du roi, considérée principalement sous le rapport de sa transmission* (Paris: Imprimerie royale, 1823). Keraudren was one of the founders of *Annales d'hygiène publique et de médecine légale* in 1829, and discussed the health of sailors in the article on "Naval Hydrography" that he contributed to the *Dictionnaire des sciences médicales* in 1818.

The overall official history of the **Egyptian Expedition** is C. de La Jonquière, ed., *L'expédition d'Egypte* (5 vols.; Paris: Charles Lanauzelle, 1899–1907). Two interesting brief articles are F. Charles-Roux, "Le but colonial de l'expédition française en Egypte," *Revue des études napoléoniennes,* 1924, *22:* 122–139, and J. Lasserre, "A l'armée d'Egypte: Discipline, récompenses diverses, et armes d'honneur," ibid., 1930, *30,* 99–121.

The literature on the medical aspects of the Egyptian campaign is very large. See A. Gerard, "Bonaparte et le service de santé au cours de la campagne d'Egypte," *Histoire des sciences médicales*, 1974, *8*: 99–129; L. Houdard, "Le service de santé de l'armée d'Egypte," *Revue des études napoléoniennes*, 1934, *38*: 84–96, 160–168, 214–226, *39*: 37–50, 180–195, 1935, *40*: 153–168, 236–246, *41*: 16–27; P. Saint-Girons, "Le service de santé pendant l'expédition d'Egypte," *Histoire de la médecine*, 1952, 7 (July): 58–64.

The literature on the expedition to the Antilles and **yellow fever** is also voluminous: see N. P. Gilbert, *Histoire médicale de l'armée française à St. Domingue en l'An X ou Mémoire sur la fièvre jaune* (Paris: Gabon, 1803); J. Lefort, *Mémoire sur la fièvre jaune* (Paris: Colas, 1809); id., *Mémoire sur la non-contagion de la fièvre jaune* (St. Pierre: Fleurot, 1823); and J. F. X. Pugnet, *Mémoire sur les fièvres de mauvais caractère du Levant et des Antilles avec un aperçu physique et médical du Sayd et un essai sur la topographie de Sainte-Lucie* (Lyon: Reymannet, 1804). For a review of the literature about the contagiousness of yellow fever, see G. D. Sussman, "From Yellow Fever to Cholera: A Study of French Government Policy, Medical Professionalism, and Popular Movements in the Epidemic Crises of the Restoration and the July Monarchy" (Ph.D. diss., Yale University, 1971).

For medical information dealing with the the the **first Italian campaign,** see L. Houdard, "La situation sanitaire au siège de Mantoue, 1796–1797," *Revue des études napoléoniennes,* 1930, *29*: 101–110; on the wars in Germany and Russia, see R. Lacronique, "Mesures d'hygiène et de prophylaxie prescrites à l'armée d'Allemagne, 1810–1812," *La France médicale,* 25 October 1904, *51*: 377–384; P. Blouin, *Service de santé et ravitaillement de la grande armée pendant la campagne de 1812* (Thèse médecine, Paris, 1955); and H. Roos, *Souvenirs d'un médecin de la grande armée* (Paris: Perrin, 1913).

There was an outpouring of **medical literature after the wars** (and not only on the French side). This includes the diaries of S. Blaze, J. R. L. de Kerckhoffs, and H. Roos; monographs, often dealing with "fevers," by F. Boussenard, Gilbert, J. .F. X. Pugnet, F. Ruette, and L. Valentin; manuals by J. J. Martin, F. V. Pallois, and E. B. Révolat; theses by Blouin, M. G. Lachese, H. Millioz, G. Pergot, and F. C. Pouqueville; and works dealing with plague, ophthalmia, and other communicable diseases during the Egyptian campaign by P. Assalini, Bayon, L. Bruant, Chevalier, and G. N. Renati. For complete citations, see D. B. Weiner, "French Doctors Face War: 1792–1815," in *From the Ancien Régime to the Popular Front: Essays in the History of Modern France in Honor of Shepard B. Clough,* ed. C. K. Warner (New York: Columbia University Press, 1969), 51–73.

No attempt is made here to analyze the problem of vaccination in depth. This has recently been done by Yves-Marie Bercé, *Le chaudron et la lancette: Croyances populaires et médecine préventive, 1798–1830* (Paris: Presses de la Renaissance, 1984), and Pierre Darmon, *La longue traque de la variole: Les pionniers de la médecine préventive* (Paris: Perrin, 1986). Darmon discusses the trials of immunization in great detail, including those at the Salpêtrière (pp. 142, 166, and 181). Bercé investigates the popular and international level of acceptance toward vaccination. The background was also explored long ago by G. Miller in *The Adoption of Inoculation for Smallpox in England and France* (Philadelphia: University of Pennsylvania Press, 1957).

American historians of medicine have contributed fundamental work on public health during this era. George Rosen delved deeply into the background and context of the topic (see "Secondary Publications," above). Turning to the nineteenth century, Rosen discussed "What Is Social Medicine? A Genetic Analysis of the Concept," *BHM*, 1947, *21*: 674–733, where he gives a wide berth to Virchow's and Pettenkoffer's Germany. In a chapter in *The Victorian City*, ed. H. J. Dyos and M. Wolff (2 vols.; London: Routledge & Kegan Paul, 1973), vol. 2, 625–667, he analyzed "Death, Debility and Death" in Edwin Chadwick's and Sir John Simon's England.

William Coleman approached the problem from the point of view of demography and public policy. See his "Inventing Demography: Montyon on Hygiene and the State," in *Transformation and Tradition in the Sciences: Essays in Honor of I. B. Cohen*, ed. E. Mendelsohn (Cambridge, Mass.: Harvard University Press, 1984); "Health and Hygiene in the *Encyclopédie*: A Medical Doctrine for the Bourgeoisie," *JHM*, 1974, *29*: 399–421; and especially his book, *Death Is a Social Disease*.

E. H. Ackerknecht is the American expert on the medical history of this period, who—apart from work noted elsewhere in this book—contributed the fundamental articles "Hygiene in France, 1815–1848," *BHM*, 1948, 117–155, and "Anticontagionism between 1821 and 1867," *BHM*, 1948, *22*: 562–593.

Ann LaBerge's published contributions to this topic include "The Paris Health Council, 1802–1848," *BHM*, 1975, *49*: 339–352; "A. J. B. Parent-Duchâtelet: Hygienist of Paris, 1821–1836," *Clio medica*, 1977, *12*: 279–301; "The Early Nineteenth-Century French Public Health Movement: The Disciplinary Development and Institutionalization of *Hygiène publique*," *BHM*, 1984, *58*: 363–379; and "Edwin Chadwick and the French Connection," *BHM*, 1988, *62*: 23–41. An overview of modern public health by Dorothy Porter is forthcoming.

The secondary literature on the Public Health Council is scarce. A sketchy outline of its structure and work is given in J. François and F. Prunet, *Le conseil d'hygiène et de salubrité de la Seine* (Paris: Préfecture de police, 1935). The best account so far is to be found in the early chapters of Anne F. La Berge, "Public Health in France and the Public Health Movement, 1815–1848" (Ph.D. diss., University of Tennessee, 1973). See also D. B. Weiner, "Public Health under Napoleon: The Conseil de salubrité de Paris, 1802–1815," *Clio medica*, 1974, *9*: 271–284.

Abbreviations and Acronyms

AAPP	Archives de l'Assistance publique
AAPP, CFNS	AAPP, Catalogue Fosseyeux, nouvelle série
AHPML	*Annales d'hygiène publique et de médecine légale*
AN	Archives nationales, Paris
AP	*Archives parlementaires, ou Moniteur universel de 1787 à 1860,* ed. J. Mavidal and E. Laurent (87 vols.; Paris: Dupont, 1862–1914), 1st ser., 1789–1799
APPP	Archives de la Préfecture de police, Paris
BHM	*Bulletin of the History of Medicine*
BhVdP	Bibliothèque historique de la Ville de Paris
BN	Bibliothèque nationale
CGAHHCP	[Seine] Conseil général d'administration des hôpitaux et hospices civils de Paris
EA	[Archives de la Seine] Enfants assistés
JHM	*Journal of the History of Medicine and Allied Sciences*
PVR	[France] Ministère de l'instruction publique, *Procès-verbaux et rapports du comité de mendicité de la Constituante, 1790– 1791,* ed. C. Bloch and A. Tuetey (Paris: Imprimerie nationale, 1911)
TA	A. Tuetey, ed., *L'Assistance publique à Paris pendant la révolution* (4 vols.; Paris: Imprimerie nationale, 1895–1987).
TM	Jacques Tenon, *Mémoires sur les hôpitaux de Paris* (Paris: Pierres, 1788)

Notes

Introduction

1. France, Ministère de l'instruction publique, *Procès-verbaux et rapports du comité de mendicité de la Constituante, 1790–1791*, ed. C. Bloch and A. Tuetey (Paris: Imprimerie nationale, 1911) (henceforth cited as *PVR*), 391.

2. Pierre Louis Prieur de la Marne in *Archives parlementaires, ou Moniteur universel de 1787 à 1860*, ed. J. Mavidal and E. Laurent (87 vols.; Paris: Dupont, 1862–1914), 1st ser. 1789–1799 (henceforth cited as *AP*), vol. 28, 489.

3. This topic was first addressed over twenty years ago in D. B. Weiner, "Le droit de l'homme à la santé: Une belle idée devant l'assemblée constituante," *Clio medica*, 1970, *5*: 209–233.

4. This has now taken shape: see the last four chapters of Jean Imbert, ed., *Histoire des hôpitaux en France* (Toulouse: Privat, 1982).

5. Revolutionary dates will be used sparingly in this book whenever reference to the sources requires them. For the Revolutionary calendar, see Appendix B.

6. In an insightful review article, Isser Woloch has recently pointed to the controlling features of the Revolution in its early stages. See "On the Latent Illiberalism of the French Revolution," *American Historical Review*, 1990, *95*: 1452–1470.

7. J. Léonard, *La médecine entre les pouvoirs et les savoirs: Histoire intellectuelle et politique de la médecine française au 19ème siècle* (Paris: Aubier Montaigne, 1981), 13.

8. Henry E. Sigerist, *Medicine and Human Welfare* (New Haven, Conn.: Yale University Press, 1941), 96.

9. Jean Imbert, "L'Assistance publique à Paris de la révolution française à 1977," in *L'administration de Paris: Colloque tenu au Conseil d'état le 6 mai 1978* (Paris: Centre de recherche d'histoire et de philosophie de la 4ème section de EPHE, 1979), 79–107.

10. Jean Imbert et al., *La protection sociale sous la révolution française* (Paris: Association pour l'étude de l'histoire de la sécurité sociale, 1990). See Bib. Ess., Secondary Publications.

11. The special role of the French capital in shaping men, ideas, and methods is well portrayed in R. C. Maulitz, *Morbid Appearances: The Anatomy of Pathology in the Early Nineteenth Century* (Cambridge: Cambridge University

Press, 1987), and in J. H. Warner, "The Selective Transport of Medical Knowledge: Antebellum American Physicians and Parisian Medical Therapeutics," *Bulletin of the History of Medicine* (henceforth cited as *BHM*), 1985, *59*: 213–231.

12. That is Erwin Ackerknecht's argument in *Medicine at the Paris Hospital, 1794–1848* (Baltimore: Johns Hopkins Press, 1967).

13. See Colin Jones, "Picking up the Pieces: The Politics and the Personnel of Social Welfare from the Convention to the Consulate," in *Beyond the Terror: Essays in French Regional and Social History, 1794–1815*, ed. G. Lewis and C. Lucas (Cambridge: Cambridge University Press, 1983), 53–91.

14. David M. Vess, *Medical Revolution in France, 1789–1796* (Gainesville: University Presses of Florida, 1975).

15. See Ann F. LaBerge, *Mission and Method: The Early Nineteenth-Century French Public Health Movement* (New York: Cambridge University Press, 1992).

16. N. J. Jewson, "The Disappearance of the Sick-Man from Medical Cosmology, 1770–1870," *Sociology*, 1976, *10*: 225–244.

17. See ch. 9, "Birth of the Asylum," in *Folie et déraison: Histoire de la folie à l'âge classique* (Paris: Plon, 1961), tr. R. Howard as *Madness and Civilization: A History of Insanity in the Age of Reason* (New York: Random House, 1973). The three other books from Foucault's large opus of particular relevance here are *Naissance de la clinique: Archéologie du regard médical* (Paris: Presses universitaires de France, 1963), tr. A. Sheridan as *Birth of the Clinic: An Archeology of Medical Perception* (New York: Random House 1975); *Surveiller et punir: Naissance de la prison* (Paris: Gallimard, 1975), tr. A. Sheridan as *Discipline and Punish: The Birth of the Prison* (New York: Random House, 1977); and Foucault et al., *Les machines à guérir* (Paris: Institut de l'environnement, Dossiers et documents d'architecture, 1976). Foucault scholarship is fraught with problems. For example, *clinique* in *Naissance de la clinique*, refers to clinical teaching, so that the translation *Birth of the Clinic* is totally misleading.

18. François Furet, *Penser la révolution française* (Paris: Gallimard, 1978), tr. Elborg Forster as *Reinterpreting the French Revolution* (Cambridge: Cambridge University Press, 1981).

19. René Dubos, *The Mirage of Health: Utopias, Progress and Biological Change* (New York: Harper & Brothers, 1959).

Chapter 1. Enlightened Innovation

1. C. L. de S. de Montesquieu, *The Spirit of the Laws,* tr. Th. Nugent (New York: Hafner, 1949), bk. 33, ch. 29, 25; emphasis added.

2. Denis Diderot, "Lettre sur les aveugles à l'usage de ceux qui voient," in *Oeuvres* (20 vols.; Paris: Brière, 1821), vol. 1, 283–382, and *Lettre sur les sourds-muets à l'usage de ceux qui entendent et qui parlent*, ed. O. Fellows, Diderot Studies, no. 7 (Geneva: Droz, 1965).

3. Denis Diderot, "Hôtel-Dieu," in *Encyclopédie, ou Dictionnaire raisonné des sciences, des arts, et des métiers* (35 vols.; Lausanne and Berne: Chez les so-

ciétés typographiques, 1782), vol. 17, 761–762. Terms such as "pestilential germs" were freely and loosely used at the time.

4. A. R. J. Turgot, "Fondation," in ibid., vol. 14, 892–899, passim.

5. P. S. Dupont de Nemours, *Idées sur les secours à donner aux pauvres malades dans une grande ville comme Philadelphie* (Paris: Moutard, 1786).

6. Claude Piarron de Chamousset, "Plan d'une maison d'association dans laquelle au moyen d'une somme très modique chaque associé s'assurera dans l'état de maladie toutes les sortes de secours qu'on peut désirer," in *Vues d'un citoyen* (Paris: Lambert, 1757), 35–77.

7. *Encyclopédie*, vol. 12, 911. The article, signed "A.," is presumably by Arnulfe d'Aumont.

8. An order-in-council of 9 February 1776 stated, for example, that instead of 742 small and 32 large boxes with 932,000 doses of drugs, a total of 2,258 boxes would be sent out that year. See France, *Recueil général des anciennes lois françaises, depuis l'an 420 jusqu'à la révolution de 1789 . . .* , ed. J. A. J. Léger et al. (29 vols.; Paris: Belin-le-Prieur, 1824–1857), vol. 22, 328.

9. Y. Knibiehler and C. Fouquet, *La femme et les médecins* (Paris: Hachette, 1983), 181.

10. G. Rosen, "Cameralism and the Concept of Medical Police," *BHM*, 1953, *27*: 21–42. On Rosen, see Bib. Ess., Secondary Publications.

11. Johann Peter Frank, *System einer vollständigen medizinischen Polizei* (6 vols.; Mannheim, Tübingen, and Vienna: Schwann, Cotta & Schaumburg, 1779–1819). See also E. Lesky, *Johann Peter Frank: Seine Selbstbiographie* (Stuttgart: Hans Huber Bern, 1969).

12. C. C. Gillispie, *Science and Polity in France at the End of the Old Regime* (Princeton: Princeton University Press, 1980).

13. A. Chéreau, s.v. "Parmentier," in A. Dechambre, ed., *Dictionnaire encyclopédique des sciences médicales*. See also Chapter 10.

14. R. Rappaport, "Lavoisier's Geological Activities," *Isis*, 1968, *58*: 375–384.

15. D. I. Duveen and H. S. Klickstein, "Antoine Laurent Lavoisier's Contribution to Medicine and Public Health," *BHM*, 1955, *29*: 164–179, esp. 164–165.

16. See Société royale de médecine, *Histoire et mémoires de médecine et de physique médicale* (10 vols.; Paris: Pierres, 1776–1789).

17. There is no full-length biography of Vicq d'Azyr. See Bib. Ess., Enlightened Innovation.

18. Société royale de médecine, *Histoire et mémoires*, vol. 9, 47–327 and 328–414.

19. Ibid., xv.

20. Pinel withdrew this essay from publication in order to use it in a book.

21. The materials for this "national medical topography," still extant in the archives of the Paris Academy of Medicine, are incomplete and have never been published. But much of the correspondence and many of the papers appeared between 1776 and 1789 in Société royale de médecine, *Histoire et mémoires*.

22. "Plumitif de la Société royale de médecine, du 24 juillet 1789 au 19 août 1793," Archives de l'Académie nationale de médecine, vol. 11 *bis*.

23. "Nouveau plan de constitution pour la médecine en France," in Société royale de médecine, *Histoire et mémoires*, vol. 9, 1–201. The manuscript is in the Archives nationales (henceforth cited as AN), F^{17}, 1310. The plan was translated into German as early as 1791 by M. J. J. Mederer von Wutwehr (Prague & Leipzig: n.p., 1791).

24. "Nouveau plan," pt. I, sec. 2, passim. Science was viewed as basic to medicine.

25. Ibid., 61 and 26.

26. Ibid., 69–70.

27. Ibid., 68, 62, 102.

28. Ibid., 143–145, passim.

29. P. J. G. Cabanis, "Rapports du physique et du moral de l'homme," in *Oeuvres philosophiques*, ed. C. Lehec and J. Cazeneuve (2 vols.; Paris: Presses universitaires de France, 1956), vol. 1, 142. See also Bib. Ess., Enlightened Innovation.

30. J. L. Moreau de la Sarthe, *Histoire naturelle de la femme, suivie d'un traité d'hygiène appliquée à son régime physique et moral aux différentes époques de la vie* (2 vols. in 3; Paris: Duprat, Letellier, 1803). See also his *Esquisse d'un cours d'hygiène, ou de médecine appliquée à l'art d'user de la vie et de conserver la santé; extrait d'une partie des leçons d'hygiène faites pour la première fois au Lycée républicain, en l'An VIII* (Paris: n.p., [1799–1800]).

31. *La décade philosophique, littéraire, et politique, par une Société de républicains* (later *gens de lettres*) (Paris: An II–1807).

32. P. J. G. Cabanis, "Observations sur les hôpitaux," in *Oeuvres philosophiques*, vol. 1, 3–31, passim.

33. N. Chambon de Montaux, *Moyens de rendre les hôpitaux plus utiles à la nation* (Paris: Hôtel Serpente, 1787); C. F. Duchanoy and J. B. Jumelin, "Mémoire sur l'utilité d'une école clinique de médecine," suivi de "Idée d'un plan d'études en médecine sous le titre d'école clinique," *Journal de physique: Observations et mémoires sur la physique, sur l'histoire naturelle et sur les arts*, 1778, *13*: 277–286; G. C. Würtz, *Mémoire sur l'établissement des écoles de médecine pratique à former dans les principaux hôpitaux civils de la France à l'instar de celle de Vienne, pour perfectionner l'art de médecine pratique et la faciliter aux jeunes médecins* (Paris: Didot Jeune, 1784; Strasbourg: Treuttel, 1784).

34. S. A. Tissot, *Essai sur les moyens de perfectionner les études de médecine* (Lausanne: Mourer, 1785); J. P. Frank, *Plan d'école clinique ou Méthode d'enseigner la pratique de la médecine dans un hôpital académique* (Vienna: Wappler, 1790).

35. Cabanis, "Observations sur les hôpitaux," 16–23, passim.

36. Ibid., 16 n. 1.

37. "Procès-verbal de ce qui s'est passé relativement à l'incendie de l'Hôtel-Dieu, le mercredi 30 décembre 1772" (MS, Archives, Musée de l'oeuvre Notre-Dame de Paris. fol. 458, 461–462). I wish to thank M. Pierre Joly, archivist, for kindly communicating this document to me. On the fire, see also A. Chevalier, *L'Hôtel-Dieu de Paris et les soeurs Augustines, 650-1810* (Paris:

Champion, 1901), 476–485, and Rondonneau de la Motte, *Essai historique sur l'Hôtel-Dieu de Paris* (Paris: Nyon, 1787).

38. C. P. Coquéau, *Mémoire sur la nécessité de transférer et reconstruire l'Hôtel-Dieu de Paris, suivi d'un projet de translation de cet hôpital, proposé par le sieur Poyet, architecte et contrôleur des bâtiments de la ville* (Paris: n.p., 1785), and id., *Essai sur l'établissement des hôpitaux dans les grandes villes* (Paris: Desenne, 1787).

39. Jacques Tenon, "Un instrument qui facilite la curation," in *Mémoires sur les hôpitaux de Paris* (Paris: Pierres, 1788) (henceforth cited as *TM*), 53 and 393.

40. In the nineteenth century this architectural layout was widely adopted, in hospitals such as St. André in Bordeaux (1821), St. Jean in Brussels (1848), and Lariboisière in Paris (1846–1854).

41. Marcel Fosseyeux, *L'Hôtel-Dieu de Paris au 17ème et 18ème siècles* (Paris: Berger-Levrault, 1912), 262.

42. Ackerknecht, *Medicine at the Paris Hospital*, 17.

43. Pierre Huard and M. J. Imbault-Huart, "De l'hospice de perfectionnement de l'Académie royale de chirurgie à l'Hôpital des cliniques de la Faculté de médecine de Paris (1775–1876)," *Bulletin de la Société française d'histoire des hôpitaux*, 1972, *27*: 37–47; the quotation appears on 37. The initiative came from the king, prodded by his first surgeon, Germain Pichaut de la Martinière (1696–1783) (but the original idea was Tenon's). Louis XV endowed the first six beds, his grandson Louis XVI six more, and La Martinière contributed an additional ten. It took ten years to bring the project to fruition.

44. *TM*, 52–53.

45. See T. Gelfand, *Professionalizing Modern Medicine: Paris Surgeons and Medical Science and Institutions in the Eighteenth Century* (Westport, Conn.: Greenwood Press, 1980).

46. The fundamental contemporary account is J. Colombier and F. Doublet, "Observations faites dans le département des hôpitaux civils: Institution de l'hospice des Enfants trouvés atteints de la maladie vénérienne faite à Paris en 1780," *Journal de médecine, chirurgie, pharmacie, etc.*, 1785, *63*: 289–336, 445–483; *64*: 3–41, 169–229. See also H. Asselin, *L'Hospice de Vaugirard: Une expérience hospitalière au 18ème siècle* (Thèse, Ecole pratique des hautes études, Paris, 1961); *PVR*, 592; *TM*, 82; A. Tuetey, ed., *L'Assistance publique à Paris pendant la révolution* (4 vols.; Paris: Imprimerie nationale, 1895–1987) (henceforth cited as *TA*), vol. 1, lv–lix and Nos. 119–120; and P. Valléry-Radot, *Deux siècles d'histoire hospitalière* (Paris: Dupont, 1947), 172–173.

47. *TA*, vol. 1, lvi.

48. *PVR*, 593.

49. See AN, F¹⁵, 397, and *TA*, vol. 1, 505–527.

50. Seine, Conseil général d'administration des hôpitaux et hospices civils de Paris (henceforth CGAHHCP), *Rapports au conseil général des hospices sur les hôpitaux et hospices, les secours à domicile, et la direction des nourrices* (Paris: Imprimerie des hospices civils, An XI [1803]), 50.

51. *PVR*, 266–267.

52. Seine, CGAHHCP, *Rapport fait au conseil général des hospices par un de*

ses membres sur l'état des hôpitaux, des hospices, et des secours à domicile, à Paris, depuis le 1er janvier 1804 jusqu'au 1er janvier 1814 (Paris: Imprimerie de Mme Huzard, 1816), 46.

53. *PVR*, 662.

54. *PVR*, 663–665; *TA*, vol. 1, 529–546; *TM*, 59; Valléry-Radot, *Deux siècles*, 151–157.

55. On Beaujon Hospital, see *TM*, 98–100;

56. *PVR*, 665–666. No reasons are given why the Poverty Committee's site visitors did not inspect the parish hospital of St. André des Arts. On St. André des Arts, see *TA*, vol. 1, cv.

57. *TM*, 48.

58. S. S. Kottek, "The Hospital in Jewish History," *Review of Infectious Diseases*, 1981, *3*: 636–639, and R. R. Marcus, *Communal Sick-Care in the German Ghetto* (Cincinnati: Hebrew Union College Press, 1947).

59. These Observations were published in the *Journal de médecine, chirurgie, et pharmacie*. On Vaugirard Hospital, see p. 37 above.

60. Paris, Hôpital général, Maison de la Salpêtrière, *Règlement provisoire pour les infirmeries* (Paris: Imprimerie royale, [internal evidence suggests 1785]). This text is found in Archives de l'Assistance publique (henceforth cited as AAPP), C 278.

61. Jean Colombier, *Traité général de médecine militaire* (7 vols.; Paris: Didot Jeune, 1778).

62. These men will all appear in Chapter 3, except for Antoine Poissonnier-Despierrières, who served in Santo Domingo for several years. He wrote *Traité des fièvres de l'île de St. Domingue* (Paris: Cavelier, 1763) and *Traité sur les maladies des gens de mer* (Paris: Lacombe, 1767).

63. Pierre Poissonnier, Parmentier, and Bayen.

64. Coste, Pierre Poissonnier, Bayen.

65. For naval medicine, see the initial chapters of J. Léonard, *Les officiers de santé de la marine française, de 1814 à 1835* (Paris: Klincksieck, 1967).

66. See, e.g, O. Keel, "The Politics of Health and the Institutionalization of Clinical Practices in Europe in the Second Half of the Eighteenth Century," in W. F. Bynum and R. Porter, eds., *William Hunter and the Eighteenth-Century Medical World* (Cambridge: Cambridge University Press, 1985), 207–258, and U. Tröhler, "Britische Spitäler und Polikliniken as Heil- und Forschungsstätten, 1720–1820," *Gesnerus*, 1982, *39*: 115–131.

67. *TM*, 94–98.

68. *TM*, 45–47, and *PVR*, 668–671.

69. *TM*, 47.

70. *TM*, 285.

71. On the Foundlings' Hospice, see Chapter 2; on the Venereal Diseases Hospital, see Chapter 5; on the deaf and the blind, see Chapter 8.

72. See Tenon's Fifth Memoir.

73. These architectural improvements are discussed further at the beginning of Chapter 6.

74. For the Religieuses hospitalières de la charité de Notre-Dame, known

as Religieuses hospitalières de la Place royale, see AN, S 6148, and *TA*, vol. 1, 641–673; for the Religieuses hospitalières de St. Joseph, known as Religieuses hospitalières de la Roquette, see AN, S 6149, and *TA*, vol. 1, 674–691; for the Religieuses hospitalières de la miséricorde, known as Religieuses hospitalières de la rue Mouffetard, see AN, S 6145, and *TA*, vol. 1, 692–717; for the Religieuses hospitalières de St. Mandé, see *TA*, vol. 1, 718–720; their inventory has not been found. See also *PVR*, 674–676.

75. *PVR*, 657–658; *TM*, 42; Valléry-Radot, *Deux siècles*, 157–162, but especially J. Couteaux, *La maison de retraite de la Rochefoucauld* (Paris: Solsona, 1926). Regarding the controversy over the initiative to undertake this project, see abbé de Boismont, *Maison de santé: Sermon pour l'assemblée extraordinaire de charité qui s'est tenue à Paris, à l'occasion de l'établissement d'une Maison royale de santé en faveur des Ecclésiastiques et Militaires malades prononcé dans l'Eglise des religieux de la Charité, le 13 mars 1782* (Paris: Imprimerie royale, 1782).

Chapter 2. The Grim Reality of the Public Hospital

1. F. Dreyfus, *Un philanthrope d'autrefois: La Rochefoucauld-Liancourt, 1747–1827* (Paris: Plon-Nourrit, 1903), 14.

2. For example, on 12 January 1791, he dictated twenty-six letters, and on the 19th, twenty-nine (*PVR*, 228–230). An overview of his wide range of humanitarian activities can be gained from *PVR*, xii–xiv.

3. The feud harks back to two factions among health reformers. One of these, grouped around Jacques Necker, wanted existing institutions renovated, not replaced. Liancourt, Colombier, and Thouret belonged to this group. The other was loyal to the baron de Breteuil, minister of the king's household and linked closely to the Academy of Sciences. Tenon was closely identified with this group, advocating new buildings and vast expenditures. Thouret and Tenon were thus at odds. See esp. L. S. Greenbaum, "Jean Sylvain Bailly, the Baron de Breteuil and the 'Four New Hospitals' of Paris," *Clio medica*, 1973, *8*: 261–284, and "Jacques Necker and the Reform of the Paris Hospitals on the Eve of the French Revolution," ibid., 1984, *19*: 216–230.

4. *PVR*, 255.

5. *PVR*, 97–98, 147–148, 282.

6. *TM*, 175–176, 300.

7. *PVR*, 5.

8. M. Möring, C. Quentin, and L. Brièle, eds., *Délibérations de l'ancien Hôtel-Dieu* (Paris: Imprimerie nationale, 1881), vol. 2, 271.

9. De Coulmiers, a Premonstrant priest, became the administrator of the Charité de Charenton and thus exerted considerable influence over the emergence of hospital psychiatry. Prieur de la Marne, a member of the Committee of Public Safety, stands out as the advocate of legislation for the handicapped, and Massieu, curate of Cergy, a juring priest, remained active all his life in education and politics.

10. Other useful experience came with the cooptation of P. F. de Boncerf

(1736–18 ?) and A. B. du Tremblay de Rubelles (1745–1819), both of them financiers and administrators, and of Lambert, the inspector of apprentices for the Hôpital général.

11. J. B. A. Villoutreix de Faye (1739–1792?), bishop of Oloron; Seignelay-Colbert de Castle-Hill (1736–1813), bishop of Rodez; and Lucien David (1730–18 ?).

12. Louis de Bonnefoy (1748–1797).

13. Jean Baptiste de Cretot (1743–1817).

14. [Guillotin], *Pétition des citoyens domiciliés à Paris, du 8 décembre 1788* (Paris: Clousier, 1788). The event that made Guillotin notorious forever, the parliamentary debate on "the mechanical device" for beheading criminals sentenced to death, occurred on 10 October 1789. For more on Guillotin, see Chapter 3.

15. The other was Henri, comte de Virieu (1754–1793).

16. Périsse du Luc will reappear in this study as a defender of the deaf and blind.

17. For more biographic data on these Poverty Committee members, see *PVR*, xiii–xix.

18. "Rapport fait au nom du Comité de mendicité des visites faites dans divers hôpitaux, hospices, et maisons de charité de Paris, par M. de la Rochefoucauld-Liancourt, député du département de l'Oise," in *PVR*, 575–693.

19. L. MacAuliffe, *La révolution et les hôpitaux, Années 1789, 1790, 1791* (Paris: Bellais, 1901), 44.

20. That is Tenon's figure. He says that Necker, the finance minister, gave "between 640- and 680,000, and he would take the mean" (*TM*, 24). Marcel Reinhard is no more precise (see "La démographie parisienne," in *La révolution française* [Paris: Hachette, 1971], 117–120). See also "Paris," in M. Marion, *Dictionnaire des institutions de la France au 17ème et 18ème siècle* (Paris: Picard, 1972).

21. *TM*, 24–25.

22. This received wisdom has recently been challenged. In a study of the Hôtel-Dieu of Nîmes, Colin Jones found hospital stays of reasonable length and an adequate number of recoveries. It may well be that size and location made the Paris Hôtel-Dieu exceptional, and that once again the example of the capital has overshadowed provincial reality and determined historians' perceptions. Our traditional notions of the hospital and hospice as one horrible *mouroir* may have to be revised in the light of scholarly evidence. C. Jones and M. Sonenscher, "The Social Functions of the Hospital in Eighteenth-Century France: The Case of the Hôtel-Dieu of Nîmes," *French Historical Studies*, 1983, *13*: 172–214.

23. *TM*, 198.

24. *TM*, 238.

25. *PVR*, 603.

26. The bishop of Rodez wrote the report. *PVR*, 637–648.

27. The board of trustees included the first presidents of the *parlement* of Paris and of the chambers of accounts and taxes, the chief prosecutor, the lieu-

tenant general of police, and the provost of merchants. In 1790, the mayor of Paris took the place of the representatives of the police and of the merchants.

28. They knew that the hospital board was trying to resign, but had stayed on at the National Assembly's request. (On 15 April 1791, its decision became final.)

29. Tenon's *Mémoires* remain the paramount source of detailed information about the Hôtel-Dieu under the old regime. See also Marcel Fosseyeux, "L'Hôtel-Dieu de Paris sous la révolution, 1789–1802," *La révolution française*, 1912, *66*: 40–85.

30. *PVR*, 638.

31. *TM*, 278, n. 45.

32. *TM*, 224.

33. *TM*, 642.

34. *TM*, preface, xix.

35. *TM*, 244.

36. *TM*, 130.

37. *TM*, 131, n.2.

38. Möring, Quentin, and Brièle, *Délibérations*, vol. 2, 12.

39. *TM*, preface, xx, 169.

40. See also F. Boinet, *Le lit d'hôpital en France. Etude historique* (Paris: Thèse médecine, 1945).

41. Möring, Quentin, and Brièle, *Délibérations*, vol. 2, 251.

42. *TM*, 314–315.

43. *PVR*, 639.

44. N. E. Clavareau, *Mémoires sur les hôpitaux civils de Paris* (Paris: Prault, 1805): see, e.g., his preface.

45. L. S. Greenbaum, "Science, Medicine, Religion: Three Views of Health Care in France on the Eve of the French Revolution," *Studies in Eighteenth-Century Culture*, ed. H. C. Payne, 1981, *10*: 380. See also *TM*, 136–137 and 152–155, and *TA*, vol. 1, 108, "Etat général des lits existant dans les différentes salles de l'Hôtel-Dieu, le 12 avril 1790."

46. Möring, Quentin, and Brièle, *Délibérations*, vol. 2, 273.

47. *PVR*, 642.

48. Möring, Quentin, and Brièle, *Délibérations*, vol. 2, 272.

49. On the history of St. Louis, see Bib. Ess., Grim Reality, and *TM*, 60–73; *TA*, vol. 1, 146–149; *PVR*, 647–648. On dermatology, see Chapter 6.

50. For a brief reference, see *PVR*, 648–649.

51. See *PVR*, 649–653; *TM*, 75–80; *TA*, vol. 1, 150–170; See also P. Bourée, "Heurs et malheurs de l'Hospice des Incurables," *Histoire des sciences médicales*, 1974, *8*: 535–539.

52. *PVR*, 652.

53. *PVR*, 653.

54. *TM*, 80.

55. Seine, CGAHHCP, *Rapports au conseil général* (1803), 113.

56. *PVR*, 653.

57. *PVR*, 575–636.

58. See the report about the maison de Scipion, dated 23 April 1790, by Regnard, printed in *TA*, vol. 1, 377–388; about Bicêtre, dated 30 April 1790, by Jean Antoine Hagnon, in *TA*, vol. 1, 230–253; about the Pitié, dated 17 May 1790, in *TA*, vol. 1, 175–188, with a cover letter from the administrators of the Hôpital général, the main report unsigned, and the accompanying report by Anne Brun; about the Salpêtrière, dated 19 May 1790, by Jean François Doumey, *TA*, vol. 1, 265–283. (The usual spelling is "Dommey," but Tuetey's index specifies "Doumey.") All the original documents are to be found in AN, F¹⁵, 1861.

59. *PVR*, 578–579. Some slaughtering, as we have seen, was done at the Hôtel-Dieu.

60. On Bicêtre, see Bib. Ess., Grim Reality, and *PVR*, 598–614, *TA*, vol. 1, lxv–lxxvi, and 196–261. The original documents are to be found in AN, F¹⁵, 1861.

61. *PVR*, 598–599.

62. Eighteen of the prisoners and thirty-two of the mentally ill had families who contributed to their upkeep; about forty pensioners lived there by choice and paid between 100 and 400 livres per year. *TA*, vol. 1, 231.

63. *PVR*, 601.

64. *PVR*, 606.

65. *PVR*, 601–602.

66. *PVR*, 604.

67. *PVR*, 610.

68. Honoré-Gabriel Riquetti, comte de Mirabeau, *Observations d'un voyageur anglais sur la maison de force appelée Bicêtre, suivies de réflexions sur les effets de la sévérité des peines et sur la législation criminelle de la Grande Bretagne; imité de l'anglais, par le comte de Mirabeau, avec une lettre de M. Benjamin Franklin* (Paris: n.p., 1788), 8.

69. See M. J. Cullerier, *Notes historiques sur les hôpitaux établis à Paris pour traiter la maladie vénérienne* (Paris: n.p., An XI [1802–1803]). The same description is given by Pastoret in Seine, CGAHHCP, *Rapport fait au conseil général . . . depuis le 1er janvier 1804 jusqu'au 1er janvier 1814* (1816), 80. See also Mirabeau, *Observations d'un voyageur anglais,* passim.

70. *TA*, vol. 1, lxxiii–lxxiv.

71. *PVR*, 611.

72. *PVR*, 603.

73. *TA*, vol. 1, 274.

74. *PVR*, 606.

75. *TA*, vol. 1, 240–241.

76. *TA*, vol. 1, 265–268. On the Salpêtrière, see Bib. Ess., Grim Reality, and *PVR*, 615–630, *TA*, vol. 1, 262–302. The original documents are to be found in AN, F¹⁵, 1861. A good brief general survey is J. Couteaux, "L'Histoire de la Salpêtrière," *Revue hospitalière de France,* 1944, *9*: 106–127, 215–242.

77. *TM*, 85.

78. *TA*, vol. 1, 268.

79. *PVR*, 622.

80. *TA*, vol. 1, lxxxvi.

81. It is interesting to note that the chief modern school of nursing is located at the Salpêtrière. For a quick retrospective appreciation, see, for example, X. Leclainche, *Quatre nouvelles années d'action hospitalière sociale et médico-sociale, 1956–1960* (Paris: Imprimerie municipale, 1960).

82. *PVR*, 296.

83. A. J. B. Parent-Duchâtelet, *De la prostitution dans la ville de Paris, de l'hygiène publique, de la morale, et de l'administration* (Brussels: Haumann & Cattoir, 1836), 92 and 527. On the medical dangers of prostitution and measures to curb it, see Chapter 6.

84. *PVR*, 624.

85. *PVR*, 617.

86. *TA*, vol. 1, 264.

87. *PVR*, 617.

88. *TA*, vol. 1, 271–272.

89. Ibid., 277.

90. Ibid., 280.

91. Seine, CGAHHCP, *Compte que rend M. Guérin, receveur général des hôpitaux et hospices civils, et secours à domicile de la Ville de Paris, de la recette et la dépense, faites au 1er janvier , sur l'exercice , et situation audit jour de chaque débiteur envers l'administration des hospices et respectivement de l'administration, envers chacun de ses créanciers.* These accounts are available in manuscript version (the folios were found, in 1982, under the eaves of the Salpêtrière's St. Louis chapel), and in published version, for the Years XI, XII, XIII, XIV–1808, and 1810, all printed under the auspices of the Imprimerie des hôpitaux.

92. *PVR*, 600, 604, 625.

93. *PVR*, 629.

94. *PVR*, 588. Camus confirms these proportions: on 22 March 1803, only 5,193 (or 10.5 percent) of the 49,264 babies brought to the Foundlings' Hospice since 1 January 1791 were still alive (Seine, CGAHHCP, *Rapports au conseil général* [1803], 157). For an excellent recent overview, although without bibliography or notes, see J. Sandrin, *Enfants trouvés, enfants ouvriers, 17ème–19ème siècles* (Paris: Aubier, 1982), ch. 2; see also Bib. Ess., Grim Reality.

95. See Chapter 7.

96. Lallemand, *Histoire des enfants abandonnés*, Appendix 3, 741. Comptroller General Jacques Necker imposed heavy penalties on 10 January 1779 in order to reduce this number. His decree proclaimed: "No one may transport infant foundlings or orphans, except to bring them to accredited wet nurses or the nearest foundlings' hospice, under penalty of a fine of 1,000 livres" (*PVR*, 11 and 348).

97. Camus provides the most complete table of children received at the Paris Foundlings' Hospice, extending from 1640 to 1808. His data originate from Tenon's work. See Seine, CGAHHCP, *Mémoire historique et instructif sur la Maternité* (Paris: Imprimerie des hospices civils, 1808), 42–43. In 1788, one-fourth of the children baptized in Paris (5,822 out of 20,708, or 29 per-

cent) were foundlings (M. Reinhard, *La révolution* [Paris: Hachette, 1971], 119). This corresponds with 5,529 in 1803 (Seine, CGAHHCP, *Rapports au conseil général* [1803], 156).

98. In the general Parisian population, 6,282 out of 18,667 children were born out of wedlock in 1806, and 8,530 out of 20,294 (that is, 42 percent) in 1812.

99. A. F. F. von Kotzebue, *Meine Flucht nach Paris im Winter 1790* (Leipzig: Kummer, 1791), 267–272.

100. The wet nurses' referral service is discussed in Chapter 7.

101. *PVR*, 405–406.

102. R. K. McClure, *Coram's Children: The London Foundling Hospital in the Eighteenth Century* (New Haven: Yale University Press, 1981), highlights some contrasts. See Bib. Ess., Grim Reality.

103. *PVR*, 580. The original documents are to be found in AN, F^{15}, 1861. Most are published in *TA, 1*, 175–188. See also O. Guillier, *Histoire de l'Hôpital Notre-Dame de la Pitié, 1612–1882* (Paris: Bureaux de la Gazette des Hôpitaux, 1882).

104. *PVR*, 581.

105. *PVR*, 584.

106. *TA*, vol. 1, 182–183.

107. *TA*, vol. 3, 11.

108. *TA*, vol. 1, 184 and 189.

109. J. P. Aron, *Essai sur la sensibilité alimentaire à Paris au 19ème siècle* , *Cahiers des Annales 25* (Paris: Armand Colin, 1967); see also the discussion of his "Histoire et biologie: Alimentation et épidémies au 19ème siècle," in *Bulletin de la Société d'histoire moderne, 13ème série*, 1965, *64*: 3–9.

110. *PVR*, 618.

111. *PVR*, 598. The Poverty Committee encountered abandoned children living in inappropriate places such as parish hospitals, charity offices, and old age homes; the babies of prostitutes living at the Salpêtrière; the "jewels" raised by the lay sisters; and the twenty-four choirboys at Bicêtre. Sometimes a mother about to give birth at the Hôtel-Dieu left older children at the Foundlings' Hospice for safekeeping. If the mother died in childbirth, how could the nuns refuse to shelter the children?

112. An entrance fee of 240 livres excluded the destitute. The orphanage's administrators waited till 1788 to invest this money in the municipal pawnshop, thus wasting large sums. *PVR*, 597.

113. *PVR*, 691.

114. *PVR*, 581.

115. *PVR*, 592.

116. *PVR*, 591.

117. *PVR*, 583, 585.

118. *TA*, vol. 1, 186–187.

119. This statement comes from the administrator of the Salpêtrière, but is equally applicable to boys from the Pitié who died at the Hôtel-Dieu (ibid., 275).

120. "Observations relatives à la partie des malades de la Pitié, Maison de l'Hôpital Général, adressées au Département des hôpitaux par M. Brun, chirurgien-en-chef de l'Hôpital général," AN, F^{15}, 1861, published in Tuetey, *TA*, vol. 1, 188–195.

121. "Oethiops [or aethiops] narcoticus" was mercury dissolved in nitric acid and precipitated with potassium sulfate to form mercuric sulfide. A narcotic used to induce sleep or allay pain, it was often thought superior to opium, which caused constipation. For this and other contemporary medications, see J. W. Estes, *Dictionary of Protopharmacology: Therapeutic Practices, 1700–1850* (Camden, Mass.: Science History Publications, 1980). Brun presented his findings about this "preparation recommended by a reputable surgeon" to the Academy of Surgery, which "concluded unanimously that exudatory remedies are safer and more useful" (Tuetey, *TA*, vol. 1, 192).

122. *PVR*, 602.

Chapter 3. The Rights and Duties of Citizen-Patients and Citizen-Doctors

1. Edmund Burke, *Reflections on the French Revolution* (1790; London: Dent, Everyman's Library, 1910), 40.

2. *PVR*, 639.

3. *TM*, 114.

4. *PVR*, 655.

5. *PVR*, 644.

6. *PVR*, 618.

7. *PVR*, 580.

8. *PVR*, 622.

9. *PVR*, 310. Liancourt had analyzed the philosophy that should underlie such assistance in his Work Plan (*PVR*, 309–327) and his first report, entitled "General Principles" (*PVR*, 327–334), read to the National Assembly on 12 June 1790. He also provided background information in his second report, "Present Charitable Legislation," read on 15 July 1790.

10. *PVR*, 328.

11. *PVR*, 437–453.

12. Law of 15 October 1793 (24 Vendémiaire, Year II), adopted only after lengthy discussion.

13. J. H. Bernardin de St. Pierre, *Etudes sur la nature* (3 vols.; Paris: Didot Jeune, 1784), 13ème étude.

14. *PVR*, 635. It is worth noting that a similar tendency toward home care is prevalent today, largely because of astronomic hospital costs, but also for psychologic reasons. See, e.g., M. Cherkasky, "The Hospital as a Social Instrument: Recent Experiences at Montefiore Hospital," in *Hospitals, Doctors, and the Public Interest*, ed. J. H. Knowles (Cambridge, Mass.: Harvard University Press, 1965), 111–124.

15. *PVR*, 391.

16. *PVR*, 38.

17. *PVR*, 545.

18. Jean Imbert, *Le droit hospitalier de la révolution et de l'empire* (Paris: Sirey, 1954), 24.

19. *PVR*, 465.

20. The figures for the annual maintenance of an impoverished invalid varied widely throughout France: 79 livres at Bicêtre, 75 livres at the Salpêtrière, 70 livres for the boys at the Pitié, 40 livres for foundlings in the countryside, 140 for Petites Maisons, and 96 livres for an infant supported by the Société de charité maternelle (*PVR*, 82).

21. *PVR*, 473.

22. On 10 October 1789, in order to advocate a beheading machine, and to his lasting misfortune, Guillotin for once turned orator and proclaimed: "The device strikes like lightning; the head flies, blood spouts, the man has ceased to live." Even though, in the subsequent discussions, both Mirabeau and the famous surgeon Antoine Louis intervened, and *mirabelle* and *louisette* thus figured among possible nicknames, the fact that *guillotine* rhymed to nicely with *machine* (in a popular ditty) eventually burdened Guillotin with lasting notoriety.

23. *AP*, vol. 18, 719.

24. Ibid., 748–749.

25. The duc de la Rochefoucauld-Liancourt and Talleyrand had both helped found the Society of 1789 on 12 April 1790. There they met regularly with Bailly, Lafayette, Sieyès, and Condorcet, to name but the most influential members. Furthermore, La Rochefoucauld-Liancourt held dinner parties at his town house on the rue de Varenne twice a week. "Twenty to forty deputies would come," and Talleyrand may well have been among them. See Dreyfus, *Un philanthrope d'autrefois*, 102.

26. *AP*, vol. 19, 588–589.

27. For the work of the Health Committee, see H. Ingrand, *Le comité de salubrité de l'Assemblée nationale constituante (1790–1791): Un essai de réforme de l'enseignement médical, des services d'hygiène, et d'essai de réforme de l'enseignement médical, des services d'hygiène, et de protection de la santé publique* (Thèse médecine, Paris, 1934), and F. Dreyfus, "Note sur le Comité de salubrité de l'Assemblée constituante," *Revue philanthropique*, 1904, *15*: 670–723. For the minutes of the committee, see Procès-verbaux par séances du Comité de salubrité, AN, AF, I²³.

28. J. G. Gallot's correspondence has been published by Dr. Louis Merle of Niort as *La vie et l'oeuvre du Dr. Jean Gabriel Gallot (1744–1794)*, in Mémoires de la Société des antiquaires de l'Ouest [Poitiers], 1962, 4th ser., vol. 5.

29. On 17 May 1789, Gallot wrote to his wife: "M. Vicq is still planning to have us to dinner, on Wednesday, together with the other doctor deputies whom I have indicated to him. . . . I dined at Vicq d'Azyr's and found there the brothers Thourec [*sic*], Cornette, de Sèze, Blin, Allart, and Discotes. M. Cornet [*sic*] invited us to dine at his house on Wednesday the 27th" (Merle, *La vie et l'oeuvre*, 70–71). The men he mentions were all doctor deputies. For a list, see Ingrand, *Comité de salubrité*, 34–35.

30. *Encyclopédie méthodique . . . Médecine,* ed. F. Vicq d'Azyr, vol. 1, 42.

31. Société royale de médecine, *Histoire et mémoires,* vol. 9, 198–199.

32. Ingrand, *Comité de salubrité,* 39.

33. For a complete list of the membership, medical as well as lay, see ibid., 34–37, or MacAuliffe, *La révolution et les hôpitaux,* 45 n. 3.

34. Seventeen members were present when the election for officers of the Health Committee were held. Guillotin obtained eleven votes, Gallot eight. "Procès-verbaux du Comité de salubrité," folio 1.

35. In August 1790 Gallot published *Vues générales sur la restauration de l'art de guérir, lues à la séance publique de la Société de médecine le 21 août 1790 et présentées au Comité de salubrité de l'Assemblée nationale le 6 octobre, suivies d'un Plan d'hospices ruraux pour le soulagement des campagnes* (Paris: Grouillebois, 1790). See also "Observations médicales," in Merle, *La vie et l'oeuvre,* 193–215.

36. Ingrand, *Comité de salubrité,* 38–39.

37. The Health Committee knew, of course, where the most useful expertise on health care problems was to be found, and lost no time asking for the Poverty Committee's help, but it is difficult to estimate the extent of real collaboration. Subsequent developments indicate that Thouret and La Rochefoucauld-Liancourt never forgave Guillotin for his treachery.

38. J. N. Biraben, "Essai sur la statistique des causes de décès en France sous la révolution et le premier empire," in *Hommage à Marcel Reinhard: Sur la population française au 18ème et au 19ème siècles* (Paris: Société de démographie historique, 1973), 61.

39. On 22 May 1781, Jacques de Horne had read a paper entitled "Projet de l'établissement d'une école de médecine dans les hôpitaux militaires" to the Royal Society of Medicine.

40. See Appendix A.

41. See Appendix A.

42. De Jussieu was then serving as deputy mayor for hospital affairs; Lavoisier and Bailly had participated in the Academy of Sciences' survey of Paris hospitals in 1786–1788, Bailly and Leroy had both contributed to the literature about replacing the Hôtel-Dieu after the fire in 1773.

43. "Nouveau plan," 94.

44. Ibid.

45. Cabanis, "Observations sur les hôpitaux," 25. For an excellent discussion of Cabanis's ideas, see M. S. Staum, *Cabanis: Enlightenment and Medical Philosophy in the French Revolution* (Princeton: Princeton University Press, 1980), ch. 4. See also Bib. Ess., Enlightened Innovation.

46. "Nouveau plan," 106.

47. "Rapport sur l'instruction publique," in *AP,* vol. 30, 447–511; for medical education, see 457–458 and 486–88.

48. C. M. de Talleyrand-Périgord, *Mémoires,* ed. P. L. and J. P. Couchoud (7 vols.; Paris: Plon, 1957), vol. 1 (1754–1807), 163–164.

49. *AP,* vol. 30, 458.

50. Owing to Talleyrand's grip on educational matters, the National Assembly never saw Vicq d'Azyr's New Plan. Indeed, the Archives parlemen-

taires indicate only that, on 25 November 1790, "one of the secretaries announced to the Assembly that the Royal Society of Medicine has the honor of presenting a plan of a new constitution for medicine in France, one copy of which is deposited on the rostrum." The Assembly directed that it be forwarded to the Constitution Committee. See *AP,* vol. 20, 744–745. In the National Archives, the manuscript of the "Nouveau plan" is indeed to be found in the files of the Constitution Committee. AN, F¹⁷, 1310.

51. *PVR,* 758–777.

52. *PVR,* 305.

Chapter 4. The Caring Professions

1. On the origins of Western nursing regulations, see T. Miller, "The Knights of St. John and the Hospital in the Latin West," *Speculum,* 1978, *53:* 709–723.

2. This information is dispersed throughout J. Boussoulade, *Moniales et hospitalières dans la tourmente révolutionnaire: Les communautés de religieuses de l'ancien diocèse de Paris de 1789 à 1801* (Paris: Letouzey & Ané, 1962).

3. The essay that best captures the spirit of French Catholic nursing, even though it deals with the nineteenth century, is Jacques Léonard, "Women, Religion, and Medicine," in *Medicine and Society in France,* ed. R. Forster and O. Ranum (Baltimore: Johns Hopkins University Press, 1980), 24–47.

4. For works on the history of nursing, see Bib. Ess., Archives and The Caring Professions.

5. The hospital administrator Camus wrote in 1803: "The nurses at the Hôtel-Dieu are mostly former nuns of that establishment, or novices who were about to take vows when the community they wanted to join was abolished. The nurses recruited several persons inclined to conform to their special rule" (Seine, CGAHHCP, *Rapports au conseil général* [1803], 37).

6. On the Augustinian nurses, see D. B. Weiner, "The French Revolution, Napoleon, and the Nursing Profession," *BHM,* 1972, *46:* 274–305; L. S. Greenbaum, "Nurses and Doctors in Conflict: Piety and Medicine in the Paris Hôtel-Dieu on the Eve of the French Revolution," *Clio medica,* 198 , *13:* 247–267; and id., "Science, Medicine, Religion," 373–391. The Augustinians followed an extremely rigorous schedule, rising at 3:30 in the morning to attend prayers from 4:15 to 5:00. Then they washed and comforted the patients, preparing them for the doctor's rounds at 6 A.M. (7 in winter). Meals were scheduled for 10 A.M. and 5 P.M., the early afternoon being reserved for visitors.

7. Marcel Fosseyeux, "Le service médical à l'hôpital de la Charité au 17ème et 18ème siècles," *Aesculape,* 1912: 3ème année, 117–121, 150–152. The reference is to 151–152.

8. AN, F¹⁵, 1861, printed in *TA,* vol. 1, 412–414. "So many patients come to the dispensary that the consumption of unguents and brandy has risen considerably" stated a report at the beginning of the Revolution. Any further demands on their funds would "deplete the subsistence of the poor" (ibid., 422–433, passim). On the role of dispensaries for outpatients, see Chapter 5.

9. C. Klein, *106 rue du Bac . . . une tradition de charité* (Paris: Editions

S.O.S., 1964). In 1790, twenty-four patients enjoyed the services of five domestics and eight religious. The annual budget was 34,000 livres.

10. See Chapter 9.

11. Boussoulade, *Moniales et hospitalières.*

12. AN, F[15], 1861.

13. On the Sisters of Charity at the welfare offices, see Marcel Fosseyeux, "Les comités de bienfaisance des sections du Finistère et du Panthéon," *La révolution française,* 1911, *40*: 505–535, and id., "Les comités de bienfaisance de Paris sous la révolution," *Annales révolutionnaires,* 1912, *5*: 192–205, 344–358.

14. See Archives, St. Thomas de Villeneuve, dossier "B." On the Children's Hospital, see Chapter 7.

15. C. Gazier, *Après Port-Royal: L'ordre hospitalier des soeurs de Ste. Marthe de Paris, 1713–1918* (Paris: Ambert, 1923), 41 and 92.

16. As a precondition to continuing their work, nurses had to swear an oath that "varied with the whim of the local authorities" (Boussoulade, *Moniales et hospitalières,* 125 n. 59). An individual sister might feel free to swear "faithfulness to the nation and allegiance to liberty and equality," the so-called "lesser oath" of 1791, but she might balk at taking the "oath of the Year II," which included "hatred of monarchy and anarchy."

17. The Revolutionaries knew that nurses were protecting priests who refused to take the oath of allegiance to the secular Republic and moved quickly after Pope Pius VI condemned the new Gallican Church as "heretical, sacrilegious, and schismatic." On 17 April 1791—that is, four days after the papal brief *Caritas*—the government declared hospital chaplains to be public servants, and thus liable to the oath. A suspicious police commissioner now had a new motive to test the political reliability of hospital nurses.

18. Dated 11 Frimaire, Year II (1 December 1793). AN, AD Archives imprimées, XIV, hôpitaux et secours, dossier 12, "Société philantropique, Sociétés charitables." Typically, the 500-page study of the loyalty oath by Bernard Plongeron, *Les réguliers de Paris devant le serment constitutionnel: Sens et conséquences d'une option* (Paris: Vrin, 1964), does not even mention the nuns.

19. Boussoulade, *Moniales et hospitalières,* 95, 145.

20. The Catholic historian Léon Lallemand attempts an impartial conclusion: "After the expulsion of the sisters, some dedicated women were found, but many were deplorably unsuited. Most of the women employed showed goodwill, but lacked experience. In many instances, the lay supervisors and nurses were conscious of their own shortcomings" (Lallemand, *La révolution et les pauvres,* 145, and "Les femmes patriotes," passim).

21. M. Bouchet, *L'Assistance publique en France pendant la révolution* (Paris: Jouve, 1908), 531.

22. In chapters 3 and 4 of *The French Revolution and the Poor* (New York: Oxford University Press, 1981), Alan Forrest depicts conditions in provincial hospitals, rather than in Paris. Even Lydie Boulle's detailed figures do not show the change in treatment or comfort over time. Also, her data pertain in large part to the period 1815–1848.

23. Jean Antoine Chaptal, an M.D. from Montpellier, turned first to in-

dustrial chemistry and successfully pursued the wholesale production of alum, saltpeter, dyed cotton, and local wines. During the Revolution, he supervised the extraction of the essential saltpeter at Grenelle, near Paris, and taught chemistry at the Polytechnic School. Napoleon Bonaparte, a fellow member of the Institut de France, invited Chaptal to join the council of state and appointed him minister of internal affairs. Having quarreled with Napoleon in 1804, Chaptal retired to his country place and presided over the prestigious "Society of Arcueil." Nevertheless, Napoleon made him a grand officer of the Legion of Honor and named him count of Chanteloup. After the Restoration, Chaptal joined the Paris Hospital Council in 1817 and the Chamber of Peers in 1819. See also Bib. Ess., The Caring Professions.

24. For the text of the decree, see Weiner, "French Revolution, Napoleon and the Nursing Profession," n. 49.

25. See ibid., 299–302.

26. The details of this story are garnered from AN, F^{19}, 6293.

27. AN, F^{19}, 6293. Internal evidence indicates that it was composed between 1811 and 1814.

28. For the history of pharmacy during this era, see Bib. Ess., The Caring Professions.

29. Marcel Fosseyeux, "Les apothicaireries de couvents sous l'ancien régime," *Bulletin de la société de l'histoire de Paris et de l'Ile de France,* 1919, *46:* 42–59.

30. Colin Jones notes, for example, that a "case with lancets and ligatures" formed part of a Sister of Charity's usual equipment. See "The Daughters of Charity in Hospitals from Louis XIII to Louis Philippe" and "Les Filles de Charité" in Jones, *The Charitable Imperative: Hospitals and Nursing in Ancien Regime and Revolutionary France* (New York: Routledge, 1989), 194, 259. For the work of the main French expert in the history of pharmacy, Maurice Bouvet, see Bib. Ess., The Caring Professions.

31. Matthew Ramsey's new book, *Professional and Popular Medicine in France, 1770–1830: The Social World of Medical Practice* (New York: Cambridge University Press, 1988), is a mine of information about nonconventional medicine.

32. M. Bouvet, *Les origines de la pharmacie hospitalière à Paris avant 1789. L'Hôtel-Dieu et ses annexes* (Poitiers: Imprimerie française, 1935), 29 and 19.

33. A retrospective overview can be obtained from A. Goris, *Centenaire de l'Internat en pharmacie des hôpitaux et hospices civils de Paris* (Paris: Imprimerie de la Cour d'Appel, 1920).

34. Nicolas Deyeux, François Chaussier, and Philippe Pinel, in Paris, Faculté de médecine, "Rapports faits dans les différentes séances de l'Assemblée des professeurs de l'Ecole de médecine de Paris" (An III–An VIII [1794–1800]), AN, AJ^{16}, 6698, fols. 44–46.

35. The first edition of Parmentier's *Pharmacopée à l'usage des hôpitaux civils, des secours à domicile, des prisons et dépôts de mendicité* (Paris: 1803) consisted of 184 pages; the second edition, the same year, of 326 pages; the third (1807) was 453 pages long; and the fourth (1811) counted 566 pages. All were published by the Imprimerie de la république.

36. A graduate school opened in 1803 under the famous Nicolas Louis Vauquelin (1763–1829), and an internship in 1814.

37. By the executive commission of the Public Aid Committee of the Convention on 17 Prairial, Year III (5 June 1795).

38. See H. Aurousseau-Guiraudet and R. Weitz, "Une carrière pharmaceutique sous la révolution, le premier empire, et la restauration: Etienne Guiraudet (1754–1839)," *Revue d'histoire de la pharmacie*, 1935, *5*: 20–33.

39. M. Bouvet, *La pharmacie hospitalière à Paris*, 43.

40. Quoted in ibid., 10, from Clavareau, *Mémoires sur les hôpitaux civils*.

41. Seine, CGAHHCP, *Rapports au conseil général* (1803), 10.

42. AAPP, Catalogue Fosseyeux, nouvelle série (henceforth cited as CFNS), dossier 129.

43. Henry's predecessor, Jacques François Demachy (1728–1803), actually served as pharmacist-in-chief from the beginning, in 1796, until his death. But he seems to have been a better poet than administrator, and from 1797 on, Henry was the real driving force. See Robert, "Notice biographique sur Demachy," autogr. MS no. 22881, Bibliothèque interuniversitaire de pharmacie, Paris.

44. Ackerknecht, *Medicine at the Paris Hospital*, 136.

45. Seine, CGAHHCP, *Rapports au conseil général* (1803), 140.

46. M. A. Thouret and N. Deyeux, "Rapport au Conseil de l'Ecole de santé de Paris sur une lettre du ministre de l'intérieur relative à l'établissement des pharmacies qui doivent être tenues par les Soeurs de Charité," *France médicale*, 1901, *48*: 419–420.

47. Ramsey, *Professional and Popular Medicine*, offers plentiful evidence.

48. The fate of the child will be discussed in Chapter 7.

49. Marie Louise Lachapelle's grandmother, Madame Josnet, had been accredited in 1730. She trained her daughter, Marie Dugès (1730–1797), who served as midwife-in-chief at the Hôtel-Dieu from 1775 until her death. Madame Dugès in turn supervised the professional training of her daughter, whom a brief three years of marriage to a surgeon left widowed and childless at twenty-six, when she was appointed her mother's assistant. On Madame Lachapelle and her mother, see A. Delacoux, *Biographies de sages-femmes célèbres, anciennes, modernes, et contemporaines* (Paris: Trinquart, 1833), "Dugès," 73–75, and "Lachapelle," 97–106, as well as F. Chaussier, "Notice historique sur la vie et les écrits de Madame Lachapelle," in M. L. Lachapelle, née Dugès, *Pratique des accouchements ou Mémoires ou observations choisies sur les points les plus importants de l'art* (Paris: Baillière, 1821; 2d ed., 1825), 1–16.

50. *TM*, 251.

51. Thus Tenon wrote of the use of the forceps at the Hôtel-Dieu that "half of the women involved survive, which means the loss of one woman out of 492 per year" (*TM*, 252) But among the affluent, wrote Chaussier in 1821, "the use of the forceps has become very frequent in recent years. Every accoucheur always has a forceps in his pocket, and he has to use it, it's the fashion, it's the art of being important, and one mustn't miss the opportunity" (Chaussier, "Notice historique," in Lachapelle, *Pratique*, 2d ed., 12).

52. Delacoux, *Biographies de sages-femmes célèbres*, 100–101.

53. In contrast, interested women gained admittance to the lectures (Seine, CGAHHCP, *Rapports au conseil général* [1803], 153). The following memorandum, addressed to the obstetrician Dr. Bourdier at the Maternité on 5 July 1808, illustrates the situation. (To judge from the handwriting, the note is from Jacques Benoît Hucherard, the administrator.) It reads: "Monsieur, This morning I noticed a young man, a stranger to this hospital service, who came and announced that he would follow your rounds. I take the liberty of drawing your attention to the fact that the administrators have always been opposed to the presence of strangers, and particularly of young men, at medical rounds or deliveries. . . . You would oblige the administration if you were good enough to inform any young men desiring to follow your rounds that the rules of the establishment do not permit this" (Archives de la Seine, Enfants assistés [henceforth cited as EA], Maternité, dossier 1).

54. Seine, CGAHHCP, *Rapports au conseil général* (1803), 150–1. In 1813 all the private amphitheaters were closed and an official, supervised one was opened near the Clamart cemetery.

55. All babies and about one hundred wet nurses were initially transferred to the Val-de-Grâce monastery, but the government changed its mind, preferring to use the Val-de-Grâce as its central military hospital, which it has remained to this day (Pierre Huard, "Eléments d'un rapport tendant à transformer le monastère du Val-de-Grâce en Maternité," *Clio medica,* 1967, 2: 249–254.

56. Two invaluable primary sources inform us about the Hospice de la Maternité. Seine, CGAHHCP, *Mémoire historique et instructif sur l'Hospice de la maternité* (Paris: Imprimerie des hospices civils, 1808) derives in large part from Seine,CGAHHCP, *Rapports au conseil général* (1803), 131–183. For an excellent, more objective treatment, see A. Dupoux, *Sur les pas de Monsieur Vincent: Trois cents ans d'histoire parisienne de l'enfance abandonnée* (Paris: Revue de l'Assistance publique, 1958), written after the author retired as director of the former Paris Foundlings' Hospice.

57. "Some hovels were cleared away and old structures repaired and whitewashed: the building is as adequate as its former use allows," wrote Camus (Seine, CGAHHCP, *Rapports au conseil général* [1803], 135).

58. Poirot, *Notice sur l'hospice de la Maternité* (Paris: Renaudière, An IX [1800–1801]), 16–19, cited—and rephrased—in Dupoux, *Sur les pas,* 140.

59. Charles François Viel, *Principes de l'ordonnance et de la construction des bâtiments: Notices sur divers hôpitaux, et autres édifices publics et particuliers* (Paris: Tilliard, 1812), 28. On Viel, see Chapter 6.

60. Dupoux, *Sur les pas,* 149.

61. Ibid., 29.

62. H. Carrier, *Origines de la Maternité de Paris: Les maîtresses sages-femmes et l'Office des accouchées de l'ancien Hôtel-Dieu, 1378–1796* (Paris: Steinheil, 1888), 217.

63. Chaptal may have known that the Poverty Committee had discussed such a project (*PVR,* 128). He had previously planned a school for nurses at the Foundlings' Hospice with twenty women and twenty men graduates a year, but that idea came to naught (J. A. Chaptal, *Mes souvenirs sur Napoleon*

[Paris: Plon Nourrit, 1893], 74). A knowledgeable overview of the midwifery school's early development by Hucherard can be found in Seine, CGAHHCP, *Mémoire historique*, 57–65.

64. "Arrêté du ministre de l'intérieur du 11 Messidor, An X," in Carrier, *Origines de la Maternité de Paris*, 244–250. The course was later lengthened to one year (17 January 1807).

65. On Baudelocque, see Bib. Ess., The Caring Professions.

66. J. L. Baudelocque, *Principes sur l'art des accouchements par demandes et réponses en faveur des sages-femmes de la campagne* (Paris: Méquignon, 1775), 2d ed., 1787, xii.

67. Paul Delaunay, *La Maternité de Paris. Port-Royal. Port-Libre. L'hospice de la Maternité. L'Ecole des sages-femmes et ses origines (1625–1907)* (Paris: Roussel, 1909), 192.

68. Dupoux, *Sur les pas*, 150.

69. These were the specific instructions from Chaussier and Madame Lachapelle. See Carrier, *Origines de la Maternité de Paris*, 259.

70. Seine, CGAHHCP, *Rapports au conseil général* (1803), 146. These regulations, reprinted in Carrier, *Origines de la Maternité de Paris*, 244–249, contrast favorably with the stern tone of "Règlement pour les élèves sages-femmes à la Maternité" dated 12 January 1803 (AAPP, B 5089 17), which specifies behavior, attendance, and penalties.

71. Delacoux, *Biographies de sages-femmes célèbres*, 100.

72. Madame Lachapelle then explained all the circumstances of the case in detail, the motivation for the procedure she had chosen, the precautions taken before and after its execution. In order not to neglect anything useful for teaching, she demonstrated the procedure on the mannequin and made all the students repeat it while adding more explanations (Chaussier, "Notice historique," in Lachapelle, *Pratique*, 2d ed., 12–13).

73. Delacoux, *Biographies de sages-femmes célèbres*, 100–101.

74. Toward the end of her life, Madame Lachapelle collected all of her observations for her book *Pratique des accouchements*. The first volume was published in 1820, a second, revised, two-volume edition appeared under the aegis of her nephew, Antoine Dugès, who obtained his M.D. from the Paris medical faculty and taught obstetrics at Montpellier. In the introduction she points out that in 1816, for example, there were 2,422 births in the maternity service: 2,386 were spontaneous, 36 called for an intervention: 25 of these were manual, and only in 11 cases did she use the forceps (p. 3). This meant a use of the forceps in only 0.5 percent of deliveries.

75. Seine, CGAHHCP, *Procès-verbal de la distribution des prix faite par le ministre de l'intérieur aux élèves sages-femmes de la Maternité le 23 Frimaire, An XII* (Paris: Imprimerie des hospices civils, [1804]).

76. Carrier, *Origines de la Maternité de Paris*, 255 n. 1.

77. Florence Nightingale, "A Proposal for Organizing an Institution for Training Midwives and Midwifery Nurses," *Introductory Notes on Lying-in Institutions* (London: Longmans Green, 1871), 105–110.

78. For a list of graduating students, beginning in 1802, see Hospices de Paris, Maison d'accouchement de Paris, "Distribution des prix," AAPP,

CFNS, 678[1]. A detailed list of the class of 1816, with their departments, shows us sixty-one women, ten with scholarships from the Ministry of Internal Affairs, ten who paid their own way, and the others financed by their departments. Twelve came from the Ile-de-France, fifteen from the north-east, and six from the region of Bordeaux. Eight were married, three widowed. See Hospices de Paris, Maison d'accouchement, "Etat général des sommes dues pour menus frais de cours des élèves sages-femmes admises à l'Ecole d'accouchements scolaire de juillet 1814 à 1815," Archives de la Seine, EA, Maternité, dossier 5.

79. Hucherard wrote to the Hospital Council on 25 July 1812, claiming that he faced an emergency:

When I had the honor of writing to you on the 2d instant to ask for authorization to install a dormitory in the attic of the pension, we already had 140 students. I worried that their number might equal that of last year; I demonstrated our difficulties, how overcrowded the dormitories were, and so forth. Today we have 185 students, and I must not only use the dormitory of the pregnant women and send them to the babies' section, but even place some students in unused beds in their infirmary.

The completion of our new dormitory, which is almost, but not quite, ready, will give us only fourteen beds [there is an obvious discrepancy in numbers with Carrier, *Origines de la Maternité de Paris,* 260].

So Hucherard suggested remodeling yet another, adjoining, attic at a cost of 2,000 francs.

80. Seine, CGAHHCP, *Rapports au conseil général* (1803), 152, and Carrier, *Origines de la Maternité de Paris,* 260.

81. Each candidate would follow two courses, then observe midwifery for nine months, or practice under supervision for six months, before taking the licensing examination (arts. 30 and 31). An archival document reveals that a national inquiry in 1804 yielded only fifteen replies. Some departments sent students to Paris: Indre, for example, decided that "a sum of 1,200 francs be taken from the savings [?] of the Years IX and X, and used to send Madame Lachapelle in Paris two young students." The department of Forêts did the same, noting: "Malicious rumors have attempted to discredit [the Paris school]. We hope to counteract these, and to promote an appreciation of the government's salutary initiative." Hautes-Alpes "very much hoped to continue its course, but asked for some assistance," and Creuse requested "a small indemnity in each canton for a woman to be appointed by the prefect, upon nomination by the mayor. This will enable her to attend the midwifery course to be established in one of the departmental hospices." See Cours gratuits d'accouchements, AN, F[15], 1874 A; the document is undated, but internal evidence suggests 1804.

82. Chaptal wrote on 28 July 1802, and again on 16 September 1803 (Carrier, *Origines de la Maternité de Paris,* 251–253).

83. Thus Minister of Internal Affairs Champagny in a circular of 1807 (Chaussier, "Notice historique," in Lachapelle, *Pratique,* 2d ed., 8n).

84. The letter reads in part: "The portion of land taken from the hospice

garden (the former Port-Royal convent) near the rues d'Enfer and Cassini is quite considerable, and this establishment will in the future be separated from its annex [the lying-in hospital, former Oratory convent] (1) by the new avenue; (2) by some fallow land whose destination I do not know; (3) by the rue d'Enfer, which has until now been the only public street one must cross to get from the babies' hospital to the lying-in hospital" (Archives de la Seine, EA, Maternité, dossier 1).

85. Archives de la Seine, EA, Maternité, 1814–1815, dossier 3.

86. This scholarship program worked only for three years, until May 1798, when it was discontinued.

87. Series AJ[16] in the Archives nationales has numerous boxes filled with documents pertaining to the nominations of doctors to these juries and their recommendations.

88. Quoted in A. Prévost, *Les études médicales sous le Directoire et le Consulat* (Paris: Champion, 1907), 5.

89. On medical student life in the early years of the nineteenth century, see M. Wiriot, *L'enseignement clinique dans les hôpitaux de Paris entre 1794 et 1848* (Thèse histoire de la médecine, Paris, 1970). The number of students is given on p. 45. See also Pierre Huard and M. J. Imbault-Huard, "Structure et fonctionnement de la Faculté de médecine de Paris en 1813," *Revue d'histoire des sciences,* 1975, *28*: 139–168. The number of students is given on p. 159. This article based on J. J. Leroux, "Compte-rendu à son Excellence le Ministre de l'intérieur," AN, F[17], 2168, Leroux was then dean of the medical school.

90. Prévost, *Les études médicales,* 39.

91. Some medical students asked for, and received, "certificates of capacity" from the Paris Health School during the ten years when medical diplomas did not exist officially. But Dr. Roselyne Rey has identified and analyzed 406 M.D. theses awarded in Paris during those ten years (communication at a seminar at the Centre Alexandre Koyré, Paris, May 1992).

92. AN, AJ[16], 6414.

93. Pierre Huard and M. J. Imbault-Huart, "La clinique parisienne avant et après 1802," *Clio medica,* 1975, *10*: 173–182.

94. Möring, Quentin, and Brièle, *Délibérations,* vol. 2, 238–239.

95. Prévost, *Les études médicales,* 7 and 21.

Chapter 5. The Outpatient: The Strategy of Medical Administrators

1. See D. B. Weiner, "Hospital Administrators in the French Revolution," *Koroth,* 1985, *8*: 181–191.

2. Marguerite Jubline, a *"tailleresse,"* belonged to the small and exclusive guild whose members cut and stamped the coin of the realm. The women enjoyed a privilege that may be unique: they transmitted to their sons the right to join the guild without either test or fee.

3. Louis François Alhoy, *Promenades poétiques dans les hospices et hôpitaux de Paris* (Paris: Trouvé, 1826).

4. See C. F. Duchanoy and J. B. Jumelin, "Mémoire sur l'utilité d'une école clinique de médecine," D. F. Duchanoy, *Projet d'organisation médicale* (Paris: n.p., n.d.); and id., *Précis de l'état des hôpitaux comparés à ce qu'ils étaient avant la révolution* (Paris: n.p., 1808).

5. For a list of the books most helpful for this chapter, see Bib. Ess., The Outpatient.

6. Imbert, *Le droit hospitalier*, 62.

7. For details, see A. Bonde, *Le domaine des hospices de Paris, 1789–1870* (Paris: Berger-Levrault, 1906), esp. ch. 1, "Le domaine immobilier productif pendant la période révolutionnaire."

8. Imbert, *Le droit hospitalier*, 80–82, and especially Louis Parturier, *L'assistance à Paris sous l'ancien régime et pendant la révolution* (Paris: Larose, 1897), pt. 2, ch. 4.

9. AN, F^{1c}, III, Seine, 13.

10. "Rapport de M. de Jussieu sur les hôpitaux de Paris, tendant à confier leur administration immédiate et directe à la municipalité" (16 Frimaire, An II), fol. 3, AN, F^{15}, 1861.

11. In December 1793, de Jussieu lost out completely, and his papers were transferred from the quai des Bernardins to the "parvis de la raison." We do not know whether they were lost in transit or burned in the fire of 1871. Only fragments remain.

12. Seine, CGAHHCP, *Rapport sur la situation generale des revenus et dépenses, 31 décembre 1811* (Paris: Imprimerie des hospices, 1812), 10, and Frochot, as quoted in J. Pigeire, *La vie et l'oeuvre de Chaptal*, 324 n. 1. Pigeire credits Chaptal with bringing about the ensuing reform.

13. *TA*, vol. 1, 96–98, and vol. 3, 133–134.

14. This conclusion agrees with that of Clive H. Church, in *Revolution and Red Tape: The French Ministerial Bureaucracy, 1770–1850* (Oxford: Clarendon Press, 1981), when he states, for example, that "by 1799, the bureaucracy was too well entrenched to be greatly disturbed, although Bonaparte's reign was greatly to affect its authority and efficiency" (p. 112).

15. Frochot served as justice of the peace in Burgundy, then as deputy in the Estates General and Directory. He remained prefect of the Seine until 1812, when he fell from favor because of his ineptitude in forestalling the attempted coup of General Malet. He was succeeded by Chabrol de Volvic (1773–1843), prefect until 1830, with the exception of the Hundred Days. See also Bib. Ess., The Outpatient.

16. Passy, *Frochot*, 464–469.

17. Decree of 2 February 1801 (13 Pluviôse, An IX)

18. Their salary of 6,000 francs was later (1811) increased by 600 francs for those commissioners who had to travel to the outlying hospices.

19. C E. J. P. Pastoret became professor of international law at the Collège de France in 1804, and of philosophy at the University of Paris in 1809, and a senator.

20. This accounts for his being made a regent of the Banque de France at the early age of thirty.

21. A. G. Camus (1740–1804), a member of the Academy of Inscriptions and a deputy active in elaborating the Civil Constitution of the Clergy, had been a member of the Committee of Public Safety. He served as "guardian of the national archives" until his death and deserves credit for collecting, classifying, and eventually saving thousands of documents. In 1794, he had been sent to inspect General Dumouriez, who was suspected of treason. Camus was seized by the general and turned over to the Austrians. While a prisoner, he translated Epictetus. In 1795, he was exchanged for Louis XVI's young daughter.

22. A. C. Duquesnoy had the unique distinction of legalizing Lucien Bonaparte's civil marriage to Madame Gauberton in 1804, whereupon Napoleon instantly dismissed him as mayor. But he remained on the Hospital Council.

23. E. C. Fieffé was married to Jacques Tenon's sister.

24. To fill vacancies, the following men were appointed during the Consulate and Empire: in 1804, to replace Camus, J. P. G. Camet de la Bonardière (1769–1842), mayor of the 11th arrondissement; in 1807, to replace Fieffé, J. A. M. Séguier (1768–1848), president of the court of appeals; in 1808, to replace Duquesnoy, H. Muraire (1750–1837), president of the court of appeals; in 1810, to replace Bigot de Préameneu, F. Barbé-Marbois (1745–1837), diplomat and legislator; in 1810, to replace Thouret, D. E. Rouillé de l'Etang (1731–1811), a financier; in 1811, to replace Rouillé, Denis Trutat (1748–1814), a lawyer. M. J. F. duc de Montmorency-Laval (1767–1826) served the council intermittently. He resigned immediately after his initial appointment in 1801, then served from 1814 to 1822, when he was sent to the Congress of Verona, then again from 1824 until his death.

25. Delessert, Pasquier, and Séguier became barons; Bigot, Chaptal, Frochot, Muraire, Pastoret, and Barbé-Marbois became counts (to this distinction the latter two, as well as d'Aguesseau, added marquisates; and Pasquier a dukedom, in 1844).

26. The documents speak of nineteen establishments. St. Antoine Hospital, the twentieth, opened in 1813.

27. Seine, CGAHHCP, *Rapports au conseil général* (1803), 19.

28. Nicolas Frochot, *Discours du préfet du département de la Seine, en prononçant l'installation du Conseil général d'administration des Hospices civils de Paris, le 5 Ventôse, An IX* (Paris: Ballard, An IX), 5–6.

29. Ibid., 12–21, passim. Frochot was referring to Bicêtre.

30. Ibid., 28–29, passim. Frochot was of course alluding to the writings of John Howard, Count Rumford, and Johann Peter Frank, as well as to practical reforms instituted at the Allgemeine Krankenhaus in Vienna, in Pavia, and elsewhere.

31. Seine, CGAHHCP, *Compte moral sur la situation des hospices civils rendu par la Commission administrative des ces mêmes hospices au Conseil général d'administration avec Tableau contenant la dénomination ancienne et nouvelle des hôpitaux et hospices de Paris, leur situation, leur population, leur destination, la raison des compagnies chargées de l'entreprise de leur service, le prix des journées allouées à chacune*

d'elles, le nombre des officiers de santé et des employés de toutes classes au compte tant de l'administration que des entreprises et le montant du traitement de chacune des dites classes d'employés (Paris: Prault, An IX [1800–1801]).

32. Ibid., 3–5, passim.

33. Ibid., 12–21. passim.

34. Seine, CGAHHCP, *Rapports au conseil général* (1803), 37, n. 1.

35. Ibid., 50.

36. Ibid., 20.

37. Imbert, *Le droit hospitalier*, 187.

38. CGAHHCP, *Comptes généraux des hôpitaux et hospices civils, enfants abandonnés, secours à domicile, et direction des nourrices de la ville de Paris, Recette, Dépense, Population* (6 vols. in folio; Paris: Imprimerie des hospices, 1805–1813). The remaining figures for the Empire can be found in Pastoret's report of 1816. The manuscript records, well over fifty folio volumes, were found in 1982 stored under the eaves of the St. Louis chapel in the Salpêtrière Hospice. A critical retrospective report on past accounting practices can be found in Seine, CGAHHCP, *Rapport . . . sur la situation générale des revenus et dépenses au 31 décembre 1811* (Paris: Imprimerie des hospices, 1812), AAPP, C 1367.

39. See Bib. Ess., Primary Printed Sources, and L. Boulle, "Hôpitaux parisiens: Malades et maladies à l'heure des révolutions, 1789 à 1848" (Paris: Ecole pratique des hautes études, 1986).

40. Clavareau, *Mémoire sur les hôpitaux civils*, 49 and 55.

41. We read in the 1806 annual report that, in the view of the authorities, this accusation was unfounded because admitting permits were issued to 12,261 persons and direct admissions numbered 10,698—a total of 22,959. Yet the total numbers of patients admitted to the hospitals was only 22,576 persons, indicating that 383 permits were not used. Seine, CGAHHCP, *Rapport . . . du bureau central d'admission . . . An XIII*, table XVI.

42. The numbers used derive from the tables in the admitting office reports; numbers given in the texts show slight discrepancies. When these outpatient consultations grew into outpatient departments in the mid nineteenth century, the physicians' case loads were astoundingly large. This corresponds to the British experience. For example, Dr. Robert Bridges at St. Bartholomew's Hospital in London in the 1870s "had to 'filter' over 30,000 patients a year, two-thirds of them new patients, *at an average rate of one every 88 seconds*" (I. S. L. Loudon, "Historical Importance of Outpatients," *British Medical Journal*, 1978, *1*: 974–977, at 976 [emphasis added]).

43. Seine, CGAHHCP, *Rapport . . . du bureau central d'admission . . . An XIII*, 3 and 27.

44. Ibid., 29; see also M. J. Imbault-Huart, "Les chirurgiens et l'esprit chirurgical en France au 18ème siècle," *Clio medica*, 1981, *15*: 143–157.

45. The regulations regarding the Children's Hospital are dated 3 November 1802.

46. Seine, CGAHHCP, *Rapport . . . du bureau central d'admission . . . An XII*, 12.

47. G. R. Siguret, *Histoire de l'hospitalisation des enfants malades de Paris*

(Paris: Thèse médecine, 1907), 53, and Seine, CGAHHCP, *Rapports au conseil général* (1803), 42.

48. Despite their neat categories, the doctors at the admitting office were sometimes baffled. Where to send a sick baby being nursed by a well mother? Or a sick mother with a healthy nursling? "We had no guidelines from the authorities," they complained, and, for lack of a logical solution, they sent thirteen mothers and babies to the Hôtel-Dieu between May and November 1802. The lack of clarity seemed unbearable, so the Hospital Council set up a committee to find a permanent solution! Seine, CGAHHCP, *Rapport . . . du bureau central d'admission . . . An XII*, 12.

49. Ibid., 21–23. It is not clear, from the documents, whether one or two physicians' certificates were required; the report mentions: "des certificats d'officiers de santé et de deux témoins attestant les actes de folie." The interdiction of mental patients is discussed further in Chapter 9.

50. Ibid., 7 and 9.

51. Tenon mentions "*bilanders,*" which he describes as "boxes surrounded by curtains and suspended on four-wheeled stretchers with lower, or lower and upper, bunks and four or eight washable horsehair mattresses, covered with leather. Each of these is fitted on a separate frame. A mattress is taken out, a patient is put on it and he is thus transported within the box. These mattresses have four handles for putting them in and taking them out" (*TM,* 416n).

52. The Hospital Council's retrospective table of admissions for 1806–1813 confirms our observations for 1801–1802: at the four small outlying all-purpose hospitals (Cochin, Necker, Beaujon, and St. Antoine), direct or "emergency" admissions regularly exceeded those sent by the central bureau. Necker remained the most extreme case. And the proportion of direct admissions even remained high at the centrally located general hospitals, e.g., at the Hôtel-Dieu, despite the fact that the admitting office was but a few steps away. For figures on emergency admissions as a percentage of total admissions at the Necker Hospital and Hôtel-Dieu in 1806–1812, see Appendix C, Table C.2.

53. In his annual report of 1805, Duchanoy commented that "it would be desirable to limit these admissions" (Seine, CGAHHCP, *Rapport . . . du bureau central d'admission . . . An XIII*, 8–9).

54. The Pitié's population was originally assigned by triage, with 1,931 patients in 1809. The big change came in 1812, when "emergency" admissions multiplied a hundredfold, jumping from 114 (in 1811) to 1,483, while referrals from the central admitting office declined by three-fifths that year, and ceased in 1813. Seine, CGAHHCP, *Rapport fait au conseil général* (1816), 232.

55. Camus reports, for example, that in Year X, 30 men and 65 women were transferred from hospitals for the acutely ill to Bicêtre and Salpêtrière hospices. And yet by the year XI, 80 more men and 179 women had similarly to be evacuated. The admitting office requested in 1804 that all transfers be promptly reported, thus revealing that this was not routinely done. Seine, CGAHHCP, *Rapport . . . du bureau central d'admission . . . An XII*, 8–9. 19.)

56. Seine, CGAHHCP, *Rapport fait au conseil général* (1816), 224.

57. Seine, CGAHHCP, *Rapport . . . du bureau central d'admission . . . An XII,* 13.

58. Seine, CGAHHCP, *Rapport fait au conseil général* (1816), 224–226.

59. Ibid., 24.

60. Seine, CGAHHCP, *Rapport . . . du bureau central d'admission . . . An XII,* 21.

61. Seine, CGAHHCP, *Rapport fait au conseil général* (1816), 235–236 and 84.

62. *TM,* 355.

63. Seine, CGAHHCP, *Rapports au conseil général* (1803), 64–65.

64. Ibid., 26.

65. Seine, CGAHHCP, *Rapport . . . du bureau central d'admission . . . An XIII,* p. 7.

66. A. C. Duquesnoy, "Rapport sur l'administration des secours à domicile à l'époque du 1er Germinal, An XI [March 21, 1803]," 8, in Seine, CGAHHCP, *Rapports au conseil général* (1803), appendix.

67. M. A. Thouret and Lallemand, "Rapport sur le bureau de la location et de la direction des nourrices," in Seine, CGAHHCP, *Rapports au conseil général* (1803), appendix.

68. Pastoret's report of 1816 brought the data up to date, without adding new thoughts. "Bureau de la direction des nourrices," in CGAHHCP, *Rapport fait au conseil général* (1816), 373–382.

69. Thouret and Lallemand, "Rapport sur le bureau de la location," 10 and 13.

70. Seine, CGAHHCP, *Rapport fait au conseil général* (1816), 381.

71. Thouret and Lallemand, "Rapport sur le bureau de la location," 11.

72. Seine, CGAHHCP, *Rapport fait au conseil général* (1816), 378.

73. Thouret and Lallemand, "Rapport sur le bureau de la location," 12.

74. Seine, CGAHHCP, *Rapport fait au conseil général* (1816), 376–377.

75. The Society for Maternal Charity was founded in 1788 by Madame de Fougeret, née Anne Françoise d'Oultremont (d. 1813), the daughter of a tax collector and hospital administrator.

76. "Rapport sur l'établissement de la charité maternelle de Paris par le Comité de mendicité," in *PVR,* 693–703. This society tried to work with great discretion and its action is therefore difficult to document. See, e.g., L. de Lanzac de Laborie, *Assistance et bienfaisance,* vol. 5 of *Paris sous Napoleon* (5 vols.; Paris: Plon, 1908), 147–154.

77. *PVR,* 96 and 720–721.

78. Sponsored by François de Neufchâteau, a collection of documents concerning establishments for public welfare in a number of European countries were then being published under the editorship of Councillor Duquesnoy. See France, Ministère de l'intérieur, *Recueil de mémoires sur les établissements d'humanité traduits de l'allemand et de l'anglais, publiés par ordre du ministre de l'intérieur* [François de Neufchâteau], ed. A. C. Duquesnoy (18 vols. in 7; Paris: Agasse, An VII–VIII [1799–1804]).

79. Seine, CGAHHCP, *Rapports au conseil général* (1803), 70.

80. B. Delessert, *Notice sur les soupes à la Rumford établies à Paris, rue du Mail No. 16* (Paris: n.p., 21 Pluviôse, An VIII [10 February 1800]).

81. See Société philanthropique de Paris, *Rapports et comptes-rendus*. These were published annually, beginning in the Year XI.

82. Société philanthropique de Paris, *Comptes-rendus et rapports . . . 1814* (Paris: Baron, 1815), 16.

83. On the soup kitchens, see A. A. Cadet de Vaux, A. P. de Candolle, and A. A. Parmentier, *Recueil de rapports, de mémoires, et d'expériences sur les soupes économiques et les fourneaux à la Rumford, suivi de deux mémoires sur la substitution de l'orge mondé et grué au riz* (Paris: Marchant, 1801).

84. On the Philanthropic Society of Paris, see D. B. Weiner, "The Role of the Doctor in Welfare Work: The Example of the Philanthropic Society of Paris, 1780–1815," in J. P. Goubert, ed., *La médicalisation de la société française, Historical Reflections / Réflexions historiques*, 1982, *9* (1 & 2): 279–304.

85. Société philanthropique de Paris, *Rapports et comptes-rendus* (Paris: Everat, 1814), 54–55.

86. Société philanthropique de Paris, *Rapports et comptes-rendus* (Paris: Everat, 1807), 16.

87. Seine, CGAHHCP, *Rapports au conseil général* (1803), 75.

88. Ibid., 76.

89. On the Petites Maisons Hospice, see *TA*, vol. 1, 389–403; M. Anderson, "Assistance to the Aged in Eighteenth-Century Paris" (unpublished senior essay, Barnard College, 1979), esp. ch. 3, "An Old Age Home: The Hospital of *Petites maisons*,"; and L. Cahen, *Le Grand bureau des pauvres de Paris au milieu du 18ème siècle* (Paris: Bellais, 1904).

90. For the conditions of such confinement, see Chapter 9.

91. *TM*, 74; see also Chapter 7.

92. *PVR*, 688.

93. Seine, CGAHHCP, *Rapports au conseil général* (1803), 104–104.

94. On the Invalides, see Isser Woloch, *The French Veteran from the Revolution to the Restoration* (Chapel Hill: University of North Carolina Press, 1979).

95. Seine, CGAHHCP, *Rapport fait au conseil général* (1816), 88–89. See also Chapter 7.

96. See Chapter 9.

97. *TM*, 43 and 85.

98. *PVR*, 628.

99. *TA*, vol. 1, 130.

100. *PVR*, 583. A more imaginative approach toward ailing seniors prevailed at Petites Maisons. The old people who lived there were not patients, but "invalid widows or widowers," who could not be left unsupervised. That is why their dormitories had traditionally been called "infirmaries." But a real infirmary was now deemed indispensable, to isolate the sick. The Council ordered it built, and added: "We also hope that a small garden next to the infirmary be replanted, for convalescents to walk in." Seine, CGAHHCP, *Rapports au conseil général* (1803), 104.

101. Philippe Pinel, *La médecine clinique rendue plus précise et plus exacte par*

l'application de l'analyse, ou Recueil et résultats d'observations sur les maladies aigües, *faites à la Salpêtrière* (Paris: Brosson, 1802), Introduction, xxxiv.

102. J. E. D. Esquirol, *Des établissements des aliénés en France* (Paris: Huzard, 1819), 12 (emphasis added).

Chapter 6. The Inpatient: The Claims of Medical Science

1. C. F. Duchanoy, *Compte moral sur la situation des hospices civils* (Paris: Prault, An IX [1800–1801]), 31–32.

2. *TM,* 56.

3. See Bib. Ess., The Inpatient.

4. N. E. Clavareau, *Mémoires sur les hôpitaux civils de Paris* (Paris: Prault, 1805), 51.

5. Seine, CGAHHCP, *Rapports au conseil général* (1803), 45.

6. Ibid., 41.

7. Ibid., 42.

8. A small segment of this structure can still be visited. On this hospice, see L. Hautecoeur, "L'architecture hospitalière et la Salpêtrière," *Médecine de France,* 1958, *96:* 21–36.

9. For details, see M. J. Imbault-Huart, "La médicalisation du quartier des Cordeliers au 18ème et 19ème siècles," *Bulletin de la société historique de Paris et de l'Ile-de-France,* 1972–1973, *99–100:* 109–137.

10. Seine, CGAHHCP, *Rapport fait au conseil général* (1816), 49.

11. Seine, CGAHHCP, *Rapports au conseil général* (1803), 53 and 59–60.

12. Ibid., 100, 109.

13. The ground rules for the contractors are recorded in France, Ministère de l'intérieur, François de Neufchâteau, *Cahier des charges pour le service des hospices de Paris, divisé en cinq entreprises* (Paris: n.p., An VII [1798–1799]).

14. Seine, CGAHHCP, *Cahier des charges pour le service des hospices de Paris* (Paris: Prault, An X [1801–1802]).

15. Seine, CGAHHCP, *Rapports au conseil général* (1803), 14.

16. Seine, CGAHHCP, *Cahier des charges,* 13.

17. Ibid., 11–12. The French text is even more specific: the mattresses were to be covered with "toile de Mamers," the wool for the mattress to be "laine de cuisse de Nangis," and the horsehair "crin d'échantillon blond."

18. Ibid., 14–26, passim.

19. Seine, CGAHHCP, *Rapports au conseil général* (1803), 47.

20. Ibid., 12–34, passim.

21. Expenses at the Charité in the Year X (1801–1802), for example, had been 48,725 francs for the first six months, when contracted for, and only 40,632 francs under "paternal" supervision. At St. Antoine, comparable sums fell from 28,582 francs to 21,259 francs, and the same was true for the Maternité. See Seine, CGAHHCP, *Rapports au conseil général* (1803), 44, 47.

22. Ibid., 20–22.

23. Passy, *Frochot,* 468.

24. Seine, CGAHHCP, *Rapports au conseil général* (1803), 62–63.

25. Seine, CGAHHCP, *Rapport fait au conseil général* (1816), 31 and 26.

26. Passy, *Frochot*, 474.

27. Seine, CGAHHCP, *Rapports au conseil général* (1803), 92, 125, and 100.

28. Ibid., 93, 92.

29. Ibid., 50, 70.

30. Seine, CGAHHCP, *Règlement pour l'admission dans les hospices de malades* (Paris: Imprimerie des sourds-muets, An X [1801–1802]).

31. AAPP, CFNS, IV, no. 1480.

32. Ibid., 192–196, passim.

33. Seine, CGAHHCP, *Règlement pour l'admission dans les hospices*, art. 40.

34. Seine, CGAHHCP, *Rapport . . . du bureau central d'admission . . . An XII*, 19.

35. Seine, CGAHHCP, *Rapports au conseil général* (1803), 108.

36. Huard and Imbault-Huart, "Corvisart et les débuts de la clinique de la Charité," *Médecine de France*, 1974, no. 253, 10–17. The reference is to p. 12.

37. The professors tried to add official clinical teaching services in obstetrics at the Maternity Hospice; that did not come about until 1834, and neither were such services ever created at the Venereal Diseases Hospital or in the vaccination service. Archival documents indicate that negotiations between the medical school and the Paris Hospital Council advanced quite far: the minister of internal affairs had asked that educators and administrators collaborate to find a solution. But the project foundered because the two parties could not agree on sharing financial and medical control. AN, F^{17}, 1145–1146, 2165.

38. Philippe Pinel, *The Clinical Training of Doctors: An Essay of 1793*, ed. and tr. D. B. Weiner (Baltimore: Johns Hopkins University Press, 1980), 85–93, passim.

39. S. A. Tissot, "Mémoire sur la construction d'un hôpital clinique," in *Essai sur les moyens de perfectionner les études de médecine* (Lausanne: Mourer, 1785).

40. G. L. Bayle's most important work is collected in his *Recherches sur la phthisie pulmonaire* (Paris: Gabon, 1810).

41. Huard and Imbault-Huart, "Structure et fonctionnement de la Faculté de médecine de Paris en 1813," 156 n. 15.

42. J. J. Leroux, *Règlement de la Société d'instruction médicale* (Paris: Migneret, 1818).

43. Laënnec's main work was *Traité de l'auscultation médiate et des maladies des poumons et du coeur* (Paris: Brossou & Chaudé, 1819).

44. Philippe Pinel and J. J. Leroux, *Rapport fait à l'Ecole de médecine de Paris sur la clinique d'inoculation* (Paris, n.p., 29 Fructidor, An VII [1798–1799]), 4.

45. Paris, Ecole de médecine, "Rapports faits dans les différentes séances de l'Assemblée des professeurs de l'Ecole de médecine de Paris" (An III–An VIII [1794–1800]), AN, AJ^{16}, 6307, fol. 131–136.

46. Ibid., 23 and 35.

47. Ibid., 36.

48. Seine, CGAHHCP, *Rapport fait au conseil général* (1816), 61.

49. Pierre Huard, *Sciences, médecine, pharmacie, de la révolution à l'empire* (Paris: Dacosta, 1970), 140.

50. M. J. Imbault-Huart, *L'école pratique de dissection de Paris de 1750 à 1852, ou l'influence du concept de médecine pratique et de médecine d'observation dans l'enseignement médical au dix-huitième siècle et du début du dix-neuvième siècle* (Lille: Service de reproductions des thèses, 1975).

51. Ackerknecht, *Medicine at the Paris Hospital,* 92. And see D. Trenel, "Bichat, voleur de cadavres," *Bull. soc. française hist. med.,* 1932, *26:* 97–106. See also X. Bichat, *Anatomie générale appliquée à la physiologie et à la médecine,* 4 vols. (Paris: Brosson, Gabon, 1801); id., *Cours de médecine opératoire ou des opérations de chirurgie* (Paris: n.p., [1801]); id., *Recherches physiologiques sur la vie et la mort* (Paris: Brosson, Gabon, 1800) id., *Traité d'anatomie descriptive* (Paris: Gabon, 1801–1803); id., *Traité des membranes en général et de diverses membranes en particulier* (Paris: Richard, Caille et Rouvier, 1800); and G. L. Bayle, *Recherches sur la phthisie pulmonaire.*

52. J. P. J. Darcet and A. J. B. Parent-Duchâtelet, "De l'influence et de l'assainissement des salles de dissection," *AHPML,* 1831, *5:* 243–329, see esp. 250–265.

53. Ibid., 250.

54. Imbault-Huart, *Ecole pratique,* 53.

55. Quoted in Huard and Imbault-Huart, "Structure et fonctionnement," 153.

56. The Venereal Diseases Hospital changed its name to "Hôpital du Midi" in 1836, and to "Hôpital Ricord" in 1893. In 1901 it became "Cochin Annex."

57. Cullerier was chief surgeon during the whole period under consideration in this book. His assistants were his nephew, François Guillaume Cullerier (1782–1841), Gilbert, and Bard, the latter being particularly assigned to wet nurses and prostitutes. Ackerknecht writes: "Neither Cullerier nor the younger Cullerier, his nephew, were great luminaries (only the son of the nephew [Adrien Auguste (1805–1874)] was outstanding" (*Medicine at the Paris Hospital,* 175). Bertin's predecessors had been François Doublet (1751–1795) and P. A. O. Mahon (1752–1799).

58. C. Berthollier, *La population de l'Hospice des vénériens entre 1792 et 1794: Situation antérieure et évolution de l'hospitalisation* (Paris: Mémoire de maîtrise, 1974), 140–141.

59. Seine, CGAHHCP, *Rapports au conseil général* (1803), 73.

60. A. J. B. Parent-Duchâtelet, *De la prostitution dans la ville de Paris, de l'hygiène publique, de la morale et de l'administration. Ouvrage appuyé de documents statistiques puisés dans les archives de la Prefecture de police avec cartes-tableaux* (Brussels: Hauman & Cattoir, 1836), 376, 32.

61. For example, the Law of 22 July 1791, ch. 2, arts. 8 and 9; and the laws of 10 March 1796 and 23 May 1802 (20 Ventôse, Year IV, and 13 Floréal, Year X).

62. Out of 4,470 women in the first group registered, Parent-Duchâtelet tells us, half—2,332—could not sign their names. In talking with their colleagues in the 1830s, he found a nagging loneliness and a wish to have babies and care for them. Parent-Duchâtelet, *De la prostitution,* 55 and 92.

63. Ibid., 398–400.

64. Ibid., 472.

65. R. J. H. Bertin, *Traité de la maladie vénérienne chez les enfants nouveau-nés, les femmes enceintes et les nourrices, dans lequel on expose les différents modes de transmission de cette maladie des parents aux enfants, des enfants aux nourrices, et réciproquement; les symptômes qui la caractérisent comparés avec ceux que présentent les femmes enceintes, les nourrices et les adultes en général, d'après un grand nombre d'observations recueillies à l'Hôpital des Vénériens, la méthode de traitement qu'on suit, etc.* (Paris: Gabon, 1810).

66. Ibid., 23.

67. Seine, CGAHHCP, *Rapports au conseil général* (1803) 72.

68. Seine, CGAHHCP, *Rapport fait au conseil général* (1816), 89.

69. F. S. Ratier, *Coup d'oeil sur les cliniques médicales de la Faculté de médecine et des hôpitaux civils de Paris* (Paris: Baillière, 1830).

70. Berthollier, *La population de l'Hospice des vénériens*, 70.

71. Seine, CGAHHCP, *Rapports au conseil général* (1803), 62.

72. Alibert had come to the new Health School in 1796 and served as the first secretary of the Society for Medical Emulation—that group of eager young medical researchers led by the brilliant Xavier Bichat. Alibert obtained his M.D. in 1799, accepted an appointment as assistant physician at St. Louis in 1801, and became chief-of-service the following year. At the medical faculty, he occupied the chair of therapeutics. He taught dermatology at St. Louis from 1801 to 1815, and again from 1829 until his death in 1837.

73. R. Sabouraud, *L'Hôpital St. Louis,* in *Les vieux hôpitaux français* (Lyon: Ciba, 1937), 34.

74. See D. B. Weiner, "A Geriatric Hospital Service at the Salpêtrière under Napoleon," *BHM,* forthcoming.

75. To establish Pinel's credentials as a geriatrician, it is imperative to consult his book *La médecine clinique rendue plus précise et plus exacte par l'application de l'analyse, ou Recueil et résultat d'observations sur les maladies aiguës, faites à la Salpêtrière* (Paris: Brosson, Gabon, 1802; 2d ed., 1804; 3d ed., 1815). Unless otherwise indicated, references are to the introduction to the first edition (1802) and to the text of the third edition (1815). The present reference is to the introduction to the first edition, xxxiv. In *La médecine clinique,* Pinel presents 256 case histories, most of them concerning elderly patients. See also the articles "Asthenia," "Adynamia," "Ataxia," and "Cachexia" that he contributed to the *Dictionnaire des sciences médicales* in 1812.

76. Pinel, *Médecine clinique,* 414–415.

77. For a definition, see R. N. Butler, "Geriatric Medicine," in *The Oxford Companion to Medicine,* ed. J. Walton, P. V. Beeson, and R. B. Scott (New York: Oxford University Press, 1986), vol. 2, 469–474.

78. Pinel, *Médecine clinique,* 229–240, 186–193.

79. In *Médecine clinique,* Pinel prints a long list of the plant remedies he used most frequently. His list of chemical products is equally long, and he acknowledges the assistance of his students C. J. A. Schwilgué (1775–1808) and Pierre Hubert Nysten (1774–1817), both outstanding pharmacists, adding that "experimentation in the infirmaries gradually determined" his preferences (Pinel, *Médecine clinique,* 513n). Pinel's list of Latin terms could not

have been made understandable without the help of Estes, *Dictionary of Proto-pharmacology*.

Chapter 7. Clinical Specialization: Children at Risk

1. Seine, CGAHHCP, *Code spécial de l'Hospice de la Maternité* (Paris: Imprimerie des sourds-muets, An X [1801–1802]), Title II, ch. 1, par. 18.

2. Seine, CGAHHCP, *Rapports au conseil général* (1803), 142. Some Catholic homes traditionally sheltered pregnant unmarried women (AN, F[15], 1861; *TA*, vol. 1, 761–766; see also Marcel Fosseyeux, "Une maison de l'Hôpital général: Le refuge de Ste. Pélagie sous l'ancien régime," *Bulletin de la société de l'histoire de Paris et de l'Ile de France,* 1912, *39*: 63–76). In this context, a manuscript register of novices who joined the Augustinians of the Paris Hôtel-Dieu between 1748 and 1797 reveals some surprising facts: 305 young women between the ages of 14 and 26 entered the novitiate; 85 of these took vows after seven years' probation; the remaining 220 left or were dismissed. The reasons given for their departure are that they found the training unbearably arduous or were homesick or "insubordinate." It is startling to find that 66 out of 304—that is, well over one-fifth of all the novices—stayed between one and nine months, one half of these between six and nine months. Is it far-fetched to conjecture that not a few young women, being in an early stage of pregnancy that no one but they were aware of, took advantage of the anonymity and safety of the cloister? The nuns would help them over a desperate moment, take their babies to the Foundlings' Hospice, and then dismiss them. See Religieuses hospitalières Augustines de l'Hôtel-Dieu de Paris, "Extraits de naissance, 1748–1787. Registre pour les novices entrées depuis le 6 juillet 1748" (folio). This register was kindly communicated to the author by the late Sister Saint Scholastica.

3. Seine, CGAHHCP, *Mémoire historique et instructif sur l'Hospice de Maternité,* xiii.

4. Seine, CGAHHCP, *Code spécial . . . de la Maternité* , Title II, ch. 1, par. 18.

5. *Recherches statistiques sur la Ville de Paris,* vol. 2, table 53, quoted in J. Tulard, *Paris, le Consulat et l'Empire* (Paris: Hachette, 1970), 272.

6. Seine, CGAHHCP, *Rapport fait au conseil général* (1816), 103.

7. Seine, CGAHHCP, *Rapports au conseil général* (1803), 136–137.

8. Seine, CGAHHCP. *Mémoire historique et instructif sur l'Hospice de Maternité,* 42–43.

9. Seine, CGAHHCP, *Code spécial . . . de la Maternité,* Title II, ch. 1, par. 28. The council evidently softened this draconic rule, for the *Mémoire historique et instructif sur l'Hospice de Maternité* explains that women were not permitted to go out "unless personal matters or arrangements for the expected child require it. But they must return by nightfall. If they stay out overnight, they are not taken back until the time for delivery" (p. 48).

10. Ibid.

11. Seine, CGAHHCP, *Rapport fait au conseil général* (1816), 96.

12. CGAHHCP, *Rapports au conseil général* (1803), 135.

13. Ibid., 147.

14. Quoted in Delaunay, *Maternité*, 104.

15. Seine, CGAHHCP, *Rapport fait au conseil général* (1816), 101.

16. *TM*, 267, n. 41. The sickest women were transferred to the crib room or to Ste. Geneviève. The Augustinians kept no registers of these assignments.

17. Seine, CGAHHCP, *Rapport fait au conseil général* (1816), 101.

18. *TM*, 242.

19. Seine, CGAHHCP, *Rapports au conseil général* (1803), 145–150.

20. Archives de la Seine, EA, Maternité, dossier 3.

21. The reader will remember that, when the sisters resumed control under the Restoration, the Hospital Council was ordered to reverse the use of the two buildings, transferring the lying-in service to Port-Royal and grouping the babies at the Oratory. This reversal did not, of course, alter the distance between the two services. Birth registers have been preserved. See Archives de la Seine, EA, Maternité (Port-Royal), dossier 288, 145 registers: "Registres naissances, Ans XI, XII, XIII; 1797–1913." It is chilling to turn their pages, with row upon row of numbers and names, with crosses added in another hand.

22. The eldest, Jean Pierre, entitled his thesis *Considérations générales sur les maladies propres aux enfants dans les premiers moments de leur vie* (Paris: Thèse médecine, 1808); the second son, Antoine, wrote *Considerations générales sur la première dentition et sur le sevrage* (Paris: Thèse médecine, 1812); the youngest, Ambroise, produced *Recherches sur les causes des convulsions auxquelles les enfants sont exposés dans le premier âge de leur vie* (Paris: Thèse médecine, 1815). He is the least original of the three.

23. Jean Pierre Auvity, *Considérations*, 8.

24. Antoine Auvity, *Considérations*, 15–16, 20.

25. Seine, CGAHHCP, *Rapport fait au conseil général* (1816), 106.

26. See, e.g., H. Bruening, *Geschichte der Methodik der künstlichen Säuglingsernährung nach medizin-, kultur-, und kunstgeschichtlichen Studien* (Stuttgart: Enke, 1908). In the Drake Collection at the Academy of Medicine of Toronto, manifold objects and documents illustrate past practices of infant care and feeding.

27. The debate over infant feeding continued throughout the nineteenth century. Pastoret reports on experiments with goat's milk, fed to four babies in July–September 1803. The first baby developed digestive troubles, and thrush on the 22d day. The goat ran out of milk and the baby, handed to a sedentary wet nurse, died at 77 days of age. The second baby developed thrush and aphthous pustules on his belly, and died after a week. The third baby died of thrush after two weeks. The fourth baby lived on goat's milk for 26 days, only to die after 7 more days with a wet nurse. These babies received a great deal of attention from two nursemaids and an apprentice midwife, who "tormented the goat: to nourish it better, they gave it unusual food to eat. Perhaps the experiment is worth repeating," concluded Pastoret, "but who will dare, after such awful results?" (CGAHHCP, *Rapport fait au conseil général* [1816],

120). The late emeritus professor of pediatrics at the Hôpital des enfants assistés, Dr. Stéphane Thieffry, still remembered the Pavillon des ânesses (asses' shed) on the hospital grounds (personal communication).

28. Jean Abraham Auvity, "Mémoire sur l'Hospice de la Maternité," *Recueil périodique de la Société de médecine de Paris*, 1797, *3*: 165–176, 173–174.

29. Archives, Ville de Paris, EA, Maternité, 1813, dossier 2.

30. Jean Pierre Auvity, *Considérations*, 27.

31. Jean Abraham Auvity, "Sur la maladie aphtheuse des nouveaux-nés, *Mémoires de la Société royale de médecine*, 1787–1788, *9*: 122–168; and "Mémoire sur l'endurcissement du tissu celullaire," ibid., 328–414. In the judgment of Dr. Stéphane Thieffry (see n. 27 above), these clinical observations are excellent and entirely valid today (personal communication).

32. Auvity, "Sur la maladie aphtheuse," 128.

33. Auvity must have diagnosed this in children held back at Port-Royal, for the signs of primary syphilis appear only one month after infection.

34. Antoine Auvity, *Considérations*, 13.

35. M. A. V. Boivin, *Mémorial de l'art des accouchements, suivi 1) des Aphorismes de Mauriceau, 2) de ceux l'Orazio Valota, 3) d'une série de 136 gravures représentant le mécanisme de toutes les espèces d'accouchements, tant naturels qu'artificiels* . . . (Paris: Méquignon, 1813; 2d ed., 1817). The first edition is dedicated to Madame Lachapelle; the second to Count Chabrol de Volvic, prefect of the Seine. Madame Boivin also published *Traité pratique des maladies de l'utérus et de ses annexes, fondé sur un grand nombre d'observations cliniques* (Paris: Baillière, 1833).

36. According to the anonymous article in Dechambre's *Dictionnaire* and to Delaunay, a close friendship between Boivin and Lachapelle turned into deadly rivalry when Boivin's book found wide acclaim. Also according to these sources, Boivin refused an invitation to move to St. Petersburg, where the empress was actively recruiting Western leaders for her charitable institutions. Boivin had a large Parisian clientèle, including the famous surgeon Dupuytren, who insisted she deliver his daughter, saying that she seemed to "have an eye at her fingertips." She was apparently considered as midwife to the empress Marie Louise, but then fashion prevailed and the "king of Rome" was delivered by the accoucheur Dubois instead. Had she agreed to head the midwifery school at the Maternité after Madame Lachapelle's death in 1821, she might have given solid academic standards to this pioneering institution for the professional education of women. Her decorations included the Gold Medal for Civil Merit of Prussia and she held honorary membership in the Academy of Medicine of Berlin, the Societies for Medicine and Natural Sciences of Brussels and Bruges, and an honorary M.D. from the faculty of Marburg. In Paris, we find her a member of the Société médicale d'émulation, the Société de médecine pratique, and the Athénée des sciences et des arts; in the provinces, a corresponding member of the Society of Medicine of Bordeaux. (This account is based on G. J. A. Witkowski, *Accoucheurs et sages-femmes célèbres: Esquisses biographiques* [Paris: Steilheil, 1891], 59–60; Delaunay, *Maternité*; and A. Dechambre, ed., *Dictionnaire encyclopédique*, s.v. "Boivin.")

37. Seine, CGAHHCP, *Rapport fait au conseil général* (1816), 122, 121.

38. Charles Michel Billard, *Traité des maladies des enfants nouveau-nés et à la mamelle* (Paris: Baillière, 1828). See B. Bianchetti, *Charles Michel Billard und sein Traité des maladies des enfants nouveau-nés et à la mamelle* (Zürich: Juris, 1963).

39. Dupoux, *Sur les pas,* 285.

40. Seine, CGAHHCP, *Rapport fait au conseil général* (1816), 116 and 126.

41. Seine, CGAHHCP, *Rapports au conseil général* (1803), 25.

42. Seine, CGAHHCP, *Mémoire historique et instructif sur l'Hospice de Maternité,* 16, 17.

43. Seine, CGAHHCP, *Rapports au conseil général* (1803), 155.

44. Seine, CGAHHCP. *Code spécial . . . de la Maternité,* Title IV, par. 17.

45. Seine, CGAHHCP, *Rapports au conseil général* (1803), 118.

46. Seine, CGAHHCP, *Mémoire historique et instructif sur l'Hospice de Maternité,* 16, and Seine, CGAHHCP, *Rapports au conseil général* (1803), 118.

47. Seine, CGAHHCP, *Rapports au conseil général* (1803), 161–162.

48. Seine, CGAHHCP, *Rapport fait au conseil général* (1816), 116.

49. See Seine, CGAHHCP, *Rapport fait au conseil général* (1816), 116, table.

50. See Table 7.5, adapted from Seine, CGAHHCP, *Code spécial . . . de la Maternité,* Title V, ch. 1, par. 3, and Seine, CGAHHCP, *Rapports au conseil général* (1803), 170n.

51. See Seine, CGAHHCP, *Code spécial . . . de la Maternité,* Title V, ch. 1, par. 2; Seine, CGAHHCP, *Rapports au conseil général* (1803), 169n; and Seine, CGAHHCP, *Rapport fait au conseil général* (1816), 116.

52. Seine, CGAHHCP, *Rapport fait au conseil général* (1816), 113. This description seems much truer than Delaunay's fanciful account: "The *meneur,* distributor of public welfare treasure, was the master of his canton, revered by peasant women, honored by tavern-keepers, popular in those hostelries by the highway where he sheltered his caravan, fed his wet nurses, talked loudly, drank hard, and caroused at the relays with the coachmen of the mail. His profession was lucrative" (Delaunay, *Maternité,* 112).

53. The drivers sometimes picked up passengers who were not welcome in Paris. On 7 October 1810, Hucherard protested against the arrival of "country women or girls who are only five to seven months pregnant . . . [who] . . . have no abode in Paris and I must therefore admit them. . . . They abandon their baby, but come back with the same driver at a later date to seek a nursling. . . . They would not blush to take back their own child and receive a salary" (Archives de la Seine, EA, Maternité, dossier 4).

54. The Code spécial de la Maternité set a limit of twenty babies. Pastoret mentions sixteen.

55. Seine, CGAHHCP, *Rapports au conseil général* (1803), 168 n. 1.

56. A circular dated 2 October 1810, reads: "Winter is approaching and . . . the administration has instructed me to notify you to recondition your wagon. This means that it should be lined with plaited straw, that the hoops for the roof be close enough together and sturdy enough to hold up the canvas. And this canvas must be strong enough to shield the children from rain. This is to inform you that I shall demand compliance with this order." Archives de la Seine, EA, Maternité, dossier 4.

57. On 18 March, the driver Dejouy wrote from Riquebourg: "Total terror reigns in my arrondissement. . . . I do not know whether my nurses will decide to undertake the trip." A more intrepid driver, Deteuf, wrote from Nancy on 4 April: "I have just returned from my trip with twenty-four nurses, but could not penetrate into Paris because of the armies. A copy of the *Moniteur* just announced that Paris, and we too, now belong to the great Alexander. . . . tell me immediately whether I should re-alert my nurses and leave again. We await your news." Archives de la Seine, EA, Maternité, dossier 3.

58. Seine, CGAHHCP, *Rapport fait au conseil général* (1816), 111.

59. The high figure is given by Pastoret in 1816. The *Code spécial . . . de la Maternité,* in 1802, gives 2–3,000 francs.

60. See "Etat du mouvement et des journées pendant l'An XIII, des enfants abandonnés placés à la campagne," Seine, CGAHHCP, *Mémoire historique,* 121–122.

61. When a *meneur* transferred an infant (which evidently happened often), confusion frequently resulted in Paris bookkeeping. Archives de la Seine, EA, Maternité, dossier 4.

62. Archives de la Seine, EA, Maternité, dossier 3.

63. Seine, CGAHHCP, *Rapports au conseil général* (1803).

64. Deteuf, for example, wrote to the Paris office in 1814: "Tell us what your situation is like, and whether we might help you out with a little flour or some other commodity that you and the other gentlemen at the hospice lack." Archives de la Seine, EA, Maternité, dossier 3.

65. Seine, CGAHHCP, *Rapports au conseil général* (1803), 170.

66. Archives de la Seine, EA, Maternité, 1059.

67. Seine, CGAHHCP, *Rapports au conseil général* (1803), 175.

68. M. Garden, *Lyon et les Lyonnais au dix-huitième siècle* (Paris: Belles lettres, 1970), 140.

69. Seine, CGAHHCP, *Rapport fait au conseil général* (1816), 113.

70. A particularly flagrant violation is portrayed in a letter dated 13 October 1810, from Trognon, mayor of Le Coudray-St.Germain, near Beauvais (Oise) where "a frightening number of children from the [Paris] hospice died" that year. He attributed eighteen deaths to the fact that some wet nurses had two, three, or even four infants in their care. Archives de la Seine, EA, Maternité, dossier 4.

71. A contemporary description of this establishment—still functioning today as the Hôpital des enfants malades at the corner of rue de Sèvres and Boulevard du Montparnasse, can be found in AN S 7051, drawn up at the time of nationalization. This is also published in *TA,* vol. 1, 733–739. See also J. Boussoulade, "La maison de l'Enfant Jésus de la rue de Sèvres, sous la révolution," *Revue de l'Assistance publique,* 1954, *5*: 425–436; P. Valléry Radot, "L'hôpital des enfants malades," *Deux siècles,* 217–224; and especially L. Lambeau, "La maison royale de l'Enfant Jésus, actuellement Hôpital des enfants malades, rue de Sèvres, 149, 1694–1908," in Ville de Paris, Commission du vieux Paris, *Annexe au procès-verbal de la séance du 16 novembre 1907,* 396–410. On the opening of the hospital, see AAPP, *Recueil manuscrit No. 42,* "Arrêté

du Conseil des hospices, 9 Floréal An X, portant que l'Hospice des orphelines, rue de Sèvres, sera consacré à recevoir les enfants malades." See also F. S. Hügel, *Beschreibung sämmtlicher Kinderheilanstalten in Europa* (Vienna: Kaulfuss & Prandel, 1849), 111–138.

72. Information about the Ladies of St. Thomas de Villeneuve is mainly derived from archival documents graciously put at the author's disposal by Sister Stanislas Kostkas, their archivist. See also G. Bernoville, *Les religieuses de St. Thomas de Villeneuve* (Paris: Grasset, 1953).

73. Seine, CGAHHCP, *Rapport fait au conseil général* (1816), 57, 62.

74. Jean François Jadelot, "Description topographique de l'Hôpital des enfants malades," *Journal de médecine, chirurgie, pharmacie, etc.*, Year XIV (1805–1806), *11:* 115–127, and id., "De la constitution de l'air et des maladies observées à l'hôpital des enfants malades dans les années XIII et XIV," ibid., Year XIV (1805–1806), *11:* 483–515. See also G. R. Siguret, *Histoire de l'hospitalisation des enfants malades de Paris* (Paris: Thèse médecine, 1907).

75. Jadelot, "Description topographique de l'Hôpital des enfants malades," 120.

76. Ibid., 122.

77. Seine, CGAHHCP, *Rapports au conseil général* (1803), 125.

78. Seine, CGAHHCP, *Rapport fait au conseil général* (1816), 60–61.

79. Jadelot annotated a famous textbook on children's diseases that one of his students had translated into French; see M. Underwood, *Traité des maladies des enfants; entièrement refondu, complèté et mis sur un nouveau plan, avec des notes de M. Jadelot*, tr. Eusèbe de Salle (Paris & Montpellier: Gabon, 1823), 45.

80. A. B. Marfan, "L'enseignement de la pédiatrie à la Faculté de médecine de Paris," *Paris médical*, 1921, *18:* 337–348.

81. N. Andry, *L'orthopédie, ou l'art de prévenir et de corriger, dans les enfants, les difformités du corps* (2 vols.; Paris: Veuve Alix, 1741).

82. A decisive stimulus seems to have come from that ancient seat of medical learning with the publication of Jacques Mathieu Delpech's *De l'orthomorphie par rapport à l'espèce humaine, ou recherche anatomico-pathologique sur les causes, les moyens de prévenir, ceux de guérir les principales difformités et sur les véritables fondements de l'art appelé orthopédique* (Paris: Gabon, 1828).

83. See Ackerknecht, *Medicine at the Paris Hospital*, 176–177.

84. Jadelot, "Description topographique de l'Hôpital des enfants malades," 126.

85. Seine, CGAHHCP, *Rapport fait au conseil général* (1816), 56–57.

86. The central office sent 1,592 children to the new establishment while 1,289, or 45 percent of the total, gained direct admission.

87. Seine, CGAHHCP, *Rapports au conseil général* (1803), 78, 64.

88. P. Lereboullet, "L'Hôpital des enfants malades, 1802–1913," *Paris médical*, 1913–1914, *14 supplément:* 3–19, p. 14.

89. The best secondary work on this topic is J. Dehaussy, *L'Assistance publique à l'enfance: Les enfants abandonnés* (Paris: Sirey, 1951).

90. The relevant decrees under the Directory are dated 27 December 1796 and 20 March 1797 (17 Frimaire and 30 Ventôse, Year V); under the Consulate the relevant law is dated 4 February 1805 (15 Pluviôse, Year XIII). The na-

tional government promising to help out, in case of extreme need. Seine, CGAHHCP, *Rapport fait au conseil général* (1816), 279–281.

91. Ibid., 25.

92. Such a turntable can be operated at the museum of the Assistance publique in Paris.

93. *PVR*, 588. For a clear and sympathetic discussion of these procedures, see Dupoux, 151–152. At the Hôpital des enfants assistés in Paris (the former Foundlings' Hospice), a door is presumed always kept open to take in unwanted babies, but it was locked on this author's visit in the summer of 1982.

94. Title II of the decree of 19 January 1811, regarding Foundlings, Abandoned Children, and Orphans proclaimed:

Article 2.. Foundlings are children of unknown father and mother, found exposed somewhere or brought to hospices designated to receive them.

Article 3.. In each hospice designated to received foundlings there shall be a turntable where they shall be deposited.

Article 4.. There shall be at most one hospice in each arrondissement where foundlings can be received. Registers shall attest to their arrival, sex, apparent age, and describe birthmarks, and swaddling clothes that may help in their identification.

95. Dehaussy, *L'Assistance publique à l'enfance*, 46.

96. Seine, CGAHHCP, *Code spécial . . . de la Maternité,* Title III, ch. 1, par. 13.

97. Seine, CGAHHCP, *Rapport fait au conseil général* (1816), 130–136. Duchanoy, in his *Compte moral*, agreed, citing Hucherard (pp. 9–10). In fact, the administrators often preferred kindness to so much legalistic logic and stringency: see EA, dossier 0122, and EA, Maternité, dossier 6.

98. On physical standards for draftees, see A. Corvisier, *L'armée française de la fin du 17ème siècle au ministère de Choiseul: Le soldat* (2 vols.; Paris: Presses universitaires de France, 1964); see also id., "La société militaire et l'enfant," *Annales de démographie historique: Enfants et sociétés* (La Haye: Mouton, 1973), 327–434.

99. Jean François Jadelot, "Topographie médicale de l'Hospice des orphelins de Paris," *Journal de médecine, chirurgie, et pharmacie,* 1807, *13*: 243–264. See p. 258.

100. Dehaussy, *L'Assistance publique à l'enfance*, 41–42.

101. Jadelot, "Topographie médicale de l'Hospice des orphelins de Paris." Anne Brun, it will be remembered, wrote a detailed medical report about the Pitié for de Jussieu in 1790. See Chapter 2.

102. Jadelot, "Topographie médicale de l'Hospice des orphelins de Paris," 248–250.

103. Seine, CGAHHCP, *Rapports au conseil général* (1803), 122.

104. *TA,* vol. 1, 181.

105. Archives de la Seine, EA, Orphelins, dossier 0122. The first month of employment always constituted a trial period; if apprentices misbehaved, the master could request punishment (Seine, CGAHHCP, *Rapports au conseil général* [1803], 130). If a parent reclaimed a youngster who was serving an

apprenticeship, the child could be returned, but "the agreement must be respected" (Seine, CGAHHCP, *Rapport fait au conseil général* [1816], 134).

106. Seine, CGAHHCP, *Rapports au conseil général* (1803), 129. Presumably all apprentices were literate. What to make, then, of a contract that stated: François Charles Edouard, aged fifteen, "declared that he knew neither how to read nor write?" (ibid.).

107. Jadelot, "Topographie médicale de l'Hospice des orphelins de Paris," 245–247, and Seine, CGAHHCP, *Rapport fait au conseil général* (1816), 129–130.

108. Seine, CGAHHCP, *Rapports au conseil général* (1803), 126.

109. Archives de la Seine, EA, Ancien numérotage, 1060.

110. *PVR*, 582.

111. Jadelot, "Topographie médicale de l'Hospice des orphelins de Paris," 251.

112. Ibid., 256.

113. Ibid., 260.

114. Ibid., 264.

115. Dupoux, *Sur les pas*, 178.

Chapter 8. The Schooling and Health of the Deaf and Blind

1. For general discussion, political background and detailed documentation, see Bib. Ess., The Deaf and the Blind.

2. The Quinze-Vingts Hospice was founded in 1260; this hospital for the blind is still functioning, and I gratefully acknowledge the generous assistance of the administrator, M. J. G. Galtier, and the archivist, Mme Charles.

3. R. Sand, *The Advance to Social Medicine* (London: Staples, 1952), 407.

4. See "Histoire de l'art d'instruire les sourds-muets," in Institution nationale des sourds-muets de Paris, *Statue de l'abbé de l'Epée, oeuvre de M. Félix Martin. Compte-rendu de la séance d'inauguration présidée, le 14 mai 1879, dans la salle des exercices de l'Institution nationale des sourds-muets de Paris, par M. Ch. Le Père, Ministre de l'intérieur et des cultes. Notices biographiques. Documents divers* (Paris: Boucquin, 1879), 69–78.

5. See Juan Pablo Bonet, *Reducciòn de las letras y arte para enseñar a hablar los mudos* (Madrid: Abarca de Angulo, 1620).

6. See D. F. Mullett, "The Arte to Make the Dumbe to Speak, the Deafe to Hear," *JHM*, 1971, *26*: 123–149.

7. Pereira met on 11 June 1749 and 13 January 1751 with a commission of the Academy of Sciences, headed by the naturalist Buffon. See "Mémoire que J. J. R. Pereire a lu dans la séance de l'Académie royale des sciences du 11 juin 1749 et dans lequel, en présentant à cette compagnie un jeune sourd et muet de naissance, il expose avec quel succès il lui a appris à parler," *Histoire de l'Académie royale des sciences*, 1749, 269–277, and "Observations sur les sourds et muets," *Mémoires de l'Académie royale des sciences*, 1768, 500–530. It seems that Jean-Jacques Rousseau often visited Pereira's school and derived some ideas for the *Emile* from that acquaintance. See (anon.,) *Jacob Rodrigues Pereire, premier instituteur des sourds-muets en France* (Paris: Didier, 1875).

8. The Museum of the Association Valentin Haüy in Paris has recently been modernized and refurbished in order better to display its rich collection of machines, maps, globes, and games for the blind, as well as the manuscripts and books in its fine library.

9. After three futile attempts, this author was finally permitted to explore the cellars of the ancient Magloire Seminary—the present Institution nationale des jeunes sourds. It took little time to locate all the children's personal dossiers, much to the director's surprise. The elements for a detailed history of the children's progress therefore now exist. Partly on the basis of these documents, Alexis Karakostas has written "L'institution nationale des sourds-muets de Paris de 1790 à 1800: Histoire d'un corps à corps" (Thèse de médecine, Paris, 1981). In 1989 an exhibition focusing on the abbé de l'Epée and the National Institution for Deaf Children was held in the chapel of the Sorbonne.

10. Philippe Ariès, *L'enfant et la vie familiale sous l'ancien régime* (Paris: Plon, 1960); see esp. pt. 1, ch. 2, and pt. 3, ch. 2.

11. Born at Versailles as the son of a royal architect, de l'Epée found his vocation by chance when he encountered two deaf girls. Their instruction blossomed into a famous school.

12. Abbé C. M. de l'Epée, *La véritable manière d'instruire les sourds-muets, confirmée par une longue expérience* (Paris: Nyon, 1784).

13. Ibid., 203.

14. For an excellent recent discussion, see Ch. Cuxac, *Le langage des sourds* (Paris: Payot, 1983).

15. De l'Epée, *La véritable manière,* 129.

16. Letter from the abbé de l'Epée to the abbé Sicard, dated 18 December 1783, quoted in Baron M. F. de Gérando, *De l'éducation des sourds-muets de naissance* (2 vols.; Paris: Méquignon, 1827), vol. 1, 480.

17. See, e.g., *Exercices que soutiendront des sourds-et-muets de naissance, les 12 et 15 septembre 1789, dans la salle du musée de Bordeaux, dirigés par M. l'abbé Sicard, instituteur royal, sous les auspices de M. Champion de Cicé, archevêque de Bordeaux et garde des sceaux de France* (Bordeaux, Racle, 1789). AN, F^{15}, 2584 A.

18. See Mme V. Celliez, *Album d'un sourd-muet: Notice sur l'enfance de Massieu, sourd-muet, suivie de poésies* (Lons-le-Saulnier: Courbet, 1851), 7. See also D. B. Weiner, s.v. "Massieu" and "Sicard" in *Gallaudet's Encyclopedia of Deaf People and Deafness,* ed. J. V. Van Cleve (New York: McGraw-Hill, 1987).

19. Abbé R. A. C. Sicard, *Cours d'instruction d'un sourd-muet de naissance, pour servir à l'éducation des sourds-muets et qui peut être utile à celle de ceux qui entendent et qui parlent* (Paris: Le Clerc, An VIII [1799–1800]; 2d ed., 1803), 5 and 20–21; emphasis added.

20. Once, in the presence of the German dramatist August von Kotzebue, Sicard talked from 11:30 until 4 P.M.! A. V. Kotzebue, *Erinnerungen aus Paris im Jahre 1804* (Berlin: Fröhlich, 1804), 469–470.

21. See, e.g., his ambivalent statement, explaining his political allegiances, in *Ami des lois,* 21 Brumaire, An IV (11 November 1797).

22. Personal letters and documents, many dating from Haüy's exile in St. Petersburg, can be found in the dossier "Valentin Haüy" at the Association

Valentin Haüy pour le bien des aveugles, 5, rue Duroc, Paris. I wish to thank M. P. Schneider-Manoury, the general secretary, and M. Gautrot, the librarian, for making these papers accessible.

23. V. Haüy. *Essai sur l'éducation des aveugles ou Exposé de différents moyens vérifiés par l'expérience pour les mettre en état de lire à l'aide du tact, d'imprimer des livres dans lesquels ils puissent prendre des connaissances de langues, d'histoire, de géographie, de musique, etc., d'exécuter différents travaux aux métiers, etc.* (Essay on the Education of the Blind: A Treatise on Various Ways, Tested by Experience, of Enabling the Blind to Read with the Help of Touch, to Print Books in Which They Can Study Languages, History, Geography, Music, etc., and to Perform Varied Tasks on Simple Machines, etc.) (Paris: Imprimé par les enfants aveugles, 1786). For correspondence regarding royal sponsorship of this book, see AN, F[17], 1145.

24. Haüy opposed the hospitalization of a seriously ill blind child on one occasion and wrote Chaptal: "There is in blind persons a suspiciousness from which it is difficult to protect them. Each time that a blind patient has to be sent even to the best-run hospital, he thinks he is dying, which aggravates his illness. Almost always, special care given here at my school leads to a speedy recovery" (17 March 1797 [27 Ventôse, Year V]). AN, F[15], 2570 B.

25. V. Haüy, *Essai,* 117 n. 21.

26. Ibid., 31–32.

27. V. Haüy, "Moyens nouveaux, propres, si l'on ne s'abuse, à étendre et peut-être même à perfectionner le service du télégraphe" (1803), which was apparently published in St. Petersburg (where Haüy then lived in exile)] as *Mémoire historique abrégé sur les télégraphes* (1810), is mentioned by A. Skrebitzki, *Valentin Haüy à St. Petersbourg* (Paris: Noizette, 1884).

28. The Museum of the Association Valentin Haüy has a rich collection of texts printed according to Haüy's method and in Braille.

29. The only account of Haüy's institution written by a participant is Galliod, *Notice historique sur l'établissement des jeunes aveugles.* After fruitless searches for this document in all the appropriate Paris libraries and archives, it was located in the Braille Library of the Institution Valentin Haüy pour le bien des aveugles in the form of a cardboard-bound volume "printed" on blank paper in relief letters—that is, by Haüy's method (Paris: Imprimé aux Quinze-Vingts, 1828). (Bracketed page references are to the long-hand transcript in my possession, kindly undertaken by M. Gautrot, the librarian.)

30. Haüy's school had previously been located on rue Coquillière.

31. Valentin's older brother, the famous crystallographer René Just Haüy, had been elected to the Academy two years earlier.

32. "Extrait des registres de l'Académie royale des sciences, 16 février 1785," reprinted in Haüy's *Essai.*

33. *Journal de Paris,* 1 and 8 January 1787.

34. L. Lallemand, *Histoire de la charité* (4 vols.; Paris: Picard, 1912), vol. 4, pt. 2, bk. 1, 48. The whole world was ready for reform of this kind: similar schools were opened within the subsequent fifteen years at Liverpool (1791), St. Petersburg (1791), Edinburgh (1792), Bristol (1793), London (1799), Vienna (1804), Berlin (1806), Prague (1807), Amsterdam (1808), Zü-

rich (1809), Copenhaguen (1817), and the Perkins Institute for the Blind in Boston, Mass. (1829). See Sand, *Advance to Social Medicine*, 408.

35. Throughout 1789 and 1790, Haüy continued anxiously to promote his cause. He arranged for the blind children to sing masses in various churches and sought commissions for their printing skills. See S. Lacroix, *Actes de la Commune de Paris* (7 vols.; Paris: Cerf & Noblet, 1894–1909), vol. 1, 508–509, and Sébastien Mercier, who commented that there is "nothing more touching than to watch [Haüy] in the midst of his students, whose sight he seems to restore by perfecting their other senses" (Mercier, *Tableau de Paris* [12 vols.; Amsterdam: n.p., 1783], vol. 12, 179).

36. Sicard presided over the French Institution for the Deaf until his death on 10 May 1822, at the age of eighty. In January 1795, he joined the faculty of the Normal School to teach grammar and was elected to the French Academy, where he chaired the committee that revises the famous Dictionary. His writings pertain to grammar, psychology, instruction of the deaf, and devotional literature.

37. *Adresse des représentants de la Commune de Paris à l'Assemblée nationale sur la formation d'un établissement national en faveur des sourds et muets présentée le jeudi 18 février 1790* (Paris: Lottin, 1790), 4–6, passim, and *AP,* vol. 11, 644–645. See also M. Tourneux, *Bibliographie de l'histoire de Paris* (5 vols.; Paris: Imprimerie nouvelle, 1900), vol. 3, nos. 15,269–15,277.

38. *PVR,* 742.

39. Laurent Clerc became a teacher at the Paris school. In 1816, when Dr. Thomas Hopkins Gallaudet (1787–1851) journeyed to Paris from the United States to inquire into European methods of instructing the deaf, Clerc became his guide. Eventually Clerc followed Gallaudet to Hartford, Connecticut, where he taught at the American Asylum for the Deaf.

40. The handwritten answers can be found in AN, F^{15}, 2584.

41. Karakostas, in "L'institution nationale," argues that Sicard and Massieu were "a couple," and that the abbé owed the deaf man his appointment as headmaster, his successes before the National Assembly, and his liberation from prison in 1792. Yet when he died, Sicard left Massieu nothing but 30,000 francs in debts.

42. Karakostas confirms this in "L'institution nationale," 39–48.

43. "Rapport sur l'établissement de l'Institution des sourds-muets de naissance, fait au nom des comités de l'extinction de la mendicité, d'aliénation des biens nationaux, des finances, et de constitution, par M. Prieur, député de Châlons, département de la Marne, à l'assemblée nationale, imprimé par les sourds-muets," *AP,* vol. 28, 489–491, followed by a speech by Sicard, 491–492. See also *PVR,* 736–745; and for a discussion of the report by the Poverty Committee, see *PVR,* 113–114, 120–121, 176.

44. "Rapport sur l'établissement . . . des sourds-muets," 743–744. In his letter to Prieur on July 29, 1791, Sicard had proposed the sum of five hundred livres and free board for the staff; the legislature refused this, and neither was Sicard granted all the domestics he asked for.

45. By Périsse du Luc, a member of the Poverty Committee.

46. *PVR,* 120 and 211.

47. Diderot, "Lettre sur les aveugles," in *Oeuvres*, vol. 1, 295.

48. *PVR*, 756–757.

49. *Arrêt du conseil d'état du roi qui ordonne que l'établissement formé pour l'instruction des sourds et muets par le Sieur abbé de l'Epée sera incessamment et irrévocablement placé et fondé dans la partie des bâtiments des Célestins de Paris à ce désignée par le Sieur Lemoigne de Couson, architecte, et commet le Sieur de St. Julien receveur général du clergé, pour recevoir provisoirement les revenus qui sont et seront à l'avenir affectés et remis audit établissement. Du 25 mars 1785* (Paris: Imprimerie royale, 1785).

50. The transfer of Haüy's school to the Célestins convent occurred gradually over two years (February 1790 to February 1792), as building renovation permitted (Karakostas, "L'institution nationale," 50 and 68).

51. Another intriguing experiment to educate handicapped persons was a school for veterans, many of them maimed, at the Hôtel des Invalides. Founded in the Year II, it was headed by Brard. Bonaparte dissolved it. See Woloch, *French Veteran*, 156–163, passim. Woloch suggests that Brard and Haüy were friends.

52. Haüy's staff totaled nineteen, against only eleven for Sicard. In spite of this discrepancy, the total budget at the institution for the blind was 13,900 livres, not much higher than Sicard's 12,700 livres. The teachers of the deaf were therefore better paid than those of the blind, and Sicard himself earned five hundred livres more than his colleague.

53. See Convention nationale, *Rapport et projet de décret sur l'organisation définitive des deux établissements fondés à Paris et à Bordeaux pour les sourds et muets, présentés à la Convention nationale au nom des trois comités d'instruction publique, des finances, et des secours publics, le 16 Nivôse, An III, par Thomas François Ambroise Jouënne, député du Calvados* (Paris: Imprimerie nationale, 1795). See also A. Cornié. *Etude sur l'institution nationale des sourdes-muettes de Bordeaux, 1786–1903* (Bordeaux: Imprimerie nouvelle, 1903).

54. The Revolutionary dates are 16–19 Nivôse and 10 Thermidor, Year III.

55. A national survey, launched under the Convention, produced incomplete results that one finds here and there in the archives. See Karakostas, "Institution nationale," Appendix O: "Départements ayant répondu au recensement avant le décret Jouënne," and "Départements ayant répondu au recensement après le décret Jouënne." Note the author's footnote: "The census is often incomplete for each department and stops after the Year V [1796–1797]" (pp. A86–87). Some replies to a questionnaire can be found in AN, F^{15}, 2583.

56. A. Dufau, *Essai sur l'état physique, moral et intellectuel des aveugles-nés, avec un nouveau plan pour l'amélioration de leur condition sociale* (Paris: Imprimerie royale, 1837), 150.

57. Jean Baptiste Massieu had argued for eight to ten schools; Etienne Christophe Maignet proposed six. See J. B. Massieu, député de l'Oise, *Rapport et projet de décret sur l'établissement d'une école de sourds-muets en la ville de Bordeaux* (Paris: Imprimerie nationale, [12 May 1793]), and E. C. Maignet, député du Puy de Dôme, *Rapport et projet de décret sur l'organisation des établisse-*

ments pour les sourds-muets indigents, décrétés le 28 juin dernier [1793], *au nom du Comité des secours publics* (Paris: n.p., [1793]). Maignet's proposal was made on 23 December 1792.

58. "There shall also be schools for the deaf-mute and for the congenitally blind," Title III of the Daunou Law of 25 October 1795 (3 Brumaire, Year IV) asserted (art. 2), adding: "The number and organization of each of these schools shall be determined by special laws, on the recommendation of the Public Education Committee" (art. 3).

59. The minister of internal affairs decreed on 29 November 1797 (9 Frimaire, Year VI), that "since the institutions for the deaf-mute and the blind pertain to both education and public aid, they shall depend on the fifth division of the ministry, for education; and for administrative and economic matter on the second division, among whose financial obligation is the past and future funding of these establishments"(AN, F¹⁵, 2500).

60. "The location of this vast property minimizes its value," the document reads, "it consists of buildings that can only serve as a public establishment, or they would have to be sold for a pittance" (AN, F¹⁵, 2584).

61. For details of a personal and political nature concerning Sicard and Haüy, see Bib. Ess., The Deaf and the Blind.

62. See, e.g., R. Bernard, "Le Séminaire St. Magloire, les Oratoriens, et l'Institut des sourds-muets," Société historique, archéologique, et artistique des 5ème, 13ème, et 14ème arrondissements, *La montagne Ste. Geneviève et ses abords,* 1 June 1940, 2–4.

63. AN, F¹⁵, 2590.

64. The Sisters of Charity moved instead to the rue du Bac, into a vast complex of buildings, still the international headquarters of their order.

65. Sicard collected manifold honors, was visited by Pope Pius VII, and received medals from King Louis XVIII, Czar Alexander I, and King Bernadotte of Sweden.

66. AN, F¹⁵, 241. By the decree of 28 July 1795 (10 Thermidor, Year III), the blind gained permanent occupancy of the "Catherinettes."

67. Galliod, *Notice historique sur l'établissement des jeunes aveugles* (see n. 29 above), [11].

68. The seminarian aspects of the regulations derived from the general plan drafted by Prieur de la Marne, prompted by Sicard. See *Règlements pour l'établissement des sourds-muets et des aveugles, fondé par les décrets de l'assemblée nationale du 21 juillet et du 28 septembre 1791, sanctionnés par le Roi,* AN, F¹⁵, 1145. These regulations are signed by Liancourt.

69. "Règlement arrêté le 18 Vendémiaire An IX par le ministre de l'intérieur pour l'Institution nationale des sourds-muets de naissance de Paris," in Karakostas, "L'Institution nationale," Annex N.

70. "Règlement pour l'établissement des sourds-muets et des aveugles-nés" (AN F¹⁵, 1145, 17). Two generations later, Maxime Du Camp still found these facilities in good working order. See "L'enseignement exceptionnel: L'institution des sourds-muets," *Revue des deux mondes,* 1873, 2ème période, *104*: 555–577.

71. Convention nationale. *Rapport et projet . . . par Maignet,* paragraphs 44–55.

72. See a government report dated 1 September 1797 (15 Fructidor, Year V), in AN, F¹⁵, 2459, and, for confirmation of the prevalent misery, AN, F 15 2569.

73. Sicard to Lucien Bonaparte, 30 August 1800.

74. Karakostas, "L'institution nationale," 134–142.

75. L. F. J. Alhoy [et Valentin Haüy], *Eclaircissements sur le projet d'assurance des écoles nationales des sourds-muets et aveugles-nés, fournis par les instituteurs en chef de ces écoles, à Paris* (Paris: Institution des sourds-muets, An VIII [1799–1800]).

76. Lucien Bonaparte appointed three seasoned administrators, de Lassalle, the duc A. J. de Béthune Charost, and Jean Louis Brousse-Desfaucherets, the assistant mayor for public works.

77. See "Réunion des jeunes aveugles-travailleurs aux Quinze-Vingts," AN, F¹⁵, 2576.

78. Haüy is often described as the chief founder of this cult. See, e.g., L. M. de La Réveillière-Lepeaux, *Mémoires* (3 vols.; Paris: Plon-Nourrit, 1895), vol. 2, 166–167. Albert Mathiez admired Haüy's "soul of an apostle, enchanted with ideals, incapable of self-doubt, at ease in vast, moral and intrepid undertakings" (*La théophilanthropie et le culte décadaire, 1796–1801, essai sur l'histoire religieuse de la révolution* [Paris: Durand, 1904], 90).

79. Manuscript reports by police spies dated June 1797 (Prairial, Year V), describe the "real purpose" of the theophilanthropists. "Our reports indicate that this attractive façade of pure and edifying morality hides a den of anarchy and terrorism. After the public speeches, the initiate[s] retire to a private room, where they applaud everything subversive and *whisper* to each other that some *firm* step will be taken. They trample on the constitution of the Year III, call each other good brothers, three by three, that is to say, good masons. . . . Observers are following the Society closely" (AN, F⁷, 7338).

80. The decree of 2 October 1801 (12 Vendémiaire, Year X), reads: "The societies known by the name of theophilanthropists shall no longer meet in public buildings. The ministers of finance and general police shall enforce this decree. Signed: Bonaparte." See J. Fouché, *Lettre du ministre de la police générale de la république qui fait défense aux théophilanthropes de s'assembler davantage dans les endroits ci-dessus indiqués par ordre du gouvernement* (BN, LD 188 33).

81. AN, F¹⁵, 2576.

82. The richest documentation for the period 1801–1815 is to be found in the Quinze-Vingts archives, particularly series B 109, dossiers 6715–6722, to be supplemented with a few documents at the Institution nationale des jeunes aveugles, 56, boulevard des Invalides, Paris.

83. Archives, Quinze-Vingts, B 109, 6722.

84. See AN, F¹⁵, 2570 A.

85. J. Frank, *Reise nach Paris, London, und einem grossen Theile des übrigen Englands und Schottlands in Beziehung auf Spitäler, Versorgungshäuser, übrigen Armen-Institute, medizinische Lehranstalten und Gefängnisse* (2 vols.; Vienna: Camesianische Buchhandlung, 1804), vol. 1, 102.

86. See, e.g., A. Rodenbach, *Lettre sur les aveugles pour faire suite à celle de Diderot* (Brussels: n.p., 1828); id., *Les aveugles et les sourds-muets: Histoire, instruction, education, biographies* (Brussels: Slingeneyer, 1855); and id., *Notice sur la phonographie ou langue musicale télégraphique inventée par V. Haüy et perfectionnée par Sudre* (Paris: n.p., n.d.).

87. Haüy's attempts to recapture the attention of Frenchmen in high places failed. See AN, F^{17}, 1445; Archives, Quinze-Vingts, B 109, dossier 6715; and Archives, Institution nationale des jeunes aveugles. Gradually one begins to wonder whether Haüy was so wrong to talk of "years of persecution" by his "enemy." See, for example, an autobiographic fragment called "Mémoire historique" (AN, F^7, 4306).

88. J. A. Zeune, *Belisar: Über den Unterricht der Blinden* (Berlin: In der Blindenanstalt, 1821), 42–47, passim.

89. The only printed document concerning this epoch is Skrebitzki, *Valentin Haüy à St. Petersbourg.* Annual certificates of residence in St. Petersburg are found in Archives, Hospice des Quinze-Vingts, B 109, 6715. A *"fonds"* exists in the St. Petersburg state archives, but repeated inquiries there have so far been fruitless. At his departure, the czar awarded Haüy a consolation prize, the order of St. Vladimir.

90. One long letter was published in "Pièces justificatives," in Maxime Du Camp, *Paris, ses organes, ses fonctions, et sa vie dans la seconde moitié du dix-neuvième siècle,* 3d. ed. (6 vols.; Paris: Hachette, 1875), vol. 5, 370–375. Just Haüy stayed on in St. Petersburg after his father returned home, married a Mlle de Forville and had a son, Valentin, born in 1822. In 1853, Dufau, then director of the National Institution for the Blind, petitioned Napoleon III to grant young Haüy a job, seeing that he bore a "famous name" (AN, F 1d H 2).

91. The other two were Mathieu Montmorency and Baron M F. de Gérando. Denying the request, the minister of internal affairs wrote on 13 May 1814: "The motives that determined M. Haüy's retirement seem entirely opposed to his reinstatement in the post he once held" (Archives, Quinze-Vingts, B 109, dossier 6715).

92. Recalling Louis XVIII's promise at Mittau, Haüy asked for three favors: (a) his reintegration into the *Almanach royal* as royal interpreter, author of the *Essay on the Education of the Blind,* and honorary instructor of the blind; (b) permission for Alexandre Fournier to reestablish and perfect Haüy's method at the Institution for the Blind in Paris; and (c) Louis XVIII's sponsorship of a second edition of Haüy's *Essay.* Archives, Institution nationale des jeunes aveugles.

93. Galliod, *Note historique sur l'établissement des jeunes aveugles (see n. 29 above),* [22].

94. Haüy died on 19 March 1822, and was buried at the Père Lachaise cemetery. A statue of the two famous brothers was erected at St. Just, Picardy, in 1903.

95. R. A. H. Bébian, *Journal de l'instruction des sourds-muets et des aveugles* (2 vols.; Paris: Au bureau du journal, 1826–1827), vol. 2, 52.

96. Ch. L. Carton wrote a *Mémoire sur l'éducation des sourds-muets mise à la*

portée des instituteurs primaires et des parents (Brussels: Goemaere, 1856) and edited the journal *Le sourd-muet et l'aveugle: Journal mensuel* (Bruges: Vandercasteele-Werbrouk, 1837–1841).

97. Paul Seignette received the M.D. degree from Montpellier in 1791; he worked as secretary to the French ambassador in Madrid from 1798 to 1800 and then in the archives of the Ministry of Internal Affairs until his appointment as administrator of the Quinze-Vingts in August 1802. He retired from that position in 1824 and died in Paris in 1835. AN, F^{15}, 2575.

98. Galliod, *Note historique sur l'établissement des jeunes aveugles* (see n. 29 above), [12]. Galliod's retrospective report was presented to Haüy when he returned to France in 1817. An attempt to put the children to work in the tobacco and weaving shops failed, essentially because of the administrators' parsimony.

99. J. Guadet, *L'institution des jeunes aveugles de Paris, son histoire et ses procédés d'enseignement* (Paris: Thunot, 1849), 58.

100. Louis XVIII restored the autonomy of Haüy's institution on 8 February 1815 and provided it with income from the maison Sainte Catherine and fifty thousand francs a year (Archives, Quinze-Vingts, B 109, 6715bis).

101. Sébastien Guillié's *Rapport fait à son excellence le ministre secrétaire d'état au département de l'intérieur sur l'état de l'Institution royale des jeunes aveugles, pendant les exercices 1815 et 1816* (Paris: Chanson, 1818) confirms this judgment.

102. Pierre Henri, *La vie et l'oeuvre de Louis Braille, inventeur de l'alphabet des aveugles (1809–1852)* (Paris: Presses universitaires de France, 1952), 22–24.

103. Guillié, *Rapport*, 38.

104. S. Guillié, *Essai sur l'instruction des aveugles, ou Exposé analytique des procédés pour les instruire* (Paris: Imprimé par les aveugles, 1817), 29–30.

105. Henri, *La vie et l'oeuvre de Louis Braille*, 14. The successive headmasters and teachers have little good to say about each other, often for political reasons. Thus Henri dismisses Haüy's book for its "thin and superficial notions" and condemns the author for his waverings between the Bourbons and Jacobins, but grudgingly admits that "in those troubled times, his work survived solely because he was adaptable and versatile." Henri condemns Guillié for refusing to invite the aged, disillusioned, paralytic, and deaf Haüy for a parting visit to his school. Ibid., 21 and 24.

106. "[Couples] are a continual source of misunderstandings and trouble," Guillié explained (*Rapport*, 17).

107. Both Guillié and his successor, Pignier, were conservative men in every sense: in school policy, choice of curriculum, students, and housing arrangements, faculty, books, and leisure-time activities. Guillié, appointed in 1814, was dismissed in 1821. Dr. Pignier, headmaster from 1821 to 1840, was succeeded by P. A. Dufau, 1840–1855, Boné de Verdier, 1855–1863, and the baron de Watteville, 1863–1871.

108. Quoted in Henri, *La vie et l'oeuvre de Louis Braille*, 15–17.

109. Alphonse de Lamartine, *Moniteur universel*, 15 May 1838.

110. Next door, at 7, rue Duroc, rises the privately endowed Institution Valentin Haüy pour le bien des aveugles, with classrooms and workshops,

counseling and placement services, and a sales organization for the goods manufactured by the blind, as well as a famous Braille library. The casualties of World War I caused a major spurt in the number of associations to aid the blind. Yet many groups were formed before that time. For France, see, e.g., J. V. Laborde, *La société d'assistance pour les aveugles et ses créations: La clinique nationale ophthalmologique des Quinze-Vingts et l'Ecole Braille* (Paris: Coupy, 1894); A. Lucis, *Valentin Haüy et son oeuvre; Les jeunes aveugles: Ce qu'on peut faire pour eux et pour préserver les enfants de la cécité* (Clermont: Daix, 1891); L. M. M. B. Monier de la Sizeranne, *La question des aveugles en 1910: Notes et documents* (Caen: Poisson,1910); and id., *Le Valentin Haüy: Revue française des questions relatives aux aveugles, 1883–1893.* See also Ministère de l'intérieur, Institution nationale des jeunes aveugles, *Compte-rendu de la fête du centenaire de la fondation de cette institution par Valentin Haüy* (Paris: Noizette, 1884).

111. Ch. Barbier, *Instruction familière d'ècriture nocturne, pour apprendre de suite aux aveugles à consigner leurs idées sur le papier, recueillir celles d'autrui, lire leur écriture et celle des autres aveugles, sans que l'on soit pour cela obligé de leur enseigner la figure des lettres, etc.* (Versailles: n.p., 1830). Barbier's method was discussed by the Academy of Sciences on 1 December 1823, the reporters being Ampère and Lacépède.

112. Louis Braille, *Procédé pour écrire les paroles, la musique, et le plain-chant au moyen de points, à l'usage des aveugles et disposés pour eux* (Paris: Imprimé à l'Institution nationale des aveugles, 1829). The musical notation is based on the system that Jean-Jacques Rousseau had invented in the 1740s (cf. Henri, *La vie et l'oeuvre de Louis Braille,* 59). The best English study is the brief, but sound, N. Wymer, *Louis Braille* (London: Oxford University Press, 1957), in the Lives of Great Men and Women series. See also the illustrated and well-documented J. Roblin, *Louis Braille* (London: Royal National Institute for the Blind, 1952), and H. Lende, "A Servant of Humanity," *Library Journal,* 1952, 77: 1027–1030. There is an abundance of sentimental trash.

I should like gratefully to acknowledge the guidance of my student David Goldstein, who explained and demonstrated old-fashioned and modern technology to my seminar and provided us with insight into the problems of daily communication, education, and work that a blind person faces in America today.

113. Pinel's "Rapport fait à la Société des observateurs de l'homme sur l'enfant connu sous le nom de sauvage de l'Aveyron" was published for the first time by G. Hervé in *Revue anthropologique,* 1911, *21*: 383–398. Since that time, the minutes of the Société des observateurs de l'Homme have been lost. Pinel's report has recently been reprinted in J. Copans and J. Jamin, *Aux origines de l'anthropologie française: Les Mémoires de la Société des Observateurs de l'homme de l'an VIII* (Paris: Le sycomore, 1978), 88–113. I have used the latter edition; the quotation is from 112–113.

114. Itard, hired by Sicard in December 1800, became famous as the teacher of the "wild boy of Aveyron." Itard had a predecessor as doctor for the deaf children, the health officer Poulard, who lived at Bicêtre and came regularly to the school. Itard occupied lodgings at the institution for the deaf. AN, F^{15}, 2586.

115. J. M. G. Itard, *De l'education d'un homme sauvage, ou des premiers développements physiques et moraux du jeune sauvage de l'Aveyron* (Paris: Goujon fils, 1801); id., *Rapport fait à S.E. ministre de l'intérieur sur les nouveaux développements et l'état actuel du sauvage de l'Aveyron* (Paris: Imprimerie impériale, 1807); and id., "Mémoire sur le mutisme produit par la lésion des fonctions intellectuelles," Académie royale de médecine, *Mémoires*, 1828, *1*: 3–18. Itard translated his first report into English (London: Richard Phillips, 1802).

116. In the end, the administrators decided on the removal of the boy from the Institution for the Deaf. He went to live with Madame Guérin, his housekeeper until his death in 1828.

117. When Itard's reports and memoirs were finally published in 1894, the anticlerical Dr. D. M. Bourneville described the author in the preface as having "created the teaching of speech for the deaf-mute . . . more than all the priests glorified for their solicitude. . . . [He] deserves to rank among the benefactors of mankind." Itard, a bachelor, endowed six scholarships for an extra year of study at the institution (a "*cours de perfectionnement*"). These were still being awarded at the end of the century.

The controversy occasioned by Victor continued lively for quite a while. See, e.g., F. Berthier, *Sur l'opinion de feu le Dr. Itard, médecin-en-chef de l'Institution nationale des sourds-muets de Paris, relative aux facultés intellectuelles et aux qualités morales des sourds-muets: Réfutation présentée aux académies de médecine et des sciences morales et politiques* (Paris: Michel Lévy, 1852).

In recent years, there has been a burst of interest in the "wild boy," in connection with the deaf as a minority, otology as a branch of medicine, child psychiatry, and mental retardation. Truffaut's film was a harbinger of these developments. See L. Malson, *Les enfants sauvages: Mythe ou realité* (Paris: Union générale d'édition, 1964); H. Lane, *The Wild Boy of Aveyron* (Cambridge: Harvard University Press, 1976); R. Shattuck, *The Forbidden Experiment: The Story of the Wild Boy of Aveyron* (New York: Farrar, Straus & Giroux, 1980); T. Gineste, *Victor de l'Aveyron: Dernier enfant sauvage, premier enfant fou* (Paris: Le sycomore, 1981). Gineste is working on a biography of Itard.

118. *TA*, vol. 2, 20.

119. (Anon.,) *Société d'assistance pour les aveugles: Son histoire, 1879–1915* (Paris: Imprimerie nouvelle, [1916]), 83.

120. See Louis XVIII's letter of 22 June 1814. AN, F[15], 2575.

121. In 1899, René Waldeck-Rousseau, then a senator, declared in the presence of the president of the republic, Emile Loubet, that "the blind of France are the creditors of the state," and that the Cardinal de Rohan's sale of their property entailed "a natural obligation contracted by the government" (Anon., *Société d'assistance pour les aveugles*, 85).

Chapter 9. Humane Treatment of Mental Patients

1. See D. B. Weiner, "The Apprenticeship of Philippe Pinel, A New Document, 'Observations of Citizen Pussin on the Insane,'" *American Journal of Psychiatry*, 1979, *136*: 1128–1134. This article was also published in *Clio*

medica, 1978, *13*: 124–133, where Pussin's tables are reproduced. The manuscript document is to be found in AN, 27 AP, dossier 8. See also Weiner, "Philippe Pinel's 'Memoir on Madness' of 11 December 1794: A Fundamental Text of Modern Psychiatry," *American Journal of Psychiatry*, 1992, *149* (6): 725–732. The printed French text is to be found in J. Postel, *Genèse de la psychiatrie: Les premiers écrits de Philippe Pinel* (Paris: Le sycomore, 1981), 233–248. The manuscript document is in the privately held Fonds Semelaigne. On Pinel, see Bib. Ess., The Mental Patient.

2. P. Sérieux and L. Libert, "Le régime des aliénés en France au 18ème siècle d'après des documents inédits," *Annales médico-psychologiques*, 1914, 10ème série, *6*: 43–76, 196–219, 311–324, 470–497, 598–627, and 1916, *7*: 74–98. The quotation appears on *6*: 319. See Weiner, "The Brothers of Charity," for an extensive bibliography on psychiatric nursing.

3. P. Sérieux and L. Libert, "Règlements de quelques maisons d'aliénés (Documents pour servir à l'histoire de la psychiatrie en France)," *Bulletin de la Société de médecine mentale de Belgique*, 1914, *172*: 209–250, and P. Sérieux, "Le traitement des maladies mentales dans les maisons d'aliénés du 18ème siècle," *Archives internationales de neurologie*, 1924, *43* (2): 97–119, 145–154, 191–203; 1925, *44* (1): 21–31, 50–63, 90–104, 121–133. The reference is to *44*: 101.

4. *TM*, 4.

5. To my knowledge, there is no documentation for "*maisons de santé*" for all of France.

6. R. Bénard, "Une maison de santé psychiatrique sous la révolution: La maison Belhomme," *Semaine des hôpitaux*, 1956, *32*: 3990–4000. This is by far the most informative and best-documented source. Bénard found a police register that lists 112 persons who entered the maison Belhomme between 5 August 1793 and 7 February 1795, APPP, AB 316 (3994 n. 2). See also A. Ferroni, *Une maison de santé pour le traitement des aliénés à la fin du 18ème siècle* (Paris: Thèse médecine, 1964), and J. Postel, "Les premières expériences psychiatriques de Pinel à la maison de santé Belhomme," *Revue canadienne de psychiatrie*, 1983, *28*: 571–576.

7. Tenon was particularly interested in the fate of the mentally ill. He discusses their condition in *TM*, art. 3, par. 3, and proposes a model asylum in Plate XV with detailed explanations. See P. Carrette, "Tenon et l'assistance aux aliénés à la fin du 18ème siècle," *Annales médico-psychologiques*, 12th ser., 1925, *2*: 365–386.

8. *TA*, 1, 435–504.

9. Ibid., 1, 479.

10. *TM*, 215.

11. See Weiner, "Apprenticeship," 1132.

12. C. Quétel and P. Morel, *Les fous et leurs médecines* (Paris: Hachette, 1979), esp. ch. 2, "Drogues et moyens physiques." Most helpful in guiding the layman is Estes, *Dictionary of Protopharmacology*.

13. Joseph Daquin, *Philosophie de la folie* (Chambéry: Gorrin, 1791; 2d ed. Chambéry: Cléaz, 1804).

14. Vincenzo Chiarugi, *Della pazzia in genere ed in specie. Trattato medico-analitico con una centuria di osservazioni* (2 vols.; Florence: Carlieri, 1793–1794).

A second edition was published in 1808 by Pagani, and there are a one-volume translation into German, by Weigel (Leipzig: n.p., 1795), and a translation into English published in 1987. See Bib. Ess., The Mental Patient.

15. William Battie, *A Treatise on Madness* (London: Whiston & White, 1758), 68.

16. L. Gautier, *La médecine à Genève* (Geneva: Jullien, 1906), 346.

17. J. P. Huber, J. P. Macher, and J. Alliez, "L'hospitalisation 'forcée' des insensés à Avignon au 18ème siècle," *Information psychiatrique,* 1980, *56*: 1257–1266.

18. *PVR,* 605.

19. Born in Lons-le-Saunier in 1745, five months younger than Pinel and also an oldest son, Pussin was by profession a tanner. We do not know what brought him to Paris, but he was admitted to Bicêtre on 5 June 1771 with scrofula and "cured." He found employment at the hospice, first as the boys' teacher, then, in 1784, as superintendent of the ward for incurable mental patients, the seventh ward or *"emploi* St. Prix." He married Marguerite Jubline, who became a valued helpmate. Now and then, Pussin has aroused a historian's passing curiosity. See, e.g., E. S. Bixler, "A Forerunner of Psychiatric Nursing: Jean Baptiste Pussin," *Annals of Medical History,* 1936, *8*: 518–519. See also J. Postel, "Un manuscrit inédit de Philippe Pinel sur 'Les guérisons opérées dans le 7ème emploi de Bicêtre, en 1794,'" *Revue internationale d'histoire de la psychiatrie,* 1983, *1*: 79–88.

20. J. Colombier and F. Doublet, "Observations faites dans le département des hôpitaux civils: Instructions sur la manière de gouverner les insensés, et de travailler à leur guérison dans les asiles qui leur sont destinés," *Journal de médecine, chirurgie, et pharmacie,* 1785, *64*: 529–583. See P. Carrette, "François Doublet et la psychiatrie au temps de Louis XVI," *Annales médico-psychologiques,* 1926, 12ème anné, *2*: 119–131.

21. Weiner, "Philippe Pinel's 'Memoir on Madness,'" 731.

22. Colombier and Doublet, "Observations . . . : Instructions sur la manière de gouverner les insensés," 539.

23. Weiner, " Apprenticeship," 1133.

24. Colombier and Doublet, "Observations . . . : Instructions sur la manière de gouverner les insensés," 539.

25. Weiner, " Apprenticeship," 1133.

26. Ibid. Emphasis added. The straitjacket has many alleged inventors. In the English literature on psychiatry, it was first described by the Scottish physician David Macbride (1726–1778). Funck-Brentano credits an upholsterer at Bicêtre, who may have re-"invented" it. Chiarugi describes and pictures it in *Della pazzia* (1793).

27. Philippe Pinel, "Introduction," *Traité,* 2d ed., xxxi.

28. The fabrication pictured in Muller's painting was perpetrated by Pinel's son Scipion. See his "Bicêtre en 1792. De l'abolition des chaînes," *Mémoires de l'Académie de médecine de Paris,* 1836, *5*: 32–40, and the definitive critique by Gladys Swain, "Les chaînes qu'on enlève," in *Le sujet de la folie: Naissance de la psychiatrie* (Toulouse: Privat, 1977), pt. 3. The discovery of this fraud is summarized in English in D. B. Weiner, "Pinel or the Zeitgeist?" in

Zusammenhang: Festschrift fur Marielene Putscher, ed. O. Baur and O. Glandien (2 vols.; Cologne: Wienand, 1984), vol. 2, 617–731.

29. See note 1 above.

30. Though Pussin speaks of a maximum of 300 inmates, the tables indicate only half as many, with an average annual census of one hundred. In those fourteen years, the admissions totaled 1,405, and 60 percent of the men entered Bicêtre in their twenties and thirties. The total of cures was highest in younger men and then declined steadily, whereas mortality rose with age.

31. Weiner, "Apprenticeship," 1132.

32. Ibid., 1132–1133. How exceptional it was to find a man like Pussin in a job like his is highlighted by this portrait of his predecessor: "Goislard . . . , sixty-four years old, native of Maine, a gendarme of the guard; he has brains, loves gambling passionately, and that is what has brought him here. In 1750, having exhausted all the means that his resourcefulness had procured, he is still gambling, and often there are parties in his lodgings until two o'clock in the morning, and for high stakes. He is polite, gentle, engaging, adaptable, and a flatterer; he likes music, and often performs with the madmen who have this talent. His character is quite similar to that of the inmates." (Anon.,) AN, F¹⁵, 1861.

33. Pinel studied at the college of the Doctrinaires of Lavaur (Tarn) from 1762 till 1766, when he transferred to the collège de l'Esquile in Toulouse to earn an M.A. in humanities. From 1767 to 1770, he was a graduate student at the Toulouse theological faculty, but in the spring of 1770, he broke with his Dominican teachers and began to study medicine. I should like to acknowledge the warm "Occitanian" hospitality of M. and Mme Michel Roudet and the expert help of Didier Rivals in Lavaur in exploring the circumstances of Pinel's early years.

34. I should like to acknowledge expert guidance through eighteenth-century medical Montpellier by Dr. Louis Dulieu.

35. In Pinel, *Clinical Training of Doctors,* 84.

36. Such questions are suggested by Pinel, *Clinical Training of Doctors,* and by the information contained in the case histories that Pinel constructed.

37. The following analysis is based on Pinel, "A Memoir on Madness."

38. Pinel, *Traité médico-philosophique,* introduction, 48–49.

39. See "Notes inédites de Pinel, présentées par R. Semelaigne," *Bulletin de la Société clinique de médecine mentale,* 1913, 6: 221–227, printed in Postel, *Genèse de la psychiatrie,* 226–229.

40. George Wilhelm Friedrich Hegel, *Encyclopedie der philosophischen Wissenschaften im Grundrisse (1830),* ed. F. Nicolin and O. Poggeler (Hamburg: Meiner, 1969), 338. I owe this reference to Gladys Swain.

41. It also seems justifiable to view Pinel's novel concept as a precursor of Freudian psychotherapy.

42. See "Procès-verbaux de la société d'histoire naturelle," Muséum national d'histoire naturelle, MS 464, 218.

43. Philippe Pinel, *Nosographie philosophique, ou Méthode de l'analyse appliquée à la médecine* (Paris: Brosson, 1798; 2d ed., 3 vols., 1802–1803; 3d ed., 1807; 4th ed., 1810; 5th ed., 1813; 6th ed., 1818). A student named

Chaude wrote a résumé in Latin of the 5th edition, *Nosographiae compendium* (Paris, 1816).

44. Philippe Pinel, "Mémoire sur la manie périodique ou intermittente," *Mémoires de la Société médicale d'émulation,* An V [1796–1797], *1*: 94–119, "Recherches et observations sur le traitement moral des aliénés," ibid., An VI [1797–1798], *2*: 215–255, "Observations sur les aliénés et leur division en espèces distinctes," ibid., An VII [1798–1799], *3*: 1–26). See G. Swain, "La nouveauté du *Traité médico-philosophique* et ses racines historiques," *Information psychiatrique,* 1977, *53*: 463–476. See also G. Dumas, "Pinel psychologue," *Annales médico-psychologiques,* 1927, *2*: 82–89.

45. Philippe Pinel, *Traité médico-philosophique sur l'aliénation mentale ou la manie* (Paris: Caille et Ravier, An VIII [1799–1800]). A second, revised and enlarged edition of the *Traité* was published in 1809 as *Traité médico-philosophique sur l'aliénation mentale entièrement refondue et très augmentée* (Paris: Caille et Ravier, 1800), with the ambiguous phrase "*ou la manie*" dropped from the title. The book was translated into German, Spanish, English, and Italian (in this order): into German by the Hungarian physician Michael Wagner as *Philosophisch-medizinische Abhandlung über Geistesverirrungen oder Manie* (Vienna: Schaumburg, 1801); into Spanish by Dr. Guarnerio y Allavena, *Tratado medico-filosòfico de la enagenaciòn del alma or mania* (Madrid: Imprenta real, 1804); into English by Dr. D. D. Davis, under the unsatisfactory title *A Treatise on Insanity* (London: Cadell & Davies, 1806); and into Italian by Dr. C. Vaghi as *Trattato medico-filosofico sopra l'alienazione mentale* (Lodi: Orcasi, 1830).

46. Pinel's *La médecine clinique* is cited in Chapter 6, n. 75.

47. Many of the major documents pertaining to this complex era of transition are now conveniently available in print as an Appendix entitled "Documents pour servir à l'histoire de la naissance de l'asile, 1797–1811" in M. Gauchet and G. Swain, eds., *Des passions considérées comme causes, symptômes, et moyens curatifs de l'aliénation mentale par D. Esquirol* (Paris: Librairie des deux-mondes, 1980).

48. Jan Goldstein's assessment of Esquirol as the creator of concepts that were politically useful and as a master of patronage rightly portrays a doctor principally interested in creating a powerful profession. In contrast, her analysis of Pinel as a "charlatan" with a new nostrum, "moral treatment," hardly does this innovative physician justice, particularly because there is so little emphasis on his role of clinician, central to his thought and personality. See Goldstein, *Console and Classify: The French Psychiatric Profession in the Nineteenth Century* (New York: Cambridge University Press, 1987), esp. chs. 3, 5, and 8.

49. This unique manuscript document was recently acquired by the Louise M. Darling Biomedical Library at UCLA: see D. B. Weiner, "Esquirol's Patient Register: The First Private Psychiatric Hospital in Paris, 1802–1808," *BHM,* 1989, *63*: 110–120.

50. J. E. D. Esquirol, *Des passions considérées comme causes, symptômes, et moyens curatifs de l'aliénation mentale* (Paris: Didot Jeune, 1805), 70.

51. AN, 27 AP 8. The whole letter is reproduced in Weiner, "Apprenticeship," 1128–1134. It is dated 18 October 1798 (27 Vendémiaire, Year VII).

52. *Comptes généraux des hôpitaux et hospices civils, enfants abandonnés, secours à domicile et direction des nourrices de la ville de Paris An XI* (Paris: Imprimerie des hôpitaux, An XIII [1804–1805]), 194. Pussin's only documented professional honor was his election as corresponding member of the Société de médecine de Bruxelles. This was recorded in 1807; the exact date of election has not been ascertained. See "Extrait des Procès-verbaux des Séances" in *Actes de la Société de médecine de Bruxelles* (Brussels: Weissenbruch, 1808), liv.

53. AAPP, CFNS, dossier 707 10.

54. *TM,* 393, and J. E. D. Esquirol, "Maisons d'aliénés," *Dictionnaire des sciences médicales* (1818), 94.

55. By decree of 27 March 1802, twenty mentally ill women were to be treated at Charenton at the expense of the Paris Hospital Council, the rest at the Salpêtrière. The total figures of mentally ill women living at the Salpêtrière do not jibe: Pinel himself mentions 1,100 in the introduction to the second edition of *La médecine clinique* in 1804 (p. xxxiv).

56. J. N. Hallé, "Séance publique de l'Ecole de médecine, 5 Brumaire, An XI," *Recueil périodique de la Société de médecine de Paris,* 7ème année (1802–1803), *16*: 98.

57. Philippe Pinel, "Recherches sur le traitement général des femmes aliénées dans un grand hospice et résultats obtenus à la Salpêtrière après trois années d'expériences," *Moniteur universel,* 30 June 1805, 1158–1160, reprinted in Gauchet and Swain, eds., *Des passions,* 104–113.

58. Philippe Pinel, "Résultats d'observations et construction de tables pour servir à déterminer le degré de probabilité de la guérison des aliénés," France, Institut national, Première classe: Sciences mathématiques et physiques, *Mémoires,* 1st ser., 1807, *8*: 169–205.

59. Ibid., 200.

60. Pinel, "Recherches sur le traitement général des femmes aliénées," 1160; Gauchet and Swain, eds., *Des passions,* 113.

61. Philippe Pinel, "Résultats de nouvelles observations faites sur les aliénées de la Salpêtrière en 1812, 1813, 1814," *Journal universel des sciences médicales,* 1816, *1*: 82–94.

62. The documentation regarding Charenton is to be found in AN, AJ^2, particularly dossiers 23, 27–28, 60, and 86–87. For the period when Charenton came under the Ministry for Internal Affairs, 2d division, Bureau "Hospices et secours," see AN, F^{15}, 378–379. A useful, detailed, and authoritative—although personal and thus unobjective—report on Charenton is J. E. D. Esquirol, "Mémoire historique et statistique sur la maison royale de Charenton," *AHPML,* 1835, *13*: 5–192.

63. AN, AJ^2, 60. Note the similarity to the brothers' pre-Revolutionary fee.

64. Dr. Ch. F. S. Giraudy later joined Esquirol's private clinic as director of convalescents.

65. In the fall of 1799, the minister of internal affairs shifted Charenton to

the new category of "welfare establishments," together with the national institutions for the deaf and the blind and the Quinze-Vingts Hospice.

66. "Avis," in AN, AJ², 87.

67. Report by Cadet de Vaux, AN, AF¹⁵, 323.

68. Gauchet and Swain, eds., *Des passions*, 77.

69. Seine, CGAHHCP, *Rapports au conseil général* (1803), 81.

70. AN, AJ², 60 and Gauchet and Swain, eds., *Des passions*, 78–80.

71. The following analysis summarizes pp. 45–54 of Esquirol's "Mémoire historique." See also P. Sevestre, "Eloge de la maison de Charenton," *Information psychiatrique*, 1976, *52*: 361–363.

72. Esquirol, "Mémoire historique," 46.

73. Ibid., 48 and 53.

74. The number of patients at Charenton dipped briefly to 722 in 1814, possibly because of the wars. Ibid., 57.

75. Ibid., 30, 59.

76. Ibid., 48.

77. After the death of de Coulmiers in 1818, two experienced and responsible men succeeded each other as directors of Charenton: Roulhac-Dumaupas, who retired in 1830, then Palluy. According to Esquirol, they elaborated and published regulations and a budget, and demanded that the personnel keep registers, records, and exact patient charts. They also undertook renovations, and built women's wards, rooms, and baths. The straitjacket remained the only means of restraint for violent patients; but provisions for the sudden cold showers on patients' heads were built into the new bathrooms as well. Ibid., 60, 70.

78. On asylum architecture, see the work of Dieter Jetter, for example, *Zur Typologie des Irrenhauses in Frankreich und Deutschland (1780–1840)* (Wiesbaden: Steiner, 1971).

Chapter 10. The Citizen-Patient and the Environment

1. For more detailed treatment and plentiful bibliography, see D. B. Weiner, "French Doctors Face War: 1792–1815," in *From the Ancien Régime to the Popular Front: Essays in the History of Modern France in Honor of Shepard B. Clough,* ed. C. K. Warner (New York: Columbia University Press, 1969), 51–73, excerpted in F. A. Kafker and J. M. Laux, eds., *Napoleon and His Times: Selected Interpretations* (Malabar, Fla.: Robert E. Krieger, 1989), 258–264.

2. D. J. Larrey (1766–1842) began his career as a naval surgeon and enlisted in the Rhine army in 1792. He served without interruption until Waterloo, as surgeon-in-chief to the consular—later imperial—guard. He received the Legion of Honor and was made an imperial baron and elected to the Academies of Medicine and of Sciences.

3. The French were ill informed about Egypt even though they had now and then shown an interest in that country. Louis XIV was urged by the philosopher Leibnitz to dig a Suez Canal, the foreign minister Choiseul sent

Baron François de Tott as emissary in the mid eighteenth century to reconnoiter the possibility of French conquest, and the Ideologue Constantin Volney (1757–1820) surveyed the area and published a description. Bonaparte's travel library on the voyage to the Middle East included the Bible and the Koran: he dreamt of harmonizing Islam and Christianity under French protection. He also issued an appeal to the Jews of the area to join his colors; in return he would restore their "kingdom of Jerusalem."

4. Trained at Montpellier and Paris, N. R. D. Desgenettes (1762–1837) took part in all of Napoleon's wars, beginning with the first Italian campaign, where he served as physician-in-chief. Decorated with the Legion of Honor in 1804 and made an imperial baron in 1809, he was elected to the Academy of Medicine in 1820 and to the Academy of Sciences, as a corresponding member, in 1832.

5. P. F. Percy (1754–1825) graduated from the faculty of Besançon at twenty-one and enlisted in the army as surgeon in 1776. Named surgeon-in-chief of the Rhine army in 1792, he served continuously from then on, except when prevented by a serious, recurrent ophthalmia. He won election to the Academy of Sciences in 1807, and Napoleon decorated him with the Legion of Honor and made him an imperial baron in 1809.

6. J. W. Estes and L. Kuhnke, "French Observations of Disease and Drug Use in Late Eighteenth-Century Cairo," *JHM*, 1984, *39*: 121–152.

7. D. J. Larrey, "Les rapports originaux de Larrey à l'armée d'Orient," in *Mémoires de l'Institut d'Egypte: Relation historique et chirurgicale de l'expédition de l'armée d'Orient en Egypte et en Syrie* (Paris: Demonville, 1803), 13–14.

8. Ibid., 19, 32.

9. M. Meyerhof, "A Short History of Ophthalmia during the Egyptian Campaigns of 1798–1807," *British Journal of Ophthalmology*, 1932, *16*: 131–145, passim.

10. Larrey, "Les rapports originaux," 24–26.

11. Ibid., 87–88.

12. Ibid., 140.

13. Ibid., 106.

14. M. C. Buquet, *Index alphabétique et biographique du personnel médical pendant l'expédition d'Orient (Egypte et Syrie 1798–1802)* (Thèse CHU Broussais–Hôtel-Dieu, Paris, 1972), cited in A. Camelin, "La succursale d'invalides d'Avignon," *Bulletin de la Société française d'histoire des hôpitaux*, 1979, *38*, 27–44n. 12; and H. P. Bayon, "Napoleon's Egyptian Expedition: Brilliant Military Victories—and Ultimate Disaster through Disease," *West London Medical Journal*, 1943, *48*: 33–45.

15. A. Moreau de Jonnès, *Monographie historique et médicale de la fièvre jaune des Antilles et recherches physiologiques sur les lois du développement et de la propagation de cette maladie pestilentielle* (Paris: Migneret, 1820), 100.

16. See, e.g., R. S. Blanco, *Wellington's Surgeon General: Sir James McGrigor* (Durham, N.C.: Duke University Press, 1974), ch. 3, "The West Indian Campaign."

17. Moreau de Jonnès, *Monographie historique,* 129, 138.

18. P. Bonnette, "Le calvaire médical du St. Domingue et de la Gouade-

loupe," *Hippocrate*, 1938, *6*: 470–490; on Santo Domingo, see esp. the report of the chief medical officer, N. P. Gilbert, *Histoire médicale de l'armée française à St. Domingue en l'An X, ou Mémoire sur la fièvre jaune* (Paris: Gabon, 1803).

19. Larrey, "Les rapports originaux," 136–137.

20. Moreau de Jonnès, *Monographie historique,* 91.

21. F. Helme, "Napoléon et la médecine: La prophylaxie et le service de santé," *La presse médicale,* 15 and 18 June 1921, *29 (Annexe)*: 853–855, 877–880; quotation from 879.

22. Not until the early years of the Third Republic—long after the creation of the excellent Prussian Army Medical Service and even after the establishment of the U.S. Surgeon General's Office—did military medicine gain independence in France, by the decrees of 28 November 1876 and 16 March 1882. See Weiner, "French Doctors Face War," 51–73.

23. J. Lasserre, " A l'armée d'Egypte: Discipline, récompenses diverses, et armes d'honneur," *Revue des études napoléoniennes,* 1930, *30*: 99–121; quotation from 106–107.

24. See, e.g. [?] Sieur, "Histoire des tribulations du corps de santé militaire depuis sa création jusqu'à nos jours," *Bulletin de la société française d'histoire de la médecine*, 1928, *22*: 92–163.

25. L. Lefort, *La chirurgie militaire et les sociétés de secours* (Paris: Baillière, 1872), 2.

26. P. F. Percy, *Journal des campagnes du baron Percy, chirurgien-en-chef de la grande armée (1745–1825)* (Paris: Plon, 1904), 3, 16.

27. Larrey, "Les rapports originaux," 92.

28. A. G. Chevalier, "Hygienic Problems in the Napoleonic Armies," *Ciba Symposia*, 1941, *3*: 974.

29. Ibid., 975.

30. Brice and Bottet, *Le corps de santé militaire en France: Son évolution, ses campagnes, 1708–1882* (Paris: 1907), xviii. "Reading those decrees," commented the authors, "one has the impression as if nothing had happened during the previous ten years; the legislation of 1781 would have been sufficient. . . . It was a total return to the past." Thus, in the view of the French army medical corps, Napoleon's reactionary military health corps policy returned them to the most discouraging days of the old regime.

31. A. G. Chevalier, "Physicians of the French Revolution," *Ciba Symposia* 1946, *7* (11): 250. In the navy, that perennial stepchild of French military efforts, the situation was worse because heavy emigration had drained its strength. To attract new medical men, a decree of 12 November 1794 (22 Brumaire, Year III) raised the rank and pay of navy doctors to the level of those of regular officers. See P. Brau, *Trois siècles de médecine coloniale française* (Paris: Vigot, 1931), 121. But this period of recognition lasted less than three years. Although the navy doctors were briefly given jurisdiction over colonial medical problems by the decree of 8 February 1798 (19 Pluviôse, Year VI), they too became part of the administrative services owing to Bonaparte's decree of 1801. "Extreme discouragement set in and led to complete anarchy in the medical establishments of the port cities" (Brau, *Trois siècles*, 125). In normal times, these coastal stations extended health care to the colonies, and

cared for sailors in the merchant fleet and the navy (Huard, *Sciences, médecine, pharmacie*, 83–105). But France was losing her possessions in Asia, Africa, and the Caribbean to British superiority on the high seas, and gradually the British blockade cut off all French overseas connections. War thus reduced the activities of French military doctors to the European continent.

32. AN, Affaires culturelles, Registres d'élèves, Ecole de santé, AJ 16 6414–6418.

33. Jean Noël Hallé, "Hygiène," in *Encyclopédie méthodique* (194 vols.; Paris: Panckoucke, 1787–1832), vol. 7 (1798), consists of an article (pp. 373–433) and the outline of his lecture course (pp. 433–437). He never wrote down his lectures. The outline was first published in A. F. Fourcroy, ed., *La médecine éclairée par les sciences physiques, ou Journal des découvertes relatives aux différentes parties de l'art de guérir*, 1792, 4: 225–235. For a condensed English version, see M. Staum, *Cabanis and Medical Philosophy in the French Revolution* (Princeton: Princeton University Press, 1980), appendix E.

34. *Recueil périodique de la société de médecine de Paris*, 1799, 6 (1B): 225.

35. "Hygiène," in *Encyclopédie ou Dictionnaire raisonné, 8:* 385–388.

36. Actually, the essays are twenty years apart. See Hallé's articles "Hygiène," in *Encyclopédie méthodique*, vol. 7 (1798): 373–437, and "Hygiène," in *Dictionnaire des sciences médicales* (60 vols.; Paris: Panckoucke, 1812–1822), vol. 22 (1818), 508–610. The latter article was written in collaboration with the hygienist P. H. Nysten (1774–1817). This argument is indebted to a stimulating article by William Coleman, "Health and Hygiene in the *Encyclopédie*: A Medical Doctrine for the Bourgeoisie," *JHM*, 1974, *29*: 399–421; see also B. P. Lécuyer, "L'hygiène en France avant Pasteur, 1750–1850," in C. Salomon-Bayet et al., *Pasteur et la révolution pastorienne* (Paris: Payot, 1986), 65–139.

37. The Egyptian Institute was revived in 1862, then reorganized in 1919, and in 1936 it published Larrey's very frank original reports to the Paris military Health Council. See P. Pallery, ed., "Les rapports originaux de Larrey à l'armée d'Orient," *Mémoires présentés à l'Institut d'Egypte*, 1936, *30*.

38. F. M. C. Richard de Hautsierck, ed., *Recueil d'observations de médecine des hôpitaux militaires*, vol. 1 (1766); vol. 2 (1772).

39. Jacques de Horne, ed., *Journal de médecine, chirurgie, et pharmacie militaire* (7 vols.; 1782–1789).

40. What Napoleon refused to see printed, the Restoration, July Monarchy, and Second Empire prized, witness the flourishing *Recueil des mémoires de médecine, chirurgie, et pharmacie militaire*, whose first series, 1817–1845, consists of 61 volumes, and the second, 1845–1858, of 23 volumes.

41. T. M. Adams's recent *Beggars and Bureaucrats: French Social Policy in the Age of Enlightenment* (New York: Oxford University Press, 1990), discusses these in detail.

42. P. F. Keraudren (1769–1857) rose to be physician-in-chief of the naval forces at Brest in 1799 even though he did not complete the M.D. degree until 1803. He served as inspector general of the naval health service from 1813 to 1845. He wrote *Mémoire sur les causes des maladies des marins et sur les soins à prendre pour conserver leur santé dans les ports et à la mer* (Paris: Imprimerie royale,

1817; 2d ed., 1824) and *De la fièvre jaune observée aux Antilles et sur les vaissaux du roi, considérée principalement sous le rapport de sa transmission* (Paris: Imprimerie royale, 1823), was one of the founders of *Annales d'hygiène publique et de médecine légale* in 1829, and contributed to the *Dictionnaire des sciences médicales.* In the authoritative article "naval hydrography" of 1818, Keraudren discussed the health of sailors; he summed up French notions by underlining the need for cleanliness on well-aired ships, pumps to dispose of seawater that might leak in, and care in getting rid of rats; he emphasized James Lind's recommendation of citrus fruit to control scurvy, and warned against typhus and dysentery. He also mentioned the vital importance of morale.

43. Anti-contagionism was welcome to military leaders and civilian health officials alike, for it freed them from the obligation to isolate the victims of plague or yellow fever and to impose quarantines and cordons sanitaires, all those expensive measures that impede administration and the conduct of war. During the first half of the nineteenth century the French medical profession remained overwhelmingly anti-contagionist. The classic treatment of this question is E. H. Ackerknecht, "Anticontagionism between 1821 and 1867," *BHM,* 1948, *22*: 562–593.

44. No attempt is made here to analyze the problem of vaccination in depth. This has recently been done by Yves-Marie Bercé and Pierre Darmon, and the background was explored long ago by G. Miller. For details, see Bib. Ess., The Citizen-Patient and the Environment.

45. (Anon.,) "Documents: Plan d'une clinique d'inoculation, 29 Floréal, An VII [18 May 1799]," *La France médicale,* 1902, *49*: 302bis. See Chapter 6, n. 45, above.

46. Edward Jenner, *Rapport sur le cowpox ou la petite vérole des vaches et sur l'inoculation de cette maladie,* tr. Antoine Aubert (Paris: n.p., An VIII [1799–1800]), see also Antoine Aubert, *Rapport sur la vaccine, ou Traité dans lequel on trouve la réponse aux questions rédigées par les commissaires de l'Ecole de médecine de Paris sur la pratique et les résultats de cette nouvelle inoculation en Angleterre. Nouvelle édition augmentée au Traité de la vaccine chez la vache* (Paris: Richard, Caille & Ravier, An IX [1800–1801]). On the *Bibliothèque britannique* of Geneva (1796–1815), which brought Frenchmen medical news from Britain, see Bib. Ess., Serials.

47. The second attempt, also by Pinel at the Salpêtrière, was made with vaccine brought from England by a Genevan, Jean Pierre Colladon. The third attempt was made by a group of medical school professors, Pinel among them, on thirty children, at the Vaugirard house of Dr. Colon. For an excellent account of this story in English, see R. G. Dunbar, "The Introduction of the Practice of Vaccination into Napoleonic France," *BHM,* 1941, *10*: 635–650; in French, see F. Colon, *Histoire de l'introduction et des progrès de la vaccine en France* (Paris: Le Normant, 1801). For recent assessments, see Bercé and Darmon, cited in Bib. Ess., The Citizen-Patient and the Environment.

48. Woodville failed at first because he used "false" or "bastard" vaccine. The difficulty, of course, arose from the fact that knowledge of the cowpox vaccine was entirely empirical. No one had ever seen the cowpox virus or knew how to transport it over long distances. The first three times "virus was

sent on cloth soaked in vaccine," either via Geneva or directly from London, once in "a vial filled with hydrogen gas over mercury and covered with a bladder." "Rapport du comité médical," *Recueil périodique de la Société de médecine de Paris*, 1799, 8: 239.

49. Quoted in Colon, *Histoire*, 39.

50. *Le Moniteur universel*, 14 Brumaire, An XII (8 November 1803).

51. France, Institut national, *Exposition des faits recueillis jusqu'à présent concernant les effets de la vaccination, et examen des objections qu'on a faites en différents temps et que quelques personnes font encore contre cette pratique, lu à la Classe des sciences physiques et mathématiques par MM. Berthollet, Percy, et Hallé, rapporteur le 17 août 1812* (Paris: Didot, 1812), 51.

52. J. Tulard, "Louis Nicolas Dubois, premier préfet de police (1758–1847)," *Revue de l'Institut Napoléon*, nouvelle série, 1956, 58: 9–14. Etienne Denis Pasquier (1767–1862) served as prefect from 1810 to 1814, and Count Jules Jean Baptiste Anglès (1778–1828) from 1815 to 1821.

53. Initially trained as a lawyer, Charles Louis Cadet de Gassicourt entered pharmacy upon his father's death in 1799. He learned chemistry from the famous Nicolas Louis Vauquelin (1753–1829) and then took over his own family's pharmacy in the rue Saint Honoré. Literate and wealthy, at home in learned societies, academies, and salons, an elegant writer (the illegitimate son of Louis XV, so gossips whispered), Cadet published a four-volume *Chemical Dictionary* in 1803, and a variety of pamphlets on foods and health; as secretary, he wrote most of the council's reports.

54. Jean Baptiste Huzard (1755–1838) was an expert on cattle and horses. He had been a member of the Société d'agriculture under the old régime and was inspector general of veterinary schools and a member of the Academies of Sciences and of Medicine. Among his numerous reports one might cite *Instruction sur la manière de conduire et de gouverner les vaches laitières* (Paris: Huzard, 1797) and *Instructions sur les soins à donner aux chevaux, pour les conserver en santé sur les routes et dans les camps, prévenir les accidents auxquels ils sont exposés et rémédier à ceux qui pourraient leur arriver et sur les moyens propres à prévenir l'invasion de la morve, à en préserver les chevaux et à désinfecter les écuries où cette maladie a regné* (Paris: Imprimerie vétérinaire, 1794).

55. Dupuytren was a brilliant surgeon, helped in his early career by Thouret. Prosector at the new medical school at seventeen, he was appointed assistant chief surgeon at the Hôtel-Dieu in 1802 and chief in 1815, having in the meantime been chosen for the professorship of surgery at the medical school (1812).

56. Deyeux was trained in botany and chemistry and entered the pharmacy of his uncle Pia, which he eventually inherited. He was a member of the Academy of Sciences and published widely in learned journals. Practically all his investigations have relevance to public health. See A. Chéreau in Dechambre's *Dictionnaire*, s.v. "Deyeux."

57. Among the works of Antoine Augustin Parmentier that are relevant to public health, one might mention *Examen chimique des pommes de terre, dans lequel on traite des parties constituantes du blé* (Paris: Didot, 1773); *Avis aux bonnes ménagères des villes et des campagnes sur la meilleure manière de faire leur pain* (Paris:

Imprimerie royale, 1777); *Recherches sur les végétaux nourrissants qui, dans les temps de disette, peuvent remplacer les aliments ordinaires, avec de nouvelles observations sur la culture des pommes de terre* (Paris: Imprimerie royale, 1781); and *Dissertation sur la nature des eaux de la Seine, avec quelques observations relatives aux propriétés physiques et économiques de l'eau en général* (Paris: Buisson, 1787).

58. The remaining four members added to the council by 1815 were the chemist Joseph Darcet (1777–1844), who had been trained by his father and by Vauquelin, and whose work focused on industrial and commercial problems; two "médecins aux épidémies," Marc Antoine Petit (1760–1840) and Etienne Pariset (1770–1841); and Charles C. H. Marc (1771–1841), whose interests were in legal medicine and psychiatry.

59. On Pariset, see G. D. Sussman, "Etienne Pariset: A Medical Career in Government under the Restoration," *JHM*, 1971, *26*: 52–74.

60. The Civil Code (or "Code Napoleon") was adopted in 1804, the Code of Civil Procedure in 1806, the Commercial Code in 1807, the Code of Criminal Instruction in 1809, and the Penal Code in 1810.

61. See Rosen, "Problems in the Application of Statistical Analysis to Questions of Health," *BHM*, 1955, *29*: 27–45, and Coleman, *Death is a Social Disease*.

62. In Fodéré's prolific output, the works most germane to the topic of this book are *Traité de médecine légale et d'hygiène publique ou de police de santé, adapté aux codes de l'empire français et aux connaissances actuelles* (6 vols.; Paris: Mame, 1813); and *Essai historique et moral sur la pauvreté des nations, la population, la mendicité, les hôpitaux, et les enfants trouvés* (Paris: Huzard, 1825).

63. Before becoming dean of the Paris Medical Faculty in 1831, M. J. B. Orfila (1787–1853), a naturalized Spaniard, was professor of legal medicine from 1819 to 1821, and then professor of medical chemistry for ten years.

64. C. C. H. Marc had joined the Société médicale d'émulation 1795 and took his M.D. degree in 1811. Educated in Germany, he regularly reported on German legal medicine in the *Annales d'hygiène*, translated some German work, and was a prolific contributor to the *Dictionnaire des sciences médicales*.

65. Esquirol also annotated J. C. Hoffbauer's treatise dealing with the legal aspects of mental illness and deaf-mutism. See Hoffbauer, *Médecine légale relative aux aliénés et aux sourds-muets ou Les lois appliquées aux désordres de l'intelligence, avec notes par MM. Esquirol et Itard* (Paris: Baillière, 1827).

66. V. de Moléon, ed., *Rapports généraux sur la salubrité publique rédigés par les conseils ou les administrations établies en France et dans les autres parties de l'Europe. 2ème partie officielle: Rapports généraux sur les travaux du Conseil de salubrité de Paris et du département de la Seine exécutés depuis l'année 1802 jusqu'à l'année 1826 inclusivement (25 ans)* (Paris: Au bureau du Recueil industriel, 1828), vol. 1, 103.

67. Ibid., 84.

68. Ibid., 75.

69. Ibid., 11–16, passim.

70. Ibid., 53.

71. Ibid., 100–101.

72. Richard Cobb, *Death in Paris: The Records of the Basse-Geôle de la Seine,*

October 1795–September 1801, Vendémiaire Year IV–Fructidor Year IX (New York: Oxford University Press, 1978).

73. See pp. 181–183 above.

74. Société philanthropique de Paris, *Rapports et comptes-rendus pendant l'année 1815*, 91 and 98.

75. Ibid., 22.

76. Seine, CGAHHCP, *Rapports au conseil général* (1803), 91 and 106.

77. See D. B. Weiner, *François Vincent Raspail: Scientist and Reformer* (New York: Columbia University Press, 1969).

Conclusion: The Politics of Health

1. The Société académique de médecine, whose first president Guillotin became by unanimous vote and acclamation on 26 November 1804, was bent on restoring tradition. The first act of the new president was the reading of the bylaws concerning the "right of supervision granted this society over all its members, to maintain the honor of the Academy and of all Academicians" ("Procès-verbaux de la Société académique de médecine," Archives de l'Académie de médecine de Paris, vol. 42, fol. 9). The society reverted to giving speeches and papers in Latin and generally considered itself the heir of the defunct Paris medical faculty.

2. Thouret's sixteen-year tenure as dean has never been studied, even though the papers of the medical faculty are now available to scholars in the series AJ[16] at the Archives nationales. For an interesting recent account of the gradual centralization of medical power during this era, see G. Weisz, "Constructing the Medical Élite in France: The Creation of the Royal Academy of Medicine, 1814–1820," *Medical History*, 1986, *30*: 419–443.

3. AAPP, CFNS, dossier 83.

4. J. F. Coste, "Hôpital," in *Dictionnaire des sciences médicales*, 401–402.

5. As is well known, Bismarck's Germany was the pioneer in protective health legislation in the 1880s. The first ministry of health was created in czarist Russia in 1907, and in Great Britain in 1919; the United States did not follow suit until 1952. The best American scholars who have written about issues of public health in nineteenth-century France are Ann LaBerge, Martha Hildreth, Robert Nye, Harry Paul, and George Weisz.

6. G. D. Sussman, "Enlightened Health Reform, Professional Medicine and Traditional Society: The Cantonal Physicians of the Bas-Rhin, 1810–1870," *BHM*, 1977, *51*: 565–584.

7. J. Imbert, "Une expérience européenne: Le droit hospitalier sous l'empire napoléonien," *Atti del primo congresso europeo di storia ospitaliera (6–12 giugno 1960)* (Reggio Emilia: Centro italiano di storia ospitaliera, 1962), 608.

8. G. Rosen, "What is Social Medicine? A Genetic Analysis of the Concept," *BHM*, 1947, *21*: 674–733.

9. Published until World War II, the *Annales d'hygiène publique et de médecine légale* gave birth in 1921 to the official journal of the Société de médecine légale de France, *Annales de médecine légale, de criminologie et de police scientifique*), and in 1923 turned into *Annales d'hygiène publique, industrielle et sociale.*

10. Or council members were soon elected to membership—namely, Adelon, Andral, Barruel, Darcet, Esquirol, Marc, Parent-Duchâtelet, and Villermé.

11. Public health councils were established in Lyon (1822), Marseille (1825), Nantes and Lille (1828), Troyes (1830), and Rouen and Bordeaux (1831). See C. C. H. Marc, "Rapport d'une commission de l'Académie royale de médecine à M. le ministre du commerce et des travaux publics sur l'établissement de conseils de salubrité départementaux," *Annales d'hygiène publique et de médecine légale* 1837, *18*: 6–36.

12. See Ann LaBerge, "The Early Nineteenth-Century French Public Health Movement: The Disciplinary Development and Institutionalization of *Hygiène publique*," *BHM*, 1984, *58*: 363–379, and "Edwin Chadwick and the French Connection," *BHM*, 1988, *62*: 23–41. The crucial publications in the case of Britain were, of course, Edwin Chadwick's *Report on the Sanitary Conditions of the Labouring Population of Great Britain* (1842) and Friedrich Engels's *Condition of the Working Class in England* (1844).

13. See LaBerge, "Edwin Chadwick and the French Connection."

14. Moléon, *Rapports généraux*, 88.

15. Ibid., ix.

Index

Designed by Glen Burris
Set in Bembo text and Centaur display by G & S Typesetters, Inc.
Printed on 50-lb. MV Eggshell Cream by Maple Press

CPSIA information can be obtained
at www.ICGtesting.com
Printed in the USA
JSHW020307100123
36033JS00001B/1